Origins and Directions of Inflammatory Bowel Disease
Early Studies of the "Nonspecific" Inflammatory Bowel Diseases

Origins and Directions of Inflammatory Bowel Disease

Early Studies of the "Nonspecific" Inflammatory Bowel Diseases

by

Joseph B. Kirsner

M.D., Ph.D., D.Sci. (hon.)

The Louis Block Distinguished Service Professor of Medicine,
Department of Medicine, University of Chicago, Chicago, IL, USA

with a contribution by

Ulrich Klotz, Ph.D.

Professor of Pharmacology, Dr. Margarete Fischer-Bosch-Institut
für Klinische Pharmakologie, Stuttgart, Germany

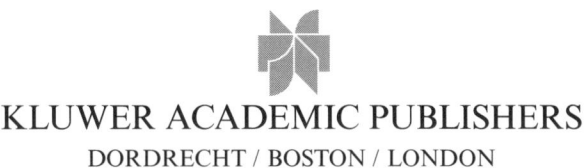

KLUWER ACADEMIC PUBLISHERS
DORDRECHT / BOSTON / LONDON

Library of Congress Cataloging-in-Publication Data is available.

ISBN (hardback) 0-7923-8777-5

Published by Kluwer Academic Publishers,
PO Box 17, 3300 AA Dordrecht, The Netherlands.

Sold and distributed in North, Central and South America
by Kluwer Academic Publishers
101 Philip Drive, Norwell, MA 02018, USA

In all other countries, sold and distributed
by Kluwer Academic Publishers, Distribution Center,
PO Box 322, 3300 AH Dordrecht, The Netherlands

Printed on acid-free paper

Supported in part by the Gastro-Intestinal Research Foundation of Chicago

This material is adapted, in part, from historical information contained in J.B. Kirsner, Inflammatory Bowel Disease – Etiology and Pathogenesis. Bockus Gastroenterology, 5th edn, W.S. Haubrich, ed., Vol. 2, Chapter 75, Part I, pp. 1293–317, W.B. Saunders Co., Philadelphia, 1995. J.B. Kirsner, Historical Aspects of Inflammatory Bowel Disease. Journal of Clinical Gastroenterology 10:288–97, 1988. J.B. Kirsner, Historical Basis of Idiopathic Inflammatory Bowel Diseases. Inflammatory Bowel Diseases 1:2–26, 1995 (with permission)

Sponsored by Falk Foundation e.V., Freiburg (Germany)

All Rights Reserved
© 2001 Kluwer Academic Publishers
No part of this publication may be reproduced or
utilized in any form or by any means, electronic, mechanical,
including photocopying, recording or by any information storage and
retrieval system, without written permission from the copyright owner.

Printed and bound in Great Britain by MPG Books Ltd., Bodmin, Cornwall.

Preface

Few human illnesses today are so challenging, medically, scientifically, and socio-economically, as the "nonspecific" inflammatory bowel diseases (IBD): ulcerative colitis and Crohn's disease. Originating several centuries ago but essentially diseases of the 20th century, often attacking children and young adults, involving all bodily systems, as well as the gastro-intestinal tract, ulcerative colitis and Crohn's disease have emerged in recent decades as among the more "glamorous," unsolved diseases, presenting unusual opportunities for insightful clinical and investigative study. Many of the prevailing concepts originated during early and mid-20th century. The purpose of *Origins and Directions of Inflammatory Bowel Disease* is to review these earlier studies and their evolution "from the mystical to the molecular;" and, like Ariadne's thread of Greek mythology, guide investigators and physicians through the challenging clinical and scientific maze of IBD. Ariadne, daughter of Pasiphae and King Minos of Crete, fell in love with the Athenian hero Theseus and with a "thread" of glittering jewels helped him escape the imprisoning Labyrinth after he had slain the evil Minotaur (half bull, half man). Metaphorically, the hope of the 21st century similarly is to slay the IBD Minotaur.

Joseph B. Kirsner
Department of Medicine
University of Chicago

Acknowledgements

I am pleased to recognize the expert assistance in editorial review by my Administrative Assistant, Mrs. Arlene Willett, and the excellent library service of my Secretary, Mrs. Diane Pieters.

I am especially grateful to Dr. Herbert Falk, President of the Falk Foundation e.V., Freiburg, Germany, for his generosity and support in making possible the publication of this book and for his long dedication to the development of knowledge of Inflammatory Bowel Disease through his more than thirty international Falk Seminars, the major channel for communication between physicians, scientists and scholars interested in inflammatory bowel disease.

Contents

Preface	v
Acknowledgements	vi
List of illustrations	ix
Introduction	1
Ulcerative colitis	13
Early IBD-related events	13
Beginnings	14
Increasing clinical recognition	24
Initial pathology of ulcerative colitis and its pathogenic implications	30
Pathology – electron microscopy – ulcerative colitis	39
"Natural" and experimental ulcerative colitis	40
References	43
Crohn's disease	55
Origins	55
Early clinical recognition	58
Animal and experimental Crohn's disease	63
Abdominal trauma	66
The early Mt. Sinai (New York) experience	67
More early 20th century reports (CD)	71
Crohn's disease of the colon – delayed recognition	77
Early pathology of Crohn's disease	81
Electron microscopy – Crohn's disease	85
Origin of eponym of Crohn's disease	87
References	90

Etiology of pathogenesis of IBD – origins and directions	103
Epidemiology	103
Psychogenic aspects (UC, CD)	112
Microbial aspects – ulcerative colitis	121
Microbial aspects – Crohn's disease	126
Immune mechanisms	133
M cell	154
Epithelial permeability	155
Inflammation (cytokines, lymphokines)	156
Genetic aspects of inflammatory bowel disease – early observations	161
Concluding commentary	167
References	173
Appendix	205
The early treatment of inflammatory bowel disease	207
References	219
Pharmacologic development of aminosalicylates for the treatment of inflammatory bowel disease – *Prof. U. Klotz*	227
References	232
Additional early publications on inflammatory bowel disease	235
Index	237

List of Illustrations

L. Wallach	6
M. Fiterman	7
J.B. Kirsner	8
S. Wilks	16
G. Moxon	17
J.P. Lockhart-Mummery	18
I. Boas	19
J.A. Bargen	22
B.N. Brooke	26
S.C. Truelove	29
S. Warren	32
V.J. McGovern	34
B.C. Morson	36
W. Fabricius Hildanus	56
G.B. Morgagni	57
T.K. Dalziel	60
G. Oppenheimer, B. Crohn, L. Ginzburg,	62
E. Moschowitz	68
A.O. Wilensky	68
A.A. Berg	72
H.E. Lockhart-Mummery	78
R. Marshak	79
H.D. Janowitz	80
A. Lesniowski	88
A.I. Mendeloff	106
C. Murray	114
J. Auer	137
C.O. Elson	153
W. Strober	160

Introduction

Inflammatory Bowel Disease at the University of Chicago – Personal Reflections (1936–2002)

My interest in inflammatory bowel disease began in January 1936 when I undertook the care of a young emaciated woman who was brought to the University of Chicago Medical Center in desperate condition with severe ulcerative colitis, a virtually unknown illness at the time. In the absence of antibacterial drugs, steroids, anti-inflammatory agents and other support measures, she succumbed to the disease several weeks later. The death of this patient had a profound impact upon me and from then on I devoted an increasing proportion of my research activities to this problem. Initially, I focused on the clinical nature of ulcerative colitis, its mode of onset, clinical manifestations, local and systemic complications, and its course. In 1948, my colleagues and I described the natural history of 120 patients with ulcerative colitis and, subsequently, the clinical course in 40 patients with regional enteritis. An important University of Chicago study later clarified the occasionally subtle distinctions between ulcerative colitis and Crohn's disease of the colon. A corollary investigation updated the definitions of "nonspecific" inflammatory bowel disease as a basis for future cooperative studies.

Many types of infection also were implicated and, though microbiological studies were negative, bacterial involvement was a major etiological consideration. The 1933–34 epidemic of amebic dysentery in Chicago had created interest in the possible role of Entamoeba histolytica in ulcerative colitis. In the 1930s, patients remained in the hospital for long periods of time; hospitalizations of 2 or 3 months were not unusual. As with other diseases of unknown etiology, numerous unsubstantiated dietary notions were advanced. Liquid, bland, milk-free, low fat, gluten-free, low fiber and high fiber diets, and even fasting were prescribed, without lasting benefit. On the other hand, increased knowledge of the metabolic and nutritional consequences of Crohn's disease of the small bowel provided the rationale for significant and helpful dietary adjustments. How then did we deal with inflammatory bowel disease in the 1930s?

As I recall those early days, we emphasized the restoration of nutritional health by the increased oral intake of food, encouraged by skilled and devoted dietitians. We also had the benefit of superior nurses who participated intelligently and caringly in the management of the IBD patient. We were aided by competent psychiatrists who helped patients and families cope with chronic, frustrating illness. In the 1930s, ulcerative colitis was widely regarded as a psychogenic illness. Many patients received formal psychotherapy and some underwent psychoanalysis. However, I cannot recall a curative effect attributable exclusively to psychotherapy in patients with severe ulcerative colitis. A curious, unexplained observation was the abrupt cessation of the diarrhea of ulcerative colitis in several patients who became temporarily psychotic. Just as curiously, the diarrhea returned when the psychosis receded. Sleep therapy was recommended by some observers. However, one patient in 1937 who, accidentally had received larger amounts of sedation than had been prescribed, slept almost continuously for seven days, without improvement in the colitis.

Limited medical approaches were available to control inflammation and infection, including dilute potassium permanganate and Dakin's solution, products of World War I research. To eliminate the anaerobic bacterial flora in ulcerative colitis, oxygen was insufflated transanally into the colon, without benefit. Small (250 ml) blood transfusions were used as a general support measure. I also recall the occasional use of small amounts of typhoid vaccine intravenously, presumably to stimulate immune defenses but this approach soon was abandoned. A few patients with ulcerative colitis had received the diplostreptococcus vaccine advocated by Dr. J.A. Bargen at the Mayo Clinic, without success. We spent many hours daily, including Saturdays and Sundays, at the bedside of each patient in an effort to be supportive and encouraging. Today's remarkable scientific and technological advances notwithstanding, I continue to regard this approach, although not tested in "controlled study," as an important part of our therapy at that time. Such was the state of treatment in the mid-1930s and 1940s; limited, empirical, symptomatic, uncertain, but with helpful personal physician and support staff involvement. The predominant form of IBD recognized in the 1930s was ulcerative colitis. Crohn's disease was not yet a major gastrointestinal problem at the University of Chicago.

The advent of sulfanilamide in 1938 initiated a completely new era in the management of disease and increased the hope of more effective control of the presumed bacterial and/or viral causes. However, the anti-microbial effects of the sulfa drugs were transient. It was impossible to characterize and to quantify or to eliminate even temporarily the vast aerobic and anaerobic flora of the gut. Antimicrobial therapy, nevertheless, appeared helpful in the management of some patients with ulcerative colitis and, lacking better therapy, it became a mainstay of treatment. The development of sulfasalazine in 1940 in Sweden, combining via an azo chemical bond the prevailing sulfonamide, sulfapyridine, and 5-aminosalicylic acid, originally developed for the treatment of arthritis, also proved effective in the management of patients with both ulcerative colitis and arthritis. In the 1970s, 5-aminosalicylic acid was found to be the active ingredient and the use of this compound alone, without sulfapyridine, became the treatment of choice. Despite the continuing obscurity of the etiology of IBD, it became possible to maintain the majority of patients with uncomplicated ulcerative colitis or with uncomplicated Crohn's disease in satisfactory health, although recurrences were frequent.

Into the 1940s, ulcerative colitis had been the predominant IBD problem at the University of Chicago but regional enteritis was increasing in frequency. My IBD studies now were interrupted by World War II. Interestingly, from the standpoint of microbial and psychogenic concepts, during my lengthy overseas duty in both the European and Pacific theaters of war, at times under stressful conditions, I saw only two American soldiers with ulcerative colitis. In each instance, the condition had preceded military service. Subsequent to the liberation of Paris in 1944, I saw two female patients with IBD at a French hospital, both originally from Poland. This was my only contact with IBD until I returned to the United States in the middle of 1946.

After visiting several gastroenterology centers in 1947, including the University of Pennsylvania (the late Dr. Thomas Machella) upon my return from overseas, my colleague, the late Dr. Leonard Scheffner, and I undertook the comprehensive investigation of protein metabolism in patients with IBD, including the development of analyses of individual amino acids. I was impressed with the tremendous losses of protein and other nutrients in the bowel movements even in patients with only moderately active ulcerative colitis and Crohn's disease.

The flow of new IBD patients to the University of Chicago increased steadily. By the 1960s as many as 100 new patients were seen within a year, and the overall numbers of patients continued to rise. More antibiotics had become available. Again, initial enthusiasm and apparent clinical success in IBD were followed by more restrained evaluations. The development of ACTH in the latter part of 1950 was a dramatic achievement in the management of human illness, including inflammatory bowel disease. In 1951 I demonstrated the adjunctive usefulness of ACTH and steroids in therapy. The excitement and the anticipation of the ACTH-steroid days (late 1950s, 1951) among patients and physicians hardly can be reconstructed today, more than 50 years later. Despite attempts at controls, the high degree of expectation with this dramatically potent medication created an atmosphere of "success," and resulted in unusual therapeutic responses. Thus, in our protein balance studies, one male patient with ulcerative colitis consumed 7000 calories including 400 g of protein daily, and another young man with ulcerative colitis, ingested 8200 calories/day during the course of almost immediate, striking clinical improvement. Most of the ingested protein was recovered as urinary nitrogen, reflecting the intense catabolic effects of the ACTH and steroid preparations. With time, the early dosage problems and the complications of steroid therapy diminished, and their use in IBD became very common. These drugs today remain an important component of medical therapy but are not recommended for long-time use. In the latter part of the 1950s and continuing to the present time, regional enteritis of the small bowel and regional enteritis (Crohn's disease) of the colon became increasingly frequent at the University of Chicago. By the late 1970s and early 1980s, Crohn's disease had become more common than ulcerative colitis in our patient population. We now were seeing at least 200 referred new patients each year and overall observing more than 3000–5000 patients. Because of the associated impairment of digestive, metabolic, and nutritional functions, Crohn's disease presented increased therapeutic problems.

During this period of nearly 50 years, we examined numerous etiological and pathogenetic aspects of IBD and a wide variety of associated clinical problems, including liver disease, cancer of the bowel, growth retardation, arthritis, and toxic dilatation of the colon. We also investigated the morphologic response of the small and large bowel in various animals to numerous damaging agents and demonstrated that the colon reacted in a similar manner in varied experimental circumstances. Considerable effort was directed to the production of colonic injury using pharmacological stimulants of bowel motility, either directly or via neurogenic stimulation. Subsequent changes in the bowel were minimal and did not reproduce IBD. Much of my laboratory research then was directed to the development of experimental models of ulcerative colitis and Crohn's disease, involving chemical, microbiological, and pharmacological injury. While these efforts did not succeed in reproducing either disease, they led me into the important, emerging field of immunology and to the study of the immunological resources and the immunological responsiveness of the gastrointestinal tract. One of the immunological techniques developed in my laboratory, the Auer–Kirsner "immune complex colitis" in the rabbit, has been utilized by other investigators. My initial observations in 1948 on the familial occurrences of IBD led to more detailed studies of larger series of patients and control populations in the 1950s, clearly indicating a genetic influence in IBD. Today, these two concepts, immunological and genetic, are receiving major emphasis.

In the 1930s, the surgical management of ulcerative colitis was in its early developmental stages. Total colectomy then was a hazardous operation. Ileostomy alone without removal of the diseased colon (diverting ileostomy), based on the uncertain concept of "resting the bowel," was performed in the hope of later restoring normal bowel continuity. Another operative procedure removed the diseased colon from its origin at the ileocecal valve to the rectum, reuniting the distal small bowel with the rectum (ileorectal anastomosis), also in an effort to maintain normal bowel continuity. Unfortunately, these techniques proved inadequate in ulcerative colitis, and infrequently successful in Crohn's disease of the colon. It became clear that, when surgery was advisable for ulcerative colitis, total removal of the colon and rectum and the establishment of an ileostomy was the most effective procedure. A major surgical advance occurred when Bryan Brooke in London and Rupert Turnbull of the Cleveland Clinic revised the ileostomy in 1951, with the folding over of the mucosal surface, an amazingly simple and yet highly effective maneuver. In the 1970s and 1980s, the continent ileostomy and various endo-anal anastomoses with J pouch, preserving the anorectal musculature, have further improved the surgical approach to ulcerative colitis. In Crohn's disease of the small intestine, narrowing of the bowel with obstruction is not uncommon, necessitating operative removal of the diseased bowel and reanastomosis of the remaining small intestine. Since the resection of diseased bowel in Crohn's disease does not necessarily cure the disease, the surgical tendency today is increasingly conservative, removing as little bowel as possible when surgery becomes necessary.

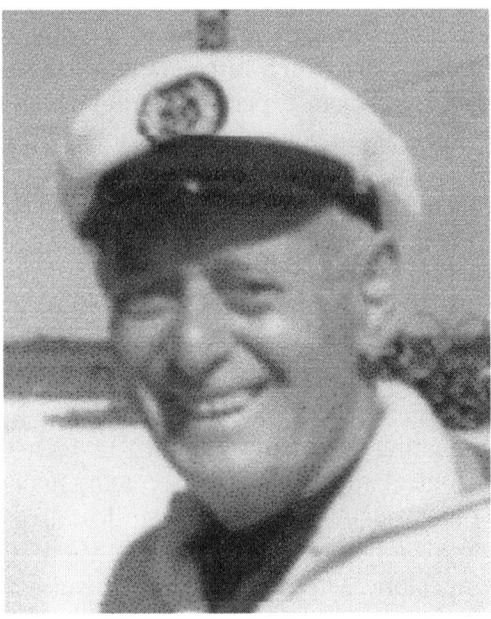

L. Wallach

The increasing numbers of patients with ulcerative colitis and with Crohn's disease, the uncertainties of medical treatment, and the growing need for surgery emphasized the importance of communication with other physicians and with patients and their families as to the nature of the IBD and the prospects for more successful management. I recall numerous conversations with interested patients and family members as to the minimal research activity in IBD. Such discussions occasionally resulted in the contribution of modest funds to initiate limited studies. The sustained generosity of the late Mr. Leo Wallach of Chicago, a prominent businessman, and of equally prominent Mr. Miles Fiterman of Minneapolis was especially helpful in the 1950s and 1960s. Mr. Wallach helped establish the first laboratories dedicated to IBD research at the University of Chicago. For many years he was our only "outside" supporter. In the mid-1950s, Mr. Fiterman, in addition to generous research support, became a key lay figure in several highly significant national developments relating to IBD, including participation with me on the Advisory Council of the National Institute for Arthritis, Metabolic and Digestive Diseases of the NIH. Beginning in 1962, the Gastro-Intestinal Research Foundation of

Introduction

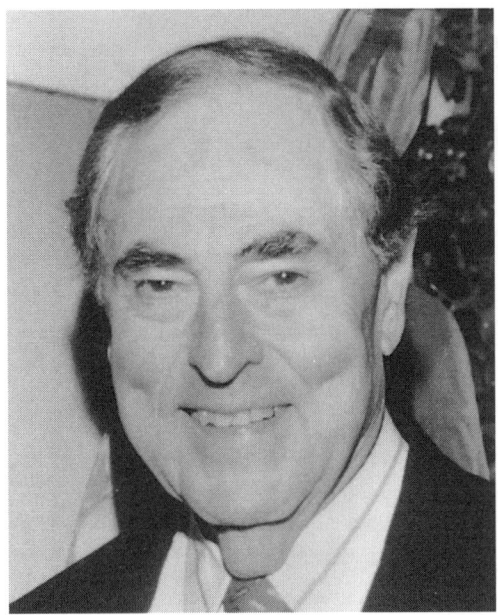

Miles Fiterman

Chicago, a group of remarkably loyal, humanitarian, and generous Chicago patients and friends, under the leadership of Mr. Joseph Valenti, Sr. and Mr. Martin Sandler, provided timely and invaluable support, a most important resource for the University of Chicago for the past 40 years.

A major development for both patients and physicians occurred when the first ileostomy club was established in Boston and a second soon thereafter in New York in the 1950s. The theme of these organizations was support for the patient requiring an ileostomy and practical information regarding its care. This movement spread throughout the country and the Chicago ileostomy club was organized by me at the University of Chicago in the 1960s. The nurse support service initiated at the Cleveland Clinic later was established at the University of Chicago and expanded to hospitals throughout the country.

Despite the increasing awareness of IBD, there continued to be relatively minimal research interest in IBD. We had endeavored in the early 1950s to bring this problem to the attention of the National Institutes of Health. Efforts by me in the mid 1950s to initiate research in IBD had been rejected by "basic scientists" (biochemists, pathologists, and physiologists) less

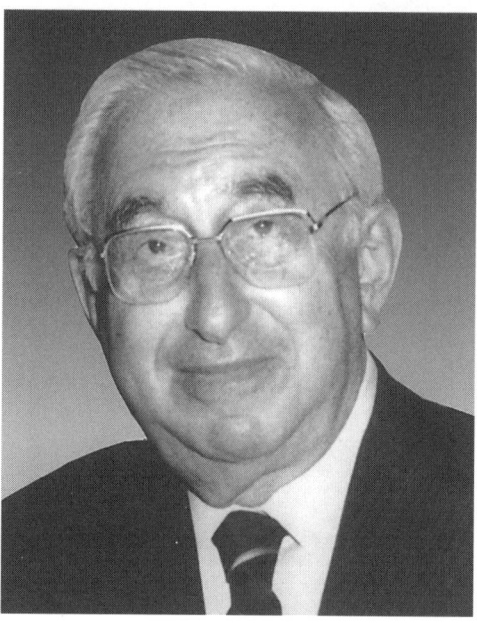

Joseph B. Kirsner

aware of the problem than clinicians. Subsequent discussion between NIH leaders, Dr. L.T. Coggeshall (Dean of the Division of Biological Sciences), and myself at the University of Chicago led to the development of the General Medicine Study Section of the NIH in the mid 1950s. Research proposals now could be reviewed by knowledgeable experts and receive informed peer review. Under the aegis of the General Medicine Study Section of the NIH, I, together with other gastroenterology members (F. Ingelfinger, Wade Volwiler, Stewart Wolf, and Julian Ruffin) organized a 1-day symposium in Washington, D.C. in January 1960, involving a small group of gastroenterologists and basic scientists. The success of this effort led to a 3-day seminar at the University of Chicago (September 1965). These meetings provided new opportunities for the interchange of ideas and stimulated some research on IBD. Dr. James A. Shannon, Director of the NIH and Drs. Floyd S. Daft and Ralph Knutti of the National Institute of Arthritis and Metabolic Diseases provided invaluable support in the implementation of these programs and in the development of NIH funds to support research in Gastroenterology during the formative years of the 1950s and early 1960s.

Mr. Fiterman's daughter suffered from ulcerative colitis and had been under my care (she is well now). Concerned with the lack of knowledge of ulcerative colitis and with the absence of significant research, Mr. Fiterman personally financed the establishment of the National Foundation for Research in Ulcerative Colitis. The Medical Advisory Committee to this foundation in the 1950s included such leaders as J.A. Bargen (Mayo Clinic), H.W. Lewis (University of Oregon), J.M. Ruffin (Duke University), C.T. Stone, Sr. (University of Texas), O.H. Wangensteen (University of Minnesota), D.L. Wilbur (Stanford), S.G. Wolf, Jr. (University of Oklahoma), and J.B. Kirsner and W.L. Palmer (University of Chicago). Mr. Fiterman also generously financed the publication of worldwide abstracts on ulcerative colitis and Crohn's disease from the world literature. These abstracts were distributed to physicians free of charge and were an important source of information on IBD. In time, this foundation, with support from the American Gastroenterological Association, expanded to include Gastroenterology as a whole, and became the Digestive Disease Foundation. Additional advisory members then included T.P. Almy (Dartmouth), A.I. Mendeloff (Johns Hopkins), and R.P. Turnbull (Cleveland Clinic). The need to communicate with patients and families on developing support for additional research as to the nature of ulcerative colitis and Crohn's disease further increased. To facilitate this campaign, Mr. Fiterman also financed the development of a publication: "The Hidden Flame – Ulcerative Colitis" by the noted science writer, Victor Cohn of Minneapolis. The introduction to this treatise was by the distinguished University of California physicist, Dr. John Lawrence, whose brother had died unexpectedly of severe ulcerative colitis. "The Hidden Flame" probably was the first publication on ulcerative colitis to be written directly for the public, and its compelling message contributed to the expanding public awareness of the IBD problem.

Public interest increased after the illness of the late President Dwight Eisenhower, who, having suffered a heart attack, later required an abdominal operation because of an intestinal obstruction resulting from an earlier regional enteritis. An intestinal bypass procedure was performed without removing the obstructed bowel loop, a wise choice since President Eisenhower subsequently had no further intestinal difficulty and he succumbed later to another heart attack. The NIH at that time became aware of the limited research activity in Crohn's disease and made available a sum of approximately $100,000.00 for this purpose. I received $10,000.00 from this block grant, a welcome addition to my fiscally struggling research program. More importantly, this action represented a beginning national interest in supporting IBD research.

As yet, there was no coordinated public or national effort in support of IBD, i.e. until the development of the National Foundation for Ileitis and Colitis in New York under the leadership of Dr. Henry D. Janowitz, Mr. and Mrs. Irwin M. Rosenthal, and Mr. and Mrs. William D. Modell in 1968. Initially active in the New York area, this foundation subsequently expanded, with numerous chapters throughout the United States. I served as Chairman of the National Scientific Advisory Committee during the 1970s. Its fund raising potential increased steadily and today, the National Foundation for Ileitis and Colitis, now the Crohn's and Colitis Foundation of America (CCFA), is the leading national organization for distributing information on IBD to patients and families, for raising funds devoted to research on IBD, for encouraging and financially assisting younger investigators in IBD, for generating new research programs, and for effective liaison with the NIH, the American Gastroenterological Association, the American College of Gastroenterology, and other gastroenterology groups.

Today (2002), the IBD situation is dramatically different from the 1930s. IBD is a significant part of the medical horizon and is a major interest of physicians and medical centers, the National Institutes of Health, pharmaceutical companies and of gastroenterological organizations everywhere. IBD now is recognized as one of the important medical problems of our time. In medical schools and medical centers, IBD also has become the prototype disease for studying a wide variety of medical problems and disease mechanisms extending anatomically beyond the gastrointestinal tract. It is worldwide in distribution, affecting millions of people in the United States and throughout the world. As a direct outcome of the activity of the CCFA, there now are many more IBD investigators than in the 1930s. Internationally, Dr. Herbert Falk, Director of the Falk Foundation e.V. in Freiburg, Germany, for many years has made very important contributions to the advancement of knowledge of IBD through the famous Falk Symposia, superbly organized and implemented symposia on various aspects of the inflammatory bowel diseases. In addition Dr. Falk has facilitated the publication of this up-to-date and highly informative scientific production. Although we have not yet identified the cause or causes of IBD, we have learned better ways of managing the patients medically and surgically. The study of IBD has led to important scientific advances in other fields; one of the more important is the role of the gastrointestinal tract in our immune defense system. We have become increasingly aware of the significance of genetic and neurohumoral mechanisms influencing the gastrointestinal tract. Many unresolved aspects of IBD require investigation: environmental factors, emerging new types of bacteria, the body's defenses against bacteria and viruses, psychoneuro-immunological, genetic and neurohormonal mechanisms mediating stress and emotional disturbances. And new highly promising therapeutic targets are being identified as "the cellular and molecular events associated with the chronic inflammatory bowel diseases are elucidated."

In meeting such a complex and compelling challenge, the cooperative efforts of physicians, surgeons, basic scientists, including epidemiologists, immunologists, pathologists, biochemists, virologists, and geneticists, together with patients and their families, governmental agencies, and the general public are indispensable. During these many years, I have been impressed with the quality, the interest, the involvement, and with the generosity of many patients and family members whom I have been privileged to count as friends. Although the etiology of ulcerative colitis and of Crohn's disease remains elusive, with such support, the outlook to me seems brighter now than ever before. I dedicate the following words of the late French writer and moralist, Albert Camus (1913–1960), slightly modified by me, to everyone involved in discovering the cause and the cure of inflammatory bowel disease:

"If you listen very carefully, you will hear, mid the uproar and tyranny of governments, the clamoring of computers, and the greed and crime of our world, the faint fluttering of wings, the gentle movement of life and the eternal stirring of hope. Some say this hope lies in a nation, others in a political system and yet others in a technology. I believe rather that hope is awakened, sustained and nourished by individuals, men and women like yourselves – whose deeds, involvement and humaneness overcome the insensitive defects of our society and the crudest implications of man's history." From this hope, from this inspiration, and from this dedication, I believe will come the solution to IBD.

Dr. Joseph B. Kirsner
University of Chicago – 2002

Part I

Ulcerative Colitis

"Natura non facit saltus"

Nature does not proceed by leaps, but rather reveals its secrets slowly, quietly and grudgingly. Notable advances of today have their background in work often carried out decades before.

Carl Linnaeus, Philosphica Botanica (Section 77), 1751

EARLY IBD-RELATED EVENTS

Introduction

Disease emerges as a "deviation from normal," with symptoms and signs observed initially in isolated instances, then in groups of patients, reappearing in larger series in increasingly identifiable clinical patterns.[1] In time, information accumulates not only on the clinical spectrum of the illness but also on its pathology, pathophysiology, and therapy. This sequence broadly defines the pattern of recognition of ulcerative colitis (UC) and Crohn's disease (CD) many years earlier. Once regarded as medical curiosities, the "nonspecific" inflammatory bowel diseases today are among the more important of human illnesses, affecting millions of people worldwide.

Nonspecific (idiopathic) ulcerative colitis (UC) begins in the rectum and advances in continuity proximally to involve the entire colon and often the terminal ileum. Crohn's disease (CD) frequently originates in the distal ("terminal") ileum but involves any part of the gastrointestinal tract (mouth to anus). Acknowledging earlier unawareness of CD and limited medical understanding, ulcerative colitis predominated during the first half of the 20th century, "Crohn's disease" during the latter half of the 20th and into the 21st century.

The currently increased knowledge of inflammatory bowel disease (IBD) has suggested that UC and CD are of recent derivation, but their origins can be re-traced several centuries. The clinical information on IBD accumulated throughout the 20th century paralleled the growth of medical knowledge. The scientific advances in IBD developing mid 20th century and accelerating during the 21st century accompanied the growth of the basic and biomedical sciences. This publication describes early clinical and scientific developments in ulcerative colitis and Crohn's disease, the background and the source of current etiopathogenetic concepts.

BEGINNINGS

The origins of ulcerative colitis are lost in the obscurities of ancient medicine. Ancient Chinese medicine based on the "yin-yang balance" between parts of the body and its environment invoked "dysharmony of the spleen and the liver" in explaining chronic diarrhea,[2] but the intriguing possibility of an "ulcerative colitis or regional ileitis" in those ancient times when the tongue and the pulse were the principal components of the clinical examination must be left to unresolvable speculation! The Yellow Emperor's canon of internal medicine (722–721 BC) referred to illnesses vaguely resembling ulcerative colitis (abdominal pain, diarrhea, rectal bleeding). Observant physicians centuries earlier: Hippocrates[3] (460–377 BC), Aretaeus[4] of Cappadocia (80–138 AD), and Soranus (Ephesus) of Rome (AD 170)[5] recognized differing forms of diarrhea but knowledge was insufficient to separate one type from another. T. Sydenham's[6] (1624–1689) "bloody flux" (1669, 1670) and the epidemics of dysentery and bloody diarrhea in Colonial America and elsewhere undoubtedly were infectious in origin. Whether or not these illnesses included instances of "chronic ulcerative colitis," such as those observed during the 20th century, is impossible to verify now. E.L. Krawitt's[7] account of W.J., a 40-year-old man, originally from Ireland, "the Mohawk Baron" of Colonial fame, illustrates the point. In 1756 he developed a persistent "bloody flux." In 1761 the patient also began to experience episodes of fever, abdominal pain and jaundice. These symptoms persisted intermittently for 13 additional years until the patient died in 1774. Recognizing the unlikelihood of a continuous specific infection causing the episodic healing and recurrence over a period of 18 years, Krawitt suggested the intriguing sequence of an initial specific bacterial infection (e.g. bacillary dysentery) followed by a "nonspecific inflammatory bowel disease," complicated by "pericholangitis and then sclerosing cholangitis," a familiar combination today but unrecognizable then. B. Morson's (London) review[8] of Matthew Baillie's[9,10] 1793 Morbid Anatomy of Some of the Most Important Parts of the Human Body concluded that patients were dying from ulcerative colitis during the latter part of the 18th century. F.T. de Dombal[11] (Leeds), cited P.J.E. Wilson[12] as "suggesting that in 1745 Prince Charles, the Young Pretender to the throne, suffered from ulcerative colitis and cured himself with a milk-free diet!"

Early discerning pathologists, such as K. Rokitansky[13,14] (Kroniggrantz, Bohemia) and R. Virchow,[15] (Berlin) also were aware of different forms of "colitis" but knowledge then was insufficient to recognize specific diseases. Rokitansky, who performed more than 30,000 autopsies, studied "the dysenteric process" in detail and described an "ulcerative colitis-like" entity ("catarrhal inflammation" of the colon). Rokitansky cited C.E. Bock (Lehrbuch des Pathologischen Anatomie. Leipzig 1864) in documenting the occurrence of "catarrhal intestinal ulcers." B. Crohn[16] credited the Surgeon General of the Union Army (American Civil War) as referring to an "ulcerative colitis," with suggestive photomicrographic evidence – a remarkble achievement for the time. The Medical and Surgical History of the Rebellion U.S.A., pubished by the Surgeon General (circular No. 4 page 143) in 1865, contains the pathologic description of an apparent ulcerative colitis (under the heading of diarrhea and dysentery), based upon the study of more than 200 pathologic specimens ... The disease is described as "originating in the 'closed follicles' or in the intestinal epithelium of the glandular layers. The enlarged follicles rupture to produce superficial ulcerations, the ulcers spreading and coalescing over vast mucosal areas ..." (See also N.K. Mottet[17]).

Earliest Recorded Cases

During the latter part of the 19th century, inflammatory bowel disease (IBD) was not in the medical lexicon and the occasional identification of patients with "simple ulcerative colitis" represented clinical curiosities, without perceived medical significance. Clinical awareness of IBD did not exist except in rare instances (Wilks and Moxon, M. Baillie) and many patients with ulcerative colitis probably were unrecognized. Interest in ulcerative colitis increased after the 1909 London Symposium and case reports from England, France, Germany, and Italy multiplied but clinical understanding was limited. Bacterial causes of disease were being discovered during the latter third of the 19th century and early in the 20th century and bacterial infection was a presumed cause of "simple ulcerative colitis."

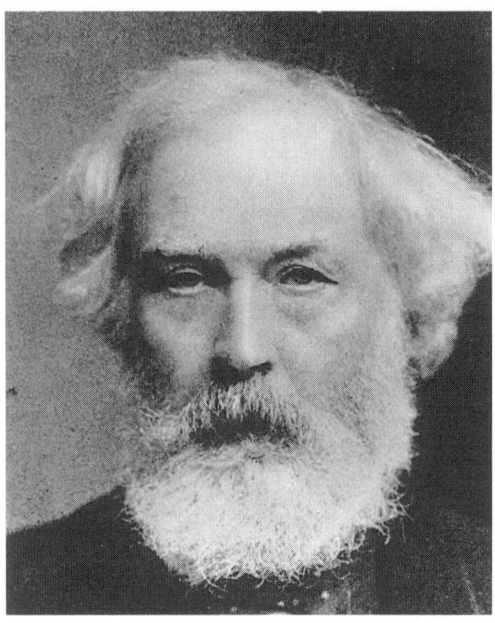

Samuel Wilks

R. Cattan et al.[18] of France cite an illustration in J.B. Cruveilhier's (1791–1874) Atlas (1829–1842) anatomically resembling ulcerative colitis. The first clinical "impact" description of "ulcerative colitis" was by Samuel Wilks[19] of London in 1859. The patient, a 42-year-old woman, (central figure in the notorious Smethurst legal trial in London[20]) had succumbed to an illness of diarrhea and fever, first mis-diagnosed as "arsenic poisoning." Autopsy demonstrated a transmural inflammation of the entire colon and terminal ileum, initially labeled ulcerative colitis but re-classified as Crohn's disease (J. Fielding[21]). Habershon[22] in 1862 described intestinal inflammatory pseudopolyps in a patient with "ulcerative colitis." "In the third stage we find ulceration, sometimes merely as minute circular ulcers, but generally of a more extensive character; the ulcers are often oval in form, placed in the transverse axis of the intestine, their edges are irregular and undermined, and their base is formed by the cellular or muscular coats. These ulcerations gradually extend and coalesce, till nearly the whole of the mucous surface is destroyed, except here and there prominent isolated portions, which become intensely congested, and resemble polypoid growths" (probably inflammatory pseudopolyps). Pathologists Wilks and Moxon[23] of London in 1875

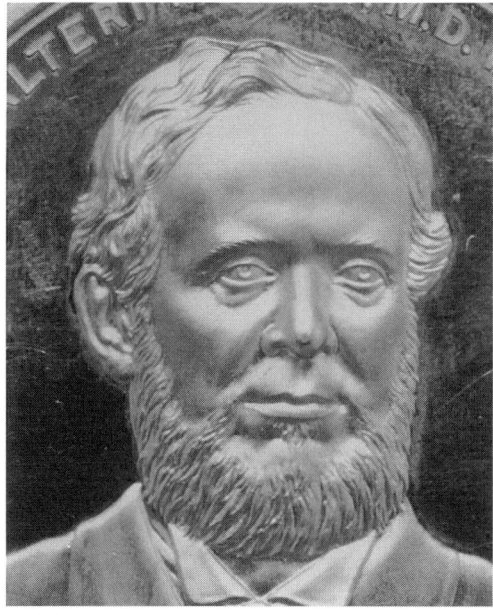

Gualteri Moxon

observed at autopsy in a young woman with a history of severe bloody diarrhea, scattered tiny ulcers in a very congested colon ("simple ulcerative colitis)," differing from "febrile epidemic dysentery." In 1881 Woodward[24] of the United States, author of the classic "Medical History of the War of the Rebellion," and, familiar with the report of Wilks and Moxon, described "pseudopolyps of the colon" in a 44-year-old man who had succumbed to a prolonged bloody diarrhea ("ulcerative colitis").

In 1885, W.H. Allchin[25] of London observed extensive denudation of the colonic mucosa in a young woman who died after six weeks of diarrhea. The opened colon contained many large ulcerations. Reports of "catarrhal ulcerative colitis" by C.H. Thomas of London,[26] W. Hale-White[27] of Guy's Hospital, London (1888), by British physicians attending the March 23, 1893 meeting of the Harvey Society of London, and from Europe (especially Germany, France, Italy), indicated the emergence of a diarrheal disease, apparently differing from the prevailing "epidemic bacillary dysentery." W. Hale-White remarked: "The condition observed is one of intense inflammation of the mucosa progressing to ulceration but the area of distribution ... and the degree of intensity vary ... from caecum to anus, occasionally even extending into the ileum, with complete destruction of

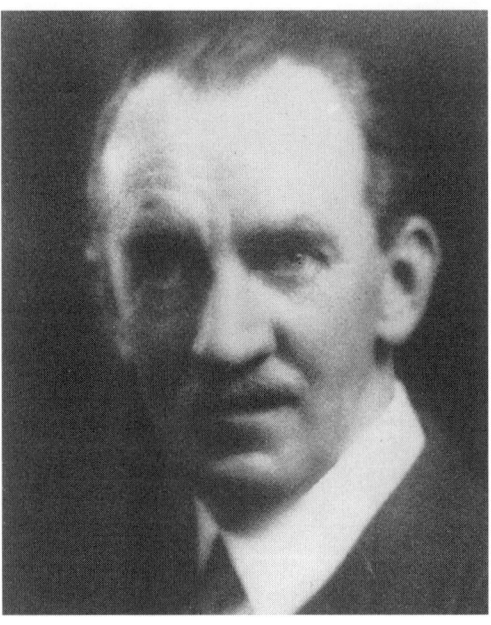

J.P. Lockhart-Mummery

the mucous membrane over large areas to merely a few discrete ulcers in the lower part of the bowel." In 1893 Mayo Robson[28] of London established an "inguinal colostomy" in a 37-year-old female with "colitis and ulceration," permitting daily irrigation of the ulcerated bowel with tincture of hamamelis and boracic acid solution, allowing later closure of the colostomy. In 1899, T.D. Lister[29] of London reported an association of ulcerative colitis with hepatitis. In 1902 R.F. Weir[30] of New York performed an appendicostomy in a patient with ulcerative colitis to irrigate the colon with a 5% solution of methylene blue and a 1:5000 solution of silver nitrate or of bismuth. In 1903, I. Boas[31] of Berlin, Germany clinically differentiated ulcerative colitis from bacillary dysentery. Ulcerative colitis was noted briefly by Wm. Osler in the 1904 edition of his Textbook of Medicine as occurring "not too rarely" in England. A.G. Wilson[32] of London in 1904 described a "simple ulcerative colitis" in a 51-year-old man, complicated by perforation and peritonitis. Discarding infectious possibilities, and, influenced by R. Bright, he emphasized the association with a "chronic granular kidney," and observed in other instances of colitis. J.P. Lockhart-Mummery[33] of St. Marks Hospital, London, aided by his new electrically-illuminated proctosigmoidoscope, in 1907 diagnosed

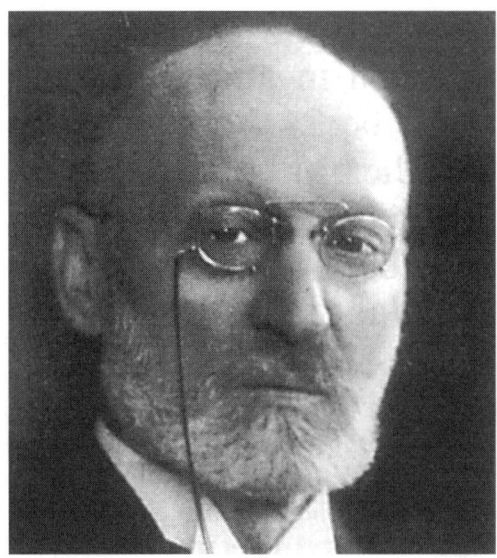

Ismar Boas

carcinoma of the colon in seven of 36 patients with ulcerative colitis, the first published report of this complication of ulcerative colitis.

The 1909 London Symposium on ("Sporadic") Ulcerative Colitis, reviewing 317 patients collected between 1888 and 1907 from seven hospitals (Guy's, London, St. Mary, St. Thomas, St. Bartholomews, St. George, Westminster), was the first cooperative effort to correlate clinical features in a substantial number of patients with ulcerative colitis.[34] The meeting opened with a detailed account of ulcerative colitis by Allchin,[35] followed by a review of the statistics from the contributing hospitals. W. Hale-White[36] described an association of ulcerative colitis with chronic interstitial nephritis and observed that in Richard Bright's original series of "100 Cases with Albuminous Urine," case no. 23, "was a very excellent instance of extensive ulceration of the intestine." Early 20th century physicians, aware of bacterial causes of disease (Entamoeba histolytica [Lösch 1875], Salmonella typhi [Ebarth 1880] and Shigella dysenteriae [Shiga 1898]), increasingly recognized the condition and implicated bacteria, especially bacillary dysentery. Treatment included: "slop diets," three pints of milk soured by lactic acid daily (Sydenham's remedy), "astringents," opium, tincture of hamamelis and rectal instillations of boracic acid, silver nitrate, "coli vaccine," or creolin, in an effort to control infection. The preferred operation was appendicostomy or, if the appendix had been removed, a "valvular cecostomy." The ulcerative colitis in a brother and sister, father and sibling, and in the father and sister of a third patient in the symposium series were considered "coincidences." One hundred forty one patients of the reported 317 died in the hospital from perforation of the colon and peritonitis, hemorrhage, septic infection, pulmonary embolism, liver disease and malnutrition.

H.P. Hawkins[37] of St. Thomas Hospital, London, in 1909 reviewed the "ulcerative colitis" in 85 patients, 41 of whom died and, implicating a bacterial pathogen, concluded: "The pedigree of this disease can be traced back nearly three hundred years to the 'bloody flux' of Sydenham[6] in 1669." He subdivided the patients as (a) acute, (b) chronic, (c) dysenteric diarrhea, (d) acute and chronic disease and, (e) hemorrhagic disease (lower bowel). He also described the surgical procedures of colostomy and ileostomy. In 1913 E. Stierlin of Basel[38] and R. Kienbock[39] of Vienna independently described the first (probably late) radiologic (bismuth or barium enema) appearances of ulcerative colitis. J.L. Kantor's[40] (New York) similar study appeared in 1927.

During the early 1900s, accounts of ulcerative colitis increased throughout Europe and it was a principal subject at the 1913 Paris Congress of Medicine. A. Bassler[41] of New York published a brief American case report in 1913. Also in 1913, J.Y. Brown[42] of St. Louis (United States), based on an experience with ten patients, only one with ulcerative colitis, recommended a temporary ileostomy to "rest" the diseased colon, a procedure that increased in "popularity" during the 1930s and 1940s and was endorsed by English surgeon R.S. Corbett (London) in 1945.[43] Actually, "colonic rest" did not ensue and the inflammatory reaction continued, as visualized proctoscopically. Other early reports were Hewitt and Howard's[44] (London) 1915 description of inflammatory polyposis in ulcerative colitis and A.H. Logan's[45] 1919 review of 117 patients (105 individuals under the age of 50), the first of many clinical studies from the Mayo Clinic.

In 1921 F.C. Yeomans[46] (New York) reported a series of 65 cases and H. Strauss[47] of Berlin published a brief paper in 1923. A. Hurst[48] (Guy's Hospital, London) in 1921 implicated an organism "closely related to B. dysenteriae," and his treatment: daily colonic irrigation of the colon with a silver nitrate solution (later a dilute solution of tannic acid), and the injection of large amounts of a "polyvalent antidysenteric serum" (four injections of 40, 60, 80 and 100 cc intravenously!) reflected this view. Hurst[48] also cited A. Mathieu and J.C. Roux[49] of France (Pathologie Gastrointestinale iii, 113, 1909) and A. Schmidt of Germany (Darmkrankheiten 1913) who had assembled the already considerable

European clinical experience with this disease. In 1926 L. Buie[50] reviewed 473 cases at the Mayo Clinic, accepting the "Bargen diplostreptococcus" as the cause (see later). During the 1920s and 1930s, reports from the United States,[51–53] Canada,[54] France,[55] Germany,[56] Russia,[57] and Italy,[58] indicated that ulcerative colitis was neither rare nor unknown early in the 20th century! A monograph on ulcerative colitis from Genoa, Italy, summarizing European case reports from the late 19th and early 20th centuries, cited approximately one thousand references.

Complications were recognized early,[26] including B. Crohn's[59] 1925 paper on the ocular complications of ulcerative colitis, attributed by Ellis and Gentry[60] to an auto-immune process and further reported from England[61] in 1967. Initial descriptions of colonic cancer complicating ulcerative colitis appeared in 1925 and 1927.[53,62] Bargen's 1928 report[63] of 20 instances of associated malignant disease comprised seventeen with adenocarcinoma of the colon and rectum, two lymphosarcomas and one lymphatic leukemia. Ive and Venables[64] (England) described polyps of the colon and a colonic stricture (probably an unrecognized carcinoma). Descriptions of other complications (hepatic abscesses, erythema nodosum, pyoderma gangrenosum) followed.[65–69] In the 1929 Mayo Clinic report,[65] 268 complications were distributed among 693 patients with chronic ulcerative colitis, including polyposis (69), stricture of the colon/rectum (59), "arteritis" (30), perirectal abscess (26) and skin lesions (17). Although listed as ulcerative colitis, the series unintentionally included instances of yet unidentified Crohn's disease of the colon (e.g. perirectal abscesses, fistulas).

In 1923 H.F. Helmholz[70] of the Mayo Clinic described the clinical features of ulcerative colitis in five children (three girls, two boys), the earliest such report in the literature. Bourne[71] (of East London Children's Hospital, England) in 1926 described one child with ulcerative colitis and reviewed the ten cases he found in the literature. He observed: "The power of the colonic mucous membrane to resist ... the heavily infected feces becomes impaired." A 1940 Mayo Clinic report enlarged the number of children with ulcerative colitis to 95[72] and in 1955 Bargen and Kennedy[73] added 139 children, concluding that "ulcerative colitis in children is not greatly unlike that in adults." The youngest recorded patient, a newborn male infant, developed an apparent ulcerative colitis at age 21 days and died after operation for rapidly deteriorating disease.[74] R. Lagercrantz[75] of Sweden (1949), Kirsner et al.[76] (1955), J. Hijmans and N. Enzer[77] (1962) Durham, N. Carolina, Korelitz et al.[78] (1962) and M. Davidson et al.[79] New York (1939, 1965) contributed early studies of IBD in children.

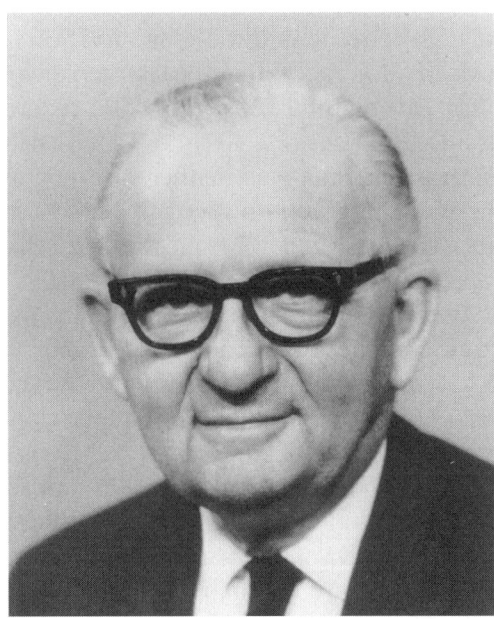

J.A. Bargen

Into the 1930s, ulcerative colitis received more attention. Hern[80] of London in 1931, reviewing 50 patients with ulcerative colitis seen between 1917 and 1926 at Guy's Hospital (mortality 40%), suggested that "the primary (etiologic) factor in ulcerative colitis acted through the blood stream with secondary infection of the mucosal surface by resident colon bacilli and streptococci ... causing deep and diffuse involvement of the submucosa and the mucous membrane."

T.L. Hardy and E. Bulmer[81] of Birmingham, England in 1933 surveyed 95 patients with ulcerative colitis seen between 1920–1932, with 31 deaths. T.E.H. Thaysen[82] of Copenhagen, Denmark in a 1934 study of 20 patients (14 women and 6 men, age range of 19–59 years) described a "simple hemorrhagic proctitis and proctosigmoiditis" which both he and H. Strauss of Berlin sought to differentiate from ulcerative colitis (diffuse congestion, ecchymoses of rectal mucosa and absence of ulceration), a recurrent issue for many years. Treatment included enemas of tannin, silver nitrate or bismuth subnitrate, and the anti-amebic compound yatren as an anti-inflammatory agent.

The impact of ulcerative colitis on pregnancy and vice versa, first mentioned at the 1909 London symposium, was not examined for thirty years. Barnes and Hayes[83] of the United States in 1931 described three patients who died after developing an ulcerative colitis during pregnancy and the puerperium. Each patient had experienced toxemia of pregnancy. Both parents of the first patient had died of Bright's disease. The second patient had severe kidney damage (chronic diffuse nephritis) and the third patient had experienced an exacerbation of chronic nephritis. Thus, the "ulcerative colitis" in these pregnant women was associated with advanced renal insufficiency, "azotemic colitis"; and, in fact, was not "idiopathic" or "simple ulcerative colitis," as earlier authors had assumed. In 1951 Abramson et al.[84] (Boston) reviewed 46 gestations in 33 patients with ulcerative colitis during pregnancy. Four of 5 patients with acute recurrences of ulcerative colitis during pregnancy died (mortality 80%); three of four patients with an acute exacerbation of ulcerative colitis during the puerperium died (mortality 75%), prompting the recommendation of therapeutic abortion in the first trimester of pregnancy in women with severe ulcerative colitis. On the other hand, MacDougall[85] of the Gordon Hospital, London (1955), reviewing 100 pregnancies in 64 women with ulcerative colitis, found that ulcerative colitis did not adversely affect pregnancy. Crohn et al.[86] (1956), analyzing the clinical status of 110 women with ulcerative colitis since the 1920s and 1930s who bore 150 pregnancies, found that the onset or recurrences of ulcerative colitis were frequent during the first trimester of pregnancy and during the puerperium. Korelitz[87] of New York later contributed authoritative information on pregnancy, fertility and inflammatory bowel disease.

Ulcerative colitis (UC) was one of the two major subjects at the 1935 International Congress of Gastroenterology in Brussels, Belgium. The five principal reports on ulcerative colitis originated in five different countries: Holland, France, Denmark, Italy and Spain. The discussants came from Germany, Sweden, Great Britain, Switzerland, Hungary, Roumania, the U.S.A. and Yugoslavia, reflecting the increased clinical interest in the disease. The 1935 program included an early instance of "familial ulcerative colitis" by M. Hamburger and A. Bensaude (France). Mones-Gallart and Sanjuan[88] of Barcelona, Spain in 1935 emphasized the inconclusive evidence for pathogenic bacteria. In the absence of modern microbiological methodology, unrecognized specific infections could not be excluded. However, the mounting clinical information indicated that "simple ulcerative colitis" was indeed a "new" entity. Indicative of today's strong interest in IBD, a 2001 Falk Symposium in Bologna, Italy, attracted abstracts from more than 40 countries and an audience exceeding 1000.

INCREASING CLINICAL RECOGNITION

Clinical recognition of ulcerative colitis increased in the United States during the 1930s to 1950s, with reports from the Mayo Clinic,[89] the most active IBD clinic in the U.S.A. at that time, Philadelphia,[90–92] and the University of Chicago,[93–95] among other U.S. centers.[96–99] T.T. Mackie[98] of New York in 1938 wrote ... "ulcerative colitis may be initiated by any of a number of bacteria, known to be pathogenic and known to produce inflammatory lesions in the colon. Once the mucosal barrier has been broken by such an agent, secondary infection necessarily occurs," a concept accepted by numerous observers today.

Brust and Bargen[100] in 1935, later Banks and Klayman[101] of Boston (1953) and Bercovitz[102] (New York) (1960) advanced the age range of patients beyond 50. In 1936 Bargen and Barker[103] reported arterial and venous thromboses complicating ulcerative colitis and in 1938 M.W. Comfort et al.[104] (Mayo Clinic) the association of ulcerative colitis with hepatic insufficiency. In 1940 Schlicke and Bargen[105] reported the combination of clubbed fingers and ulcerative colitis; later noted by Fielding and Cooke[106] also in regional enteritis (1971). In 1941 Lindahl and Bargen[107] reported the increased frequency of nephrolithiasis in ulcerative colitis, principally uric acid and calcium oxalate stones. A 1962 Mt. Sinai study[108] documented an increased nephrolithiasis in both ulcerative colitis and regional enteritis; ascribed by Gelzayd, Breuer and Kirsner[109] in 1968 to the increased concentration and excretion of urinary crystalloids and the excretion of an acid urine.

The significant nutritional impact of ulcerative colitis upon the growth and sexual development in children was recognized in the 1930s. In 1939 M. Davidson[110] of the Bronx Memorial Hospital, New York recorded three instances of retarded growth and development in children with ulcerative colitis. Benson and Bargen[111] in 1943 described fourteen young patients with ulcerative colitis, severe growth retardation and delayed sexual maturation, attributable to multiple nutritional deficiencies. In 1945 Ricketts, Benditt and Palmer[112] (University of Chicago) reported the association of ulcerative colitis with "infantilism" (growth retardation) and carcinoma of the colon. Welch, Adams and Wakefield[113] of the Mayo Clinic in 1937 had demonstrated substantial fecal losses of proteins and electrolytes in patients with active ulcerative colitis, findings confirmed by Sappington and Bockus[114] of Philadelphia (1949) and documented in detailed protein (amino acid) balance studies by Kirsner and Sheffner (University of Chicago) in 1950.[115] The 1950 Posey and Bargen[116] study of 43 patients with chronic ulcerative colitis (seen initially during the

1920s and 1930s) also emphasized the excessive losses of nutrients and minerals (sodium, potassium, calcium, chloride) in the stools.

The number and diversity of the complications steadily rose. In 1942 Jankelson et al.[117] of Boston described numerous systemic problems among 145 patients with chronic ulcerative colitis, including iron deficiency anemia, urinary problems, 10 instances of bronchopneumonia, arthritis, dermatologic disorders and psychogenic problems. Chisholm[118] of Boston in 1946 reported an acute fulminating ulcerative colitis with multiple bowel perforations and peritonitis, similar to Wilson's 1904 case description; a problem later related by Norland and Kirsner[119] to the use of opiates and anticholinergic medication in severely ill, malnourished patients with extensive disease. Jalan, Sircus, and Card et al.[120] of Edinburgh further clarified this complication in 1969.

Ricketts, Kirsner and Rothman[121] in 1948 described pyoderma gangrenosum complicating nonspecific ulcerative colitis. A.G. Leishman,[122] St. James Hospital, London (England) (1949), reporting a similar instance, cited E.C. Butler[123] in implicating "epithelial hypersensitivity" as the mechanism. In 1949 Z. Maratka and M. Spellberg,[124] comparing 52 patients from Prague and 19 patients from Chicago respectively, confirmed the similarity of symptoms and clinical course, observed also in a comparison of Australian IBD patients with IBD patients at the Cleveland Clinic.[125] Therapy during the 1930s and early 40s had been limited to nutritional supplements, small blood transfusions, "elimination diets," and occasionally fecal bacterial vaccines. The advent of sulfanilamide in 1935[126] and penicillin in the 1940s,[127] introduced the antibacterial era and adrenocorticotropic hormone (ACTH) in 1940,[128] the steroid era; developments that changed IBD therapy significantly (see treatment section in appendix).

Ulcerative colitis by the 1950s had acquired other names: nonspecific colitis, idiopathic proctocolitis, indeterminate ulcerative colitis, "streptococcal colitis," rectocolite haemorrhagique, colitis gravis, granular proctitis, mucosal colitis, thrombo-ulcerative colitis, and rectocolitis ulcerosa criptogenetica. Morson commented: "the name ulcerative colitis" is in some ways imperfect because the disease almost invariably involves the rectum and ulceration of the mucosa is by no means always present. The term "mucosal colitis," emphasizing the primary inflammation of the mucous membrane of the colon, originated in publications from the Cleveland Clinic (USA).

The geographic distribution of the disease extended to countries bordering the Mediterranean[18] (Greece, Turkey), to the middle East, Iran,

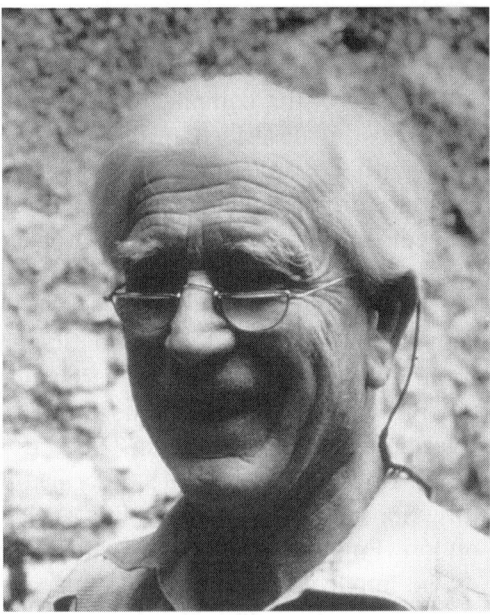

B.N. Brooke

Syria, and Kuwait, to South Africa, Australia and New Zealand,[129] India,[130] increased in Sweden[131] and appeared in Asia. At the Washington D.C. World Congress of Gastroenterology in 1958, F. Matsunaga[132] reported on 300 patients with ulcerative colitis in Japan, previously considered a rare entity in that country. Today, the number of patients with ulcerative colitis in Japan exceeds 60,000. Subsequent surveys documented the occurrence of ulcerative colitis also among the Chinese in China.[133]

Early in the 20th century, etiologic considerations had included food and pollen allergy, deficiency of an (undefined) "intestinal protective agent" and bacterial infection. Beginning in the 1930s, psychosomatic and psychiatric concepts dominated etiologic considerations, a controversial issue for many years (see later). In 1953 B.N. Brooke[134] (England) concluded that the colon could be affected by three distinct conditions: ulcerative colitis, ileocolitis and proctosigmoiditis, "all of which are customarily diagnosed as 'ulcerative colitis'. It is suggested that ulcerative colitis is not a specific disease but a pathological state ... with numerous causes." Brooke continued: "The situation is in every way analogous to a burn of the skin, except that in the colon secondary infection always supervenes rendering healing more difficult." In 1954 Kirsner and Palmer[135] advanced the concept of an "individual vulnerability to the disease," later revised to a genetically-influenced individual disease susceptibility.

Kirsner, Palmer and Klotz[136] in 1951 had documented the potential clininal reversibility and in six patients also the radiologic reversibility of ulcerative colitis in a series of 24 patients who had responded promptly to medical therapy and had maintained an uninterrupted favorable course for many years. This trend was confirmed in a larger group of patients in 1964.[137] Lennard-Jones et al.[138] of St. Marks Hospital, London in 1969 similarly reported reversibility of radiologic changes in 11 patients with colonic Crohn's disease, observations encouraging continued medical therapy in severe ulcerative colitis rather than "early" surgery (total colectomy and ileostomy); a controversial issue during the 1950s and 1960s.

The large Mayo Clinic experience continued to identify complications: pancreatic lesions[139] (interstitial pancreatitis, acinar dilatation, fibrosis) venous thrombosis,[140] and thromboembolic phenomena.[141] Beginning in 1948,[142] numerous papers documented the complication of hepatic disease in ulcerative colitis.[143-145] A 1958 report by Brooke and Slaney[146] of England on portal bacteremia suggested a possible factor in the development of sclerosing cholangitis, an important hepatic complication, preceded by pericholangitis.[147,148] Sclerosing cholangitis is of added interest as a possible risk factor for colorectal neoplasia.[149] In 1955 F.G. Wheelock and R. Warren[150] of Boston noted that 232 (68%) of 343 patients with ulcerative colitis at the Massachusetts General Hospital (Boston), since 1915 had required surgery. Carcinoma of the colon had developed in 31 patients. Hence, colectomy and ileostomy were recommended in all UC patients at the end of three years of treatment. In 1956 Bacon et al.[151] of Philadelphia described their successful surgical experience with chronic ulcerative colitis, adding to the ongoing debate on "early" colectomy and ileostomy vs. medical treatment for severe ulcerative colitis.

Seeking a physiologic basis for the psychogenic hypothesis of ulcerative colitis, Kern et al.[152] of Cornell University, New York, utilizing a balloon technique, studied the motility of the sigmoid colon in 45 patients with chronic ulcerative colitis. "The most striking abnormality of the motility pattern was a marked diminution or absence of phasic activity, correlated with severe diarrhea and attributed to 'continued ("psychogenic-induced") autonomic bombardment' of the colon." Chaudhary and Truelove[153] of

Oxford in 1961, utilizing three open-end water-filled polyethylene tubes placed in the sigmoid colon and connected to photo-electric transducers, found that in patients with mild disease, colonic motility was normal when symptom-free but with sigmoidoscopic evidence of inflammation, there was reduced motility; colonic hyperactivity was noted during moderate or severe diarrhea. The response of patients with ulcerative colitis to a standard dose of prostigmine was the same as in normal subjects. Some patients manifested colonic hyperactivity during an emotionally charged interview but the proportion of UC individuals responding positively was the same as in normal individuals and in patients with irritable colon.[154,155]

Throughout the 1950s and 60s, the number and variety of complications increased. P. Hench (1935),[156] Bywaters and Ansell (1958),[157] Fernandez-Herlihy[158] (1959), Wright and Watkinson[159] (1959) and McEwen et al.[160] (1962) described the arthritis accompanying ulcerative colitis, first mentioned by Bargen in 1929. Bywaters and Ansell studied 37 patients with mild to moderately severe arthritis, noting a high incidence of sacro-iliac involvement. The Fernandez-Herlihy study from the Lahey Clinic, Boston, comprised 555 patients seen from 1926 to 1955 and included: rheumatoid spondylitis, arthralgias, rhuematoid arthritis, erythema nodosum and "acute toxic arthritis." Wright and Watkinson, University of Leeds, England[159] described a "colitic arthritis" characterized by recurrent acute monarticular synovitis of short duration, unaccompanied by residual deformity. In the McEwen (New York University)–Kirsner study, 84 patients with ulcerative colitis were studied. Fifty-four had involvement of peripheral joints and twenty had spondylitis. Steinberg and Storey (London Hospital)[161] reported six cases of ankylosing spondylitis, four with ulcerative colitis and two with Crohn's disease, and cited Romanus[162] (author of a 368 page monograph on the subject in 1953), attributing the association to the vascular progression of infection from the pelvic veins to the vertebral veins. McBride et al.[163] (Edinburgh) added familial (genetic) disposition as a risk factor for the spondylitis.

Beal et al.[164] of Sydney, Australia, utilizing radioisotopic techniques, reaffirmed blood loss and iron deficiency as the most common cause of anemia in ulcerative colitis. F.W. Wasserman et al.[165] of Philadelphia reported a necrotizing angiitis in ulcerative colitis and M. Lehtinen et al.[166] of Finland microangiopathic hemolytic anemia in a patient with ulcerative colitis, prompting speculation on a systemic immune vulnerability in ulcerative colitis. In 1963, McCarthy and Shklar[167] of Tufts University Dental School, Boston, described a rare syndrome of pyo-

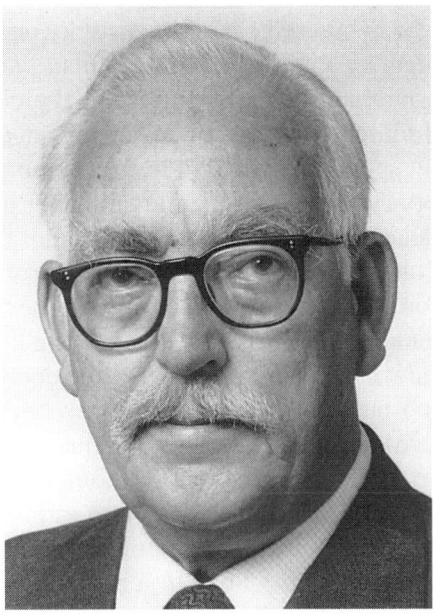

S.C. Truelove

stomatitis vegetans associated with "ulcerative colitis" in six patients. The oral lesions consisted of multiple small vegetations containing purulent exudate, resembling miliary abscesses. The most consistent organism cultured from the oral lesions was a streptococcus (hemolyticus or viridans) but the authors discounted its etiologic significance.

Analysis of the course and prognosis of ulcerative colitis by Edwards and Truelove[168] of Oxford in 1963 and 1964 included 624 patients with an impressive 100% follow-up of patients admitted to the Radcliffe Infirmary or to the Churchill Hospital (Oxford) from 1938 to March 1962. The principal factors influencing mortality in the first referred attack included severity of illness, extent of disease and age (>60 years). The course was characterized by frequent relapses within the first year of observation. "Radical" surgery was necessary in 14% and "conservative" surgery in an additional 6%. Noteworthy, however, were such local complications as aphthous ulceration of the mouth, ischio rectal abscess, fistula in ano, rectovaginal fistula, rectal and colonic stricture, evidence of the unintended (and unrecognized) inclusion of Crohn's disease of the colon in the "ulcerative colitis" series. Other gastroenterologic complications included inflammatory polyposis, acute dilatation of the colon (detected clinically by decreased peristaltic activity on abdominal auscultation and confirmed by plain abdominal films),[169] perforation of the colon, massive hemorrhage and carcinoma of the colon. The systemic complications, including erythema nodosum, pyoderma gangrenosum, arthritis, ankylosing spondylitis, ocular, liver and renal disorders, venous thromboses, pulmonary embolism, anemia and other blood disorders, and osteoporosis, paralleled the experience at other major medical centers.

Into the 1960s, colorectal cancer complicating chronic ulcerative colitis had become a major concern. Dawson and Pryse-Davies[170] in 1959 and Goldgraber and Kirsner[171] in 1964 documented the increased colo-rectal cancer risk. Devroede et al.[172] of the Mayo Clinic documented the higher cancer risk in young patients with chronic ulcerative colitis with longer duration of the IBD. MacDougall[173] of St. Bartholomew Hospital, London in 1954 had reported 5 instances of carcinoma of the large intestine among 126 patients with ulcerative colitis and estimated the risk as five times higher than for the general population. Also in 1954, Bargen, Sauer, Sloan and Gage[174] of the Mayo Clinic, in a review of 1564 patients with ulcerative colitis, had recorded 98 instances of colorectal carcinoma, 20 to 30 times more commonly a cause of death than in the general population.

Periodic literature reviews,[175-178] useful in summarizing clinical and occasional research efforts, did little to clarify etiology and pathogenesis. R. Wright[178] of Oxford, England realistically concluded in 1970: "... Clear evidence that autoimmune or allergic mechanisms are directly concerned with its (ulcerative colitis) pathogenesis has not been forthcoming ... Psychological factors are important but defy measurement or understanding."

INITIAL PATHOLOGY OF ULCERATIVE COLITIS AND ITS PATHOGENETIC IMPLICATIONS

The pathologic appearance of ulcerative colitis was early recognized as a diffuse, predominantly mucosal/submucosal disease characterized by vascular congestion, superficial ulcers, and histologically by increased cellular infiltration and crypt abscesses in the lamina propria. Pathologist P.H. Manson Bahr[179] at the 1909 London symposium had concluded: "Ulcerative colitis was merely a name for a phase or a class of diseases which hitherto had been included under the name dysentery." In 1936 he published a detailed three-type classification of the dysenteries (I. Dysenteries, II. Pseudodysenteries and III. Resembling Dysenteries) and placed idiopathic ulcerative colitis in the third category. From his observations at the London Hospital for Tropical Diseases Manson Bahr stated: "The initial lesions in the mucous membrane of the bowel would seem to be a large number of small hemorrhages ... followed by a peculiar plush-like congestion of the mucosa. Next, a layer of granulative tissue forms in the mucous surface which is extremely friable and is easily traumatized ... The whole natural history of the disease marks it out definitely as a specific infection ..." In 1933 Buie and Bargen[180] implicated vascular "thrombotic phenomena" as the pathological basis of ulcerative colitis, and in 1938 Bargen et al.[181] proposed the term "thrombo-ulcerative colitis."

In 1939 Lium[182] of the Mallory Institute of Pathology, Boston City Hospital, after describing the preparation of colonic explants in dogs and a method for quantitating the secretion of mucus by the explants, found that muscular spasm greatly increased the secretion of mucus, whether the spasm was induced by mechanical stimulation, parasympathomimetic drugs or dysentery toxin. The end result was damage to the epithelium with hemorrhage and ulceration. The regenerating epithelium was more vulnerable to trauma than the normal epithelium of the colonic graft.[183] In 6 patients with ulcerative colitis who had died, R. Lium,[184] at autopsy, found the most severe lesions in the rectum. The ulcers were linear in distribution and located over the taenial bands, indicative of intense spasm of the colonic musculature; a concept supported by other clinicians[185] and often cited in support of psychogenic mechanisms.

A review of 120 surgically treated patients and 60 autopsied cases (total 180 patients) by pathologists S. Warren and S.C. Sommers[186,187] of the New England Deaconess Hospital, Boston in 1949 and 1954, discounting spasm, re-emphasized the mucosal involvement and implicated an etiologic agent in the fecal stream, reminiscent of B. Dawson's[188] 1909 "intestinal toxin." Local "vasculitis" (necrosis of vascular walls, arteritis, thrombosis) was held responsible for colonic ulcerations in 11% of cases. Focal granulomas were present in 11 of the 17 crypt abscess cases. Complications included malnutrition, bowel perforation, peritonitis (the major cause of death), fatty liver and a "pancreatic dystrophy." None of the prevailing etiologic hypotheses, bacterial infection, psychogenic stress, locally damaging intestinal digestive enzymes and the "mucosal release of a proteolytic enzyme," was acceptable to Warren and Sommers. Early implication of the fecal stream as a cause of ulcerative colitis encouraged experiments at the University of Chicago on the local effects of prolonged instillation of filtrates of fecal discharges from patients with severe active ulcerative colitis into surgically-designed self-retaining ileocolonic pouches in dogs, with negative results.[189] R.B. Stoughton[190] of the

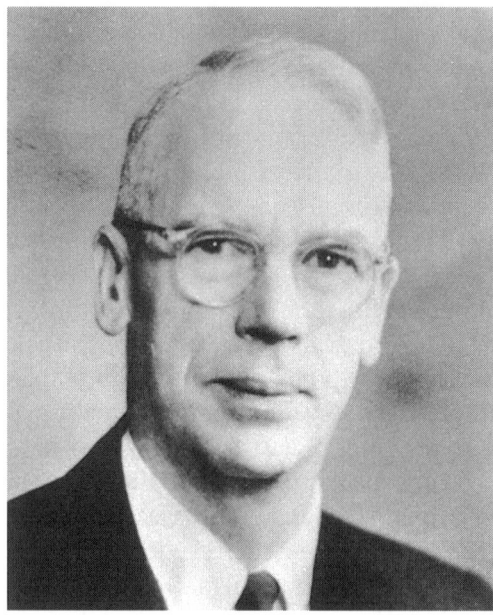

Shields Warren

University of Chicago in 1952 isolated a "proteolytic substance" from fecal filtrates of patients with ulcerative colitis capable of digesting epidermal cells, a possible contributory factor in the tissue reaction. However, while "acantholysis" was noted in three of eight patients with ulcerative colitis, it also was found in fecal filtrates from three individuals without ulcerative colittis."[191]

A mucinase capable of attacking mucus was identified in the feces of patients with ulcerative colitis by H.G. Sammons of Birmingham, England[192] as early as 1951 but the colonic mucus layer in IBD was not studied until the late 1960s, 1970s and 1980s.[193–198] In the 1967 Greco et al. (Rome, Italy)[194] investigation, histochemical and histophotometric studies of the colonic goblet cells, demonstrated a decrease or absence of the neutral goblet cells and the presence of weakly acid goblet cells, indicative of a secondarily altered cellular turnover rate. Studies of colonic mucus in 1983 and 1984 by Podolsky and Isselbacher[199,200] and in 1987 by Neutra and Forstner[201] demonstrated thinning of the surface mucus layer in ulcerative colitis and depleted of goblet cells; whereas in Crohn's disease the mucosal layer was thick and goblet cells were retained. The mucus layer in the normal human colon consists of a complex mixture of sulfated and nonsulfated mucins but the alterations in glycosylation and sulfation in ulcerative colitis apparently were considered nonspecific. In the 1983 Podolsky–Isselbacher (Boston) study of eight patients with ulcerative colitis "... a pronounced and selective reduction of one component, mucin subclass designated species IV," was noted and not found in patients with Crohn's disease of the colon. J.M. Rhodes[202] of Liverpool in 1989 could not confirm loss of mucin fraction IV but emphasized that "alterations in mucus glycoprotein biochemistry may have consequences not only on its resistance to bacterial enzymatic attack but also in the physical properties of colonic mucus as a protective barrier against the excessive localisation of bacteria in colonic mucus."

The clinical and pathologic mimicry of ulcerative colitis by colonic infections led B. Brooke[203] in 1954 to reinforce his earlier suggestion that ulcerative colitis represented a nonspecific morphologic response of the colon to multiple causes; hence, the term "nonspecific," utilized also by Goldgraber and Kirsner,[204] among others. F. Gallart-Mones[205] (Barcelona, Spain) (1953), describing "desquamation of endothelial cells in the submucosal blood vessels," implicated an undefined submucosal vascular lesion. Rachet and Busson[206] of Paris, France (1950), comparing ulcerative colitis to eczema and asthma, considered the mucosal vascular congestion as pathogenetically significant. Busson and LeQuintrec[207] (1954), re-emphasizing the intense vascular congestion of the mucosa in six patients with left sided colitis, proposed "superficial capillary angiectasia" as the earliest histologic change and implicated an unspecified "congenitale ou acquisé regional mesenteric neuro-vascular abnormality: Tous ces elements plaident en faveur de l'existence d'une dystonie neurovegetative regionale dans la zone intestinale, contrastant avec l'absence de symptomes neuro-vegetatifs dans les autres territoires."

In 1957 McGovern and Archer[208] of Sydney, Australia, ascribed the colonic vascular congestion to a histamine-release phenomenon originating in submucosal and muscular layer mast cells and added: "Augmented barrages of nervous impulses during stress may give rise to the excessive production of acetylcholine in the colon, which then reacts with the tissue mast cells causing the phenomenon of histamine-release," a "physiologic" explanation for the psychosomatic hypotheses of ulcerative colitis, of interest in relation to current views of an autonomic nervous system imbalance. McGovern states:[209] "Mast cells, in response to injury (or perhaps neurogenic stimulation), secrete histamine, a permeability factor and heparin. Histamine increases the local blood-supply, increasing capillary permeability, and fluid passes into the surrounding tissues.

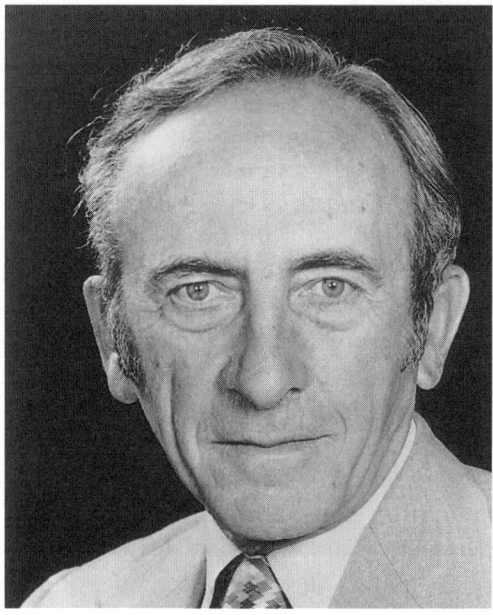

V.J. McGovern

Heparin is liberated at the same time. It is thought that heparin, which bears a negative electrical charge, is normally held in solution in the capillary endothelial cement film, thus constituting an electrostatic barrier which repels the negatively charged leukocytes. With severe injury, however, the mast cells become exhausted and if the endothelium is damaged so that it cannot restore an adequate cement film, leukocytes accumulate on the intimal surface. When the liberated heparin has become dissipated, the tissues become positively charged and leukocytes, attracted by the positive charge, migrate from the capillaries, there being no electrically-charged cement barrier to their passage."

L. Mirvish[210] of Johannesburg, South Africa (without supporting data) related the mucosal hyperemia and edema in ulcerative colitis to an immune "hypersensitivity reaction" mediated by mast cells, an interest also of S.C. Sommers[211] of New York. Binder and Hvidberg[212] of Copenhagen in 1967 reported an elevated histamine content in rectal mucosal biopsies in 17 of 36 patients with ulcerative colitis compared with control biopsies. The rectal inflammatory exudate in all 17 patients contained large numbers of eosinophils. The increased histamine content and the many eosinophils were considered "reflections of an allergic reaction in the mucosa," but this hypothesis was not pursued. In 1975 G. Lloyd et al.[213] of Manchester, England reported slightly increased numbers of mast cells and normal numbers of IgE-containing immunocytes in surgically resected bowel or rectal biopsies from patients with ulcerative colitis. In Crohn's disease, stainable mast cells were almost totally absent and IgE-containing immunocytes were decreased, suggesting an immediate hypersensitivity reaction as part of a local immunological response. However, therapy of ulcerative colitis with disodium chromoglycate, appropriate medication for immediate hypersensitivity reactions, proved ineffective. Balaza, Illyes and Vadasz[214] (1989) of Budapest, Hungary, also reported increased numbers of mast cells in active ulcerative colitis, closely associated with capillary blood vessels, neural fibers, myofibroblasts and collagenous fibers. Stead et al.[215] of McMaster University, Hamilton, Ontario, Canada (1989) similarly described the close apposition of mast cells to nerves in the human gastrointestinal mucosa. Increased numbers of mast cells were found also in white, male patients with microscopic colitis.[216] The early emphasis upon mast cells in the pathogenesis of ulcerative colitis is of interest in relation to the current recognition of human mast cells as important sources of nitric oxide and multiple cytokines mediating allergic and inflammatory reactions (IL-4, IL-5, IL-13, TNF-α),[217] including the finding of "significantly increased rates of mast cell tryptase secretion both in non-inflamed and inflamed tissue of ulcerative colitis" by M. Raithel et al.[218] of Erlangen-Nurenberg, Germany and the important role of mast cells in chronic stress-induced colonic epithelial barrier dysfunction in the rat, demonstrated by M.H. Perdue[219] and her associates at McMaster University, Hamilton, Ontario, Canada.

Lumb[220] and Lumb and Protheroe, Central Middlesex Hospital, London[221] (1958), in a study of 152 fresh surgical specimens, localized the earliest lesions of ulcerative colitis to the bases of the crypts of Lieberkuhn where neutrophils accumulated, with early necrosis of the basal cells, progressing to crypt abscesses formation. In 22 of 29 cases they also noted "small focal abnormalities ... in areas of resected colon which initially had appeared normal." A study of 130 surgical specimens and 271 rectal biopsy specimens did not identify significant vascular abnormalities. Lumb, dismissing extrinsic causes, speculated that, "a variety of stimuli, both intrinsic and extrinsic, may be sufficient to produce spreading ulceration of the colonic mucosa in an individual with intrinsic failure of normal epithelial regeneration."

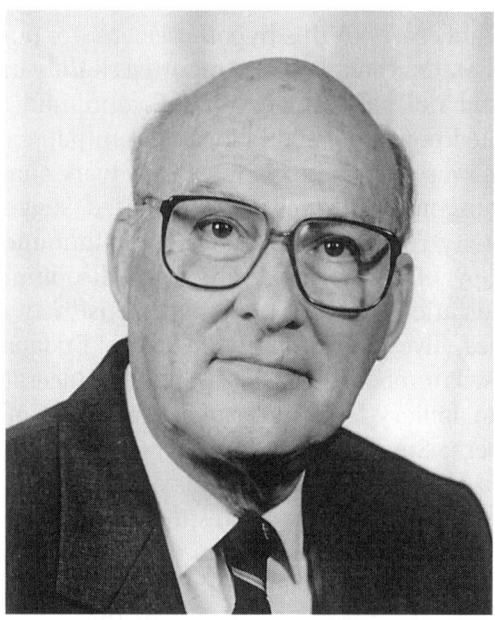

Basil C. Morson

B. Morson[222,223] (St. Marks Hospital, London) in the 1970s emphasized the continuity of the mucosal inflammation beginning in the rectum. "The initial abnormality is dilatation and congestion of the capillaries in the mucous membrane. This is immediately followed by cell death probably because of local anoxia. Further changes are likely to be the result of secondary infection of the damaged mucous membrane by organisms from the faeces and include crypt abscess formation, inflammatory cell infiltration and mucosal ulceration" ... "In active ulcerative colitis, the mucous membrane shows diffuse infiltration with chronic inflammatory cells, mainly lymphocytic and plasma cells but also eosinophiles. There also is a variable degree of capillary dilatation, vascular congestion and intramucosal hemorrhage (perhaps caused by a 'histamine-release mechanism, itself the result of "hypersensitivity" to unknown antigenic stimuli'). The epithelium shows necrosis of epithelial cells, goblet cell depletion and reactive hyperplasia, and some of the tubules contain an accumulation of polymorphonuclear leukocytes, so-called crypt abscesses. With remission, the first change is restoration of the goblet cell population, accompanied by a reduction in inflammation and the disappearance of crypt abscesses. The mucous membrane can return entirely to normal but if there have been repeated attacks of severe colitis, it is likely that the mucosa will show permanent signs of atrophy as judged by a reduction in the number of epithelial tubules per unit area, loss of parallelism of the tubules and failure of the base of the crypts to reach right down to the muscularis mucosae. Although none of these features individually is specific for ulcerative colitis, together they create a characteristic histologic picture." Morson, persuaded that "the colonic mucosa can be rendered anoxic by the squeezing action of the muscularis mucosae," considered ulcerative colitis a neuromuscular disorder caused by an imbalance of the autonomic nervous system, a concept also emphasized currently. Riis, Valdorf-Hansen and Anthonisen (Gentofte Hospital, Hellerup, Denmark) in 1966[224] identified latent chronicity as a distinguishing feature of the ulcerative colitis inflammatory reaction but did not elaborate on the factors involved.

P.B. Counsell and C.E. Dukes, St. Marks Hospital, London,[225,226] in 1952 and 1954, reviewing the surgical pathology of ulcerative colitis, cited R.S. Corbett,[43] who also emphasized vascular hyperemia and edema of the mucosa as the earliest change in ulcerative colitis. Dukes focused on histological changes related to carcinoma and noted that, during the process of epithelial regeneration and repair, detached fragments of glandular epithelium were buried in the submucosa or the muscular layer; one of the features of the epithelial dysplasia described by Morson and Pang[227] thirteen years later (1967). Intestinal cancer was found in seven of Dukes 120 patients (5.8%). Cook and Goligher[228] of Leeds, England, Riddell et al.[229] and Blackstone et al.[230] of the University of Chicago later expanded the dysplasia concept, which, with fiberoptic colonoscopy, constituted the basis of colon cancer screening programs in IBD.

Kirsner et al.[231] in 1951 had observed disorganization of the ground substance of the connective tissue of the bowel and loss of the basement membranes beneath the colonic epithelial cells in active ulcerative colitis, reappearing after successful therapy with ACTH, changes considered consistent with "collagen type disease," a disease mechanism popular during the 1950s. Utilizing the McManus and Mowry sulfuric acid-hematoxylin stain for basement membranes, in surgical pathology specimens of regional enteritis, ulcerative colitis, diverticulosis and diverticulitis, Sommers et al.[232] two years later failed to demonstrate dissolution or absence of basement membranes except in the presence of inflammatory exudate. Streicher, Catchpole and Pirani[233] of the University of Illinois in 1956 confirmed Kirsner's observations. However, additional studies by Kirsner and Jacobson[234] indicated that, while such abnormalities were indeed more severe in ulcerative colitis and were absent in one patient with active amebic colitis, they also were seen in several individuals with carcinoma of the colon.

The eosinophil, described by P. Ehrlich in 1879, characterized by avid staining of its granules when exposed to the acidic dye eosin, is increased in the rectal mucosa of ulcerative colitis and also in the lamina propria and submucosa of Crohn's disease intestine. The interrelationship between eosinophils and tissue mast cells is of interest since eosinophils often are associated with mast cells and both are involved in the immunology of the gut mucosal immune system. Mast cells elaborate a potent eosinophil chemotactic agent; the eosinophil ingests mast cell granules and neutralizes histamine, a mast cell product. The tissue mast cell can liberate a powerful chemotactic agent of anaphylaxis and is a significant modulator of immune responses.[235] During the 1960s, Riis and Anthonisen[236] of Copenhagen had been impressed with the increased numbers of eosinophils in the rectal discharges of patients with ulcerative colitis, "consistent with an allergic pathogenesis," as had been proposed for Crohn's disease by Tallroth in 1943. Forty years later, the eosinophil has been further identified as the source of important biological mediators not only in IBD but also in asthma, allergy and eosinophilic gastroenteritis.[237] Asking the question in 1999 "Activated Eosinophils in IBD: Do They Matter?," Desreumaux, Nutten and Colombel[238] of France stated: "Increased numbers of tissue eosinophils with ultrastructural evidence of activation have been noted in patients with ulcerative colitis and with Crohn's disease. In reference to eosinophil granule proteins, increased concentrations of cationic proteins have been found in jejunal effluent from patients with CD and in whole gut lavage fluid and feces from patients with IBD."

In 1938, Robertson and Kernohan,[239] during a study of the myenteric plexus in congenital megacolon, noted hypertrophy of the myenteric nerve plexus and increased numbers of ganglion cells in the colon of two patients with chronic ulcerative colitis. Fifteen years later (1953), a threefold increased number of parasympathetic ganglion cells was reported by Storsteen, Kernohan and Bargen[240] of the Mayo Clinic in the myenteric plexus of the ulcerative colitis colon, unrelated to the duration of the disease and the age or sex of the patient. Although fibrotic shortening of the colon may have contributed to the increased number of ganglion cells per unit of tissue examined, the increase appeared to be valid and was confirmed by P. Steiner at the University of Chicago one year later (unpublished data) (see also [241]). Studying rectal mucosal biopsies from 13 patients with ulcerative colitis, 7 with irritable colon and 7 control individuals, Kyosola, Penttila and Salaspuro[242] of Helsinki, Finland, in 1977 observed a "significantly pronounced" density of the adrenergic nerve network in the ulcerative colitis (also in the irritable colon) and implicated "biogenic amines" in the tissue reaction. Today, neurogenic-immune interactions are recognized participants in the IBD tissue reaction[243] and the local anesthetic lidocaine enemas have been used therapeutically.

PATHOLOGY – ELECTRON MICROSCOPY – ULCERATIVE COLITIS

Electron microscopic studies of the IBD tissue reaction demonstrated important alterations in the intestinal epithelium and submucosa of the ulcerative colitis bowel of uncertain pathogenetic significance. Having previously (1965) described the electron microscopic structure of the normal colonic mucosa in biopsies obtained at sigmoidoscopy (8 patients) and at operation in two individuals,[244] W.L. Donnellan of Northwestern University (Chicago) endeavored to identify "early histologic changes" in 27 patients with chronic ulcerative colitis studied by light and electron microscopy.[245] Unfortunately, most patients had taken various medications prior to examination, including corticosteroids in five individuals prior to the initial biopsy. The tissue sampling was confined to the "least involved bowel," arbitrarily estimated in the sigmoid at a level of 18 cm proximal to the anal verge. Degeneration of the reticulin fibers of the basement membrane beneath the surface columnar epithelium (resembling the changes described by Kirsner et al. in 1951), originated in tiny areas of the mucosa. "Changes" in the fibroblasts and histiocytes of the colonic mucosa and dilation of subepithelial capillaries were constant and "early" findings in ulcerative colitis, followed by a progressive infiltration of the lamina propria with plasma cells and lymphocytes and, in some cases, eosinophils and polymorphonuclear cells. Ulceration of the mucosa appeared to be directly related to platelet agglutination of small mucosal vessels. Etiologic emphasis was upon "the role of the fibroblast and histiocytes of the colonic mucosa and related collagen abnormalities," in accord with the observations of Movat and Ferando.[246]

The widespread axonal necrosis of enteric autonomic nerve fibers and ganglion cells in Crohn's disease noted at electron microscopy by A. Dvorak[247] of Boston was not seen in ulcerative colitis. "Nonspecific" loss of "mucosal neuropeptide innervation" in the surgically resected colon both in ulcerative colitis and in Crohn's disease, were considered consequences of severe inflammation contributed to the "disruption of local neuro-immunoregulation."[248] A comparative ultrastructural study of the mucosa in ulcerative colitis, Shigellosis and other human colonic disease by Yardley et al. of Johns Hopkins University in 1966 indicated the non-specificity of such findings as cytosegresomes, dilated endoplastic reticulum, altered mitochondria and of the intracellular spaces.[249,250] Electron microscopy of a rectal biopsy from a young patient with chronic ulcerative colitis for five years disclosed a "labyrinthine system of clefts and compartments between columnar mucosal epithelial cells ... clusters of small clavate fimbriae projected from the tips of microvilli" ... Their significance was not known. The vascular dilatation, congestion, and hyperemia and edema of the colonic mucosa emphasized by the early pathologists should be of interest to today's vascular endothelial biologists.[251]

"NATURAL" AND EXPERIMENTAL ULCERATIVE COLITIS

A 1946 literature review by R.S. Ginsberg and A.C. Ivy[252] considered the etiological implications of earlier efforts to produce an experimental ulcerative colitis, including bacterial agents, allergy, mechanical trauma, vascular ischemia and "neurogenic factors." Discarding emotional disturbances, the authors were impressed with experiments implicating diplostreptococci in ulcerative colitis but the review had little impact upon the direction of IBD research.

Investigative interest during the 1950s turned to possible animal counterparts of ulcerative colitis as new sources of information on IBD. Actually, veterinarians long have been aware of colitides in animals (e.g. dogs) and numerous inflammatory diseases of the colon, caused by bacteria or viruses, have been described in the veterinary literature (dogs, cat, horse, cattle, sheep, swine, rodents,[253] quails,[254] apes[255]). None duplicated human IBD in clinical course and complications.[256,257] The changes in rat colitis[253] (actually a "cecitis") today would be compared to Crohn's disease rather than ulcerative colitis (involvement of the cecum, chronic lymphangitis, obstructive lymphedema and lymphoid hyperplasia of mesenteric lymph nodes). The changes in the colonic mucosa in two young gorillas (Gorilla gorilla) and an orangutan (Pongo pygmaeus) were "virtually identical to those of the active phase of human ulcerative colitis" but non-specificity limits the interpretation. Only the colitis developing in captive cotton top tamarins (Saguinus oedipus),[258] when removed from their natural habitat in the rain forests of Colombia, South America and housed in the United States, resembled human ulcerative colitis in clinical and histologic features, therapeutic response to sulfasalazine and in the later development of colonic carcinoma.[259] Since tamarin colitis does not occur among the wild cotton top tamarins of Colombia, an environmental etiology for the "tamarin colitis" is likely ("cold stress," ?infection).

Early attempts to induce ulcerative colitis in animals (rabbit, guinea pig, hamster, dog, mouse, rat) included nutritional deficiencies (vitamin A[260]) pantothenic acid,[261] pyridoxine, folic acid deficiency,[262] local vasoconstriction induced by adrenalin hydrochloride injected intraperitoneally in dogs,[263] the intravenous injection of staphylococcus toxin in rabbits, the administration of enzymes, collagenase and lysozyme intrarectally and intraarterially, and later the topical (colonic) application of 4–10% acetic acid and other chemical agents; e.g. trinitrobenzene sulfonic acid in 50% alcohol, dextran sulfate sodium, peptidoglycan polysaccharide and indomethacin.[264–266] The bowel was readily injured but human ulcerative colitis with its persistent, recurrent and complicated course was not reproduced. In 1944 Portis, Block and Necheles of Chicago,[267] noting the large content of trypsin in rectal and ileostomy discharges of IBD patients, implicated pancreatic enzymes (e.g. trypsin) acting upon the colonic epithelium. Perfusion of the colon in dogs with a 1 to 2% trypsin solution increased mucus secretion and induced hemorrhages; findings that were quickly refuted by other investigators.[268,269]

Unsuccessful experiments at the University of Chicago during the 1950s included the repeated and prolonged instillation of human pancreatic juice and bile into canine ileocolonic pouches and the repeated intrarectal instillation of concentrated solutions of gram-negative bacterial endotoxins but colitis did not develop. Animal experiments involving psychogenic, immunologic and transgenic mechanisms are noted elsewhere in the text. In early studies elsewhere, ulcerations in the right colon were produced in guinea pigs and rabbits given a 5% aqueous solution of a common food additive carrageenan (a sulfated polysaccharide of high molecular weight extracted from red sea weed – species chondrus crispus and Eucheuma spinosum) in drinking water.[270,271] Experimental carrageenan colitis was enhanced by a component of the outer cell wall of the anaerobe B. vulgatus, inhibited by the antibiotic metronidazole,[272] and non-reproducible in germfree animals, an early indication of the determinant role of the intestinal microflora. Carrageenans are present in infant foods, ice cream, canned fruit, jams, soups, toothpaste and tablet binders and temporarily were implicated in the development of ulcerative colitis.

W.E. Roediger of Australia, then at the Radcliffe Infirmary, Oxford, in 1980 noted decreased oxidation of N. butyrate in isolated colonic epithelial cells from the mucosa of the descending colon in patients with ulcerative colitis.[273] In 1986 he induced a colitis via the inhibition of mitochondrial short chain fatty acid (butyric acid) oxidation in the colonic mucosa by sodium 2-bromo-octanoate rectally.[274] These findings prompted the therapeutic use of butyrate enemas in ulcerative colitis with unimpressive results. While observations such as the abnormal release of ^{51}CR by ulcerative colitis colonic epithelial cells suggested "an underlying (undefined) abnormality" in the colonic epithelium of ulcerative colitis,[275] and while the intestinal epithelium obviously participates in the IBD inflammatory reaction, the precise nature of the presumed epithelial dysfunction is yet to be determined.

Other exogenous agents inducing ulcerative colitis included peptido-glycan-polysaccharide, dextran sodium sulfate and Freund's adjuvant. In the early 1990s, intestinal inflammation became more readily reproducible in mice and rats, via many novel methods, including not only chemical, microbial and polymer-induced models, but also via genetically engineered[276] (transgenic, gene "knockout" [e.g. IL-2, IL-10] models, a heritable colitis in C3H/HEj Bir mice, developed by Elson and his colleagues, in conjunction with the Jackson Laboratories (Maine, U.S.A.) SCID mice following reconstitution with naive CD45RB^{h1} T cells and the NOD/it mouse model of diabetes which develops a spontaneous autoimmune discontinuous colitis, providing a diverse array of experimental models for biologic investigation. As pointed out by F. Cominelli et al.,[277] the newer models have produced important information on mucosal immunoregulation and IBD inflammation, including the key role of regulatory T cells, specifically CD^{4+} T cells, proinflammatory and immunoregulating cytokines, the role of susceptibility genes and the essentiality of the indigenous bacterial flora in the experimental disease.

W. Strober and his colleagues[278] (National Institutes of Health) observed: "two broad categories of animal models of mucosal inflammation have been discovered: (a) a mucosal inflammation, IL-12 driven, with the appearance of Th$_1$ T cells producing proinflammatory cytokines, such as IFN-γ and TNF-α and (b) a second type of mucosal inflammation, IL-4 driven, with the appearance of Th$_2$ T cells. The Th$_1$ model clearly resembles the Crohn's disease tissue reaction. The Th$_2$ model resembles the ulcerative colitis type of inflammation." Strober further notes, "that in both the Th$_1$ and Th$_2$-type models, a variety of very different immunologic defects can lead to the same basic immunopathology." Strober concluded his important overview of mucosal immunoregulation and inflammatory bowel disease: "The ... new and emerging knowledge of IBD derived from the study of murine models represents a significant advance in our understanding of this disease. It is safe to say, however, that the models have hardly been exhausted; on the contrary, they remain storehouses of information that can be visited again and again for new information concerning the mechanisms of mucosal homeostasis."

REFERENCES

Early IBD Related Events – Ulcerative Colitis Origins

1. Cohen H. The evolution of the concept of disease. Proc Roy Soc Med 1955;48: 156–60.
2. Yanchi L. The essential book of traditional Chinese medicine. Translated by Tingyn F and Laidi C. Vol. 1, New York: Columbia University Press, 1988.
3. The genuine works of Hippocrates translated by Adams F for the Sydenham Society, London, 1849, 2 Volumes cited by Guthrie D – A History of Medicine. Philadelphia: JB Lippincott Co. (2 Volumes), 1946.
4. Aretaeus. On the causes and symptoms of chronic diseases. (ca 300 AD) cited by de Dombal FT. Ulcerative colitis: definition, historical background, aetiology, diagnosis, natural history, and local complications. Postgrad Med J 1968;44: 684–92.
5. Soranus of Ephesus. Cited by Mettler CC. History of medicine. Philadelphia, PA: Blakiston, 1947.
6. Sydenham T. Medical observations concerning history and cure of acute diseases, 3rd edn, Vol. 1. London: Greenhill, 1898.
7. Burch W, Gump DW, Krawitt EL. Historical case report of Sir William Johnson, The Mohawk Baronet. Am J Gastroent 1992;87:1023–25.
8. Morson BC. Current concepts of colitis. The 1970 Lettsomian Lectures. Trans Med Soc London 1970;86:159–76.
9. Baillie M. The morbid anatomy of some of the most important parts of the human body. Printed for London: J Johnson and G Nicol, 1793.
10. Rodin AE. The influence of Matthew Baillie's morbid anatomy. Diseased appearances in the intestines. Springfield, IL: CC Thomas, Chapter viii, 1973:146–8.
11. de Dombal FT. Ulcerative colitis: definition, historical background, aetiology, diagnosis, natural history and local complications. Postgrad Med J 1968;44:684–92.
12. Wilson PJE. The young pretender. Br Med J 1961;ii:1226.
13. Rokitansky K. Der dysenterische prozess auf dem dickdarms und der ihmgleiche. Med Jahrb K K Staates 1839;29:88.
14. Rokitansky K. A manual of pathologic anatomy. 4 Volumes. London: Sydenham Society, 1849–54.
15. Virchow RLD. Die krankheiten geshwultste. 3 Volumes. Berlin: Hirschwald, 1863.
16. Crohn BB. An historic note on ulcerative colitis. Gastroenterology 1962;42:366–7.
17. Mottet NK. Histopathologic spectrum of regional enteritis and ulcerative colitis. Philadelphia: WB Saunders Co., 1971.
18. Cattan R, Bucaille M, Carasso R. La rectocolite hemorragique et purulente. Paris: Editions Medicales Flammarion, 1959.
19. Wilks S. Morbid appearances in the intestine of Miss Bankes. London Medical Times and Gazette 1859;2:264–8.

20. Stanford E. Thomas Addison and his times – the tragic last year 1859–1860. History of Medicine 1973;5:3–10.
21. Fielding JF. Inflammatory bowel disease. Br Med J 1985;290:47–8.
22. Habershon S. Diseases of the abdomen. London: J Churchill, 1862.
23. Wilks S, Moxon W. Lectures on pathological anatomy, 2nd edn. London: Lindsay and Blackiston, 1875:408.
24. Woodward JJ. Pseudopolyps of the colon: An anomalous result of follicular ulceration (of the colon). Am J Med Sci 1881;81:142–5.
25. Allchin WH. A case of extensive ulceration of the colon. Trans Path Soc London 1885;36:199–202.
26. Thomas CH. Ulceration of the colon with a much enlarged fatty liver. Trans Path Soc Philadelphia 1874;4:87–8.
27. Hale-White W. On simple ulcerative colitis and other rare intestinal ulcers. Guy's Hosp Rep 1888;45:131–62.
28. Robson M. Case of colitis with ulceration. Treated by inguinal colostomy and local treatment of the ulcerated surfaces with subsequent closure of the artificial anus. Trans Clin Soc London 1893;26:213–5.
29. Lister TD. A specimen of diffuse ulcerative colitis with secondary acute interstitial hepatitis. Trans Path Soc London 1899;50:130–3.
30. Weir RF. A new use for the useless appendix in the surgical treatment of obstinate colitis. Med Record 1902;62:201–2.
31. Boas I. (1903) cited by Lups S, Baker AK. Vaccine therapy in ulcerative colitis. Am J Dig Dis 1935;21:65–90.
32. Wilson AG. A case of ulcerative colitis with multiple perforations. Lancet 1904;2:1208–9.
33. Lockhart-Mummery JP. The causes of colitis: with special reference to its surgical treatment, with an account of 36 cases. Lancet 1907;1:1638–43.
34. Cammeron HC, Rippman CH. Statistics of ulcerative colitis from London hospitals. Proc Roy Soc Med 1909;2:100–6.
35. Allchin WH. Ulcerative colitis. Proc Roy Soc Med 1909;2:59–82.
36. Hale-White W. Discussion – 1909 London symposium on ulcerative colitis. Proc Roy Soc Med 1909;2:59–156. (Total symposium. Many discussants.)
37. Hawkins HP. An address on the natural history of ulcerative colitis and its bearing upon treatment. Br Med J (Clin Res) 1909;1:765–70.
38. Stierlin E. Zur rontgen diagnostik der colitis ulcerosa. Z Klin Med 1913;75:486–93.
39. Kienbock R. Zur rontgendiagnose der colitis ulcerosa. Fortschr Geb Rontgenstrahlen 1913;20:231–9.
40. Kantor JL. Colon studies. IV. The roentgen diagnosis of colitis. Am J Roentg Radium Ther 1927;17:405–16.
41. Bassler A. Ulcerative colitis. Interstate Med J 1913;20:705–6.
42. Brown JY. The value of complete physiological rest of the large bowel in the treatment of certain ulcerative and obstructive lesions of this organ. Surg Gynecol Obstet 1913;16:610–3.
43. Corbett RS. A review of the surgical treatment of chronic ulcerative colitis. Proc Roy Soc Med 1945;38:277–90.
44. Hewitt JH, Howard WT. Chronic ulcerative colitis with polyps. Arch Int Med 1915;15:714–23.
45. Logan AH. Chronic ulcerative colitis: A review of one hundred and seventeen cases. Northwest Med 1919;18:1–9.
46. Yeomans FC. Chronic ulcerative colitis. JAMA 1921;77:2043–8.
47. Strauss H. Ueber kolitis-probleme. Dtsch Med Wochschr 1923;49:1568–70.
48. Hurst AF. Ulcerative colitis. Guy's Hosp Rep 1921;71:26–41.

49. Mathieu A, Roux JC. Pathologie gastrointestinale. A. Schmidt. VII Colitis chronica mucosa et membranacea. VIII Colitis Chronica Suppurativa (Colitis Gravis, Colitis Ulcerosa). Darmkrankheiten Wiesbaden, Clinique et Therapeutique. Paris: O'Dorn, 1909:325 and 486–94. Cited by Hurst AF (48).
50. Buie LA. Chronic ulcerative colitis. JAMA 1926;87:1271–4.
51. Einhorn M. Chronic ulcerative colitis and its treatment. New York Med J 1923; 117:214–8.
52. Crohn BB, Rosenberg H. The medical treatment of chronic ulcerative colitis (nonspecific). JAMA 1924;83:526–31.
53. Crohn BB, Rosenberg H. The sigmoidoscopic picture of chronic ulcerative colitis (nonspecific). Am J Med Sci 1925;170:220–8.
54. Thorlakson PHT. Primary ulcerative colitis. Can Med Assoc J 1924;14:1168–73.
55. Bensaude R, Oury P. Quelques remarques sur les rectocolites hemorrhagiques et purulentes et leurs traitements. J Med Chir Prat 1927;98:761–72.
56. Schur H. Ueber die ursachen der colitis ulcerosa und ihre behandlung. Wien Klin Wochnschr 1927;40:756–9.
57. Alekesiev A. Etiology and therapy of chronic ulcerative colitis. Klin Med 1927; 5:863–71.
58. Debenedetti E. La colite ucerosa cronica. Rassegna Internaz Clin erap 1930; 11:459–80.
59. Crohn BB. Ocular lesions complicating ulcerative colitis. Am J Med Sci 1925;169: 260–7.
60. Ellis PP, Gentry JH. Ocular complications of ulcerative colitis. J Ophthalmol 1964;58:779–85.
61. Billson FA, de Dombal FT, Watkinson GA, Goligher JC. Ocular complications of ulcerative colitis. Gut 1967;8:102–6.
62. Yeomans FC. Carcinomatous degeneration of rectal adenomas. JAMA 1927;89: 852–5.
63. Bargen JA, Dixon CF. Chronic ulcerative colitis associated with carcinoma. Arch Surg 1928;17:561–76.
64. Ive C, Venables JF. Some cases of ulcerative colitis. Cited by Hurst AF. Colitis. Br Encyclopedia Med Pract 1937;3:292–316.
65. Bargen JA. Complications and sequelae of ulcerative colitis. Ann Int Med 1929;3: 335–52.
66. Brunsting LA, Goeckerman WH, O'Leary PA. Pyoderma (echthyma) gangrenosum. Arch Dermatol 1930;22:655–80.
67. Lansbury J, Bargen JA. The association of multiple hepatic abscesses and chronic ulcerative colitis. Med Clin North Am 1933;16:1427–31.
68. Brooke PA. Erythema nodosum-like lesions in chronic ulcerative colitis. New Eng J Med 1933;209:233–5.
69. Jankelson IR, Massell BF. Pyogenic skin lesions accompanying chronic ulcerative colitis; report of 5 cases. Am J Digest Dis 1936;3:19–22.
70. Helmholz HF. Chronic ulcerative colitis in childhood. Am J Dis Child 1923;26: 418–30.
71. Bourne G. Chronic ulcerative colitis in children. Arch Dis Children 1926;1:175–81.
72. Jackman RP, Bargen JA, Helmholz HF. Life histories of ninety-five children with chronic ulcerative colitis: A statistical study based on comparison with a whole group of eight hundred and seventy-one patients. Am J Dis Children 1940;59: 459–67.
73. Bargen JA, Kennedy RLJ. Chronic ulcerative colitis in children. Postgrad Med 1955;17:127–31.

74. Beranbaum SL, Waldron RJ. Chronic ulcerative colitis in a newborn infant. Pediatrics 1952;9:773–8.
75. Lagercrantz R. Ulcerative colitis in children. Acta Paediatr Uppsala Suppl 1949;75:89–151.
76. Kirsner JB, Raskin HF, Palmer WL. Ulcerative colitis in children – observations in selected patients. Am J Dis Child 1955;90:141–52.
77. Hijmans JC, Enzer NB. Ulcerative colitis in childhood. Pediatrics 1962;29:389–403.
78. Korelitz BI, Grobits D, Danziger I. The prognosis of ulcerative colitis with onset in childhood. Ann Int Med 1962;57:582–93.
79. Davidson M, Bloom AA, Kugler MM. Chronic ulcerative colitis of childhood. J Pediatr 1965;67:471–90.
80. Hern JRB. Ulcerative colitis. Guy's Hosp Rep 1931;81:322–74.
81. Hardy TL, Bulmer E. Ulcerative colitis – a survey of ninety five cases. Br Med J 1933;2:812–5.
82. Thaysen TEH. Simple haemorrhagic proctitis and proctosigmoiditis. Acta Med Scand 1934;84:1–24.
83. Barnes CS, Hayes HH. Ulcerative colitis complicating pregnancy and the puerperium. Am J Obstet Gynecol 1931;22:907–12.
84. Abramson D, Jankelson IR, Milner LR. Pregnancy in idiopathic ulcerative colitis. Am J Obstet Gynecol 1951;61:121–9.
85. MacDougall I. Ulcerative colitis and pregnancy. Lancet 1955;2:641–3.
86. Crohn BB, Yarnis H, Crohn EB, Walter RI, Gabrielove LJ. Ulcerative colitis and pregnancy. Gastroenterology 1956;30:391–403.
87. Korelitz BI. Pregnancy, fertility and inflammatory bowel disease. Am J Gastroenterol 1982;80:365–374.
88. Mones-Gallart E, Sanjuan PD, eds. Colitis ulcerosa graves non amibianas – etiologia, diagnostica, y tratamiento, salvat. Barcelona: LA Barcelone, 1935.

Increasing Clinical Recognition

89. Sloan WP, Bargen JA, Gage RP. Life histories of patients with chronic ulcerative colitis: a review of 2,000 cases. Gastroenterology 1950;16:25–38.
90. Bockus HL, Roth JLA, Buchman E, Kalser M, Staub WR, Finkelstein A, et al. Life history of nonspecific ulcerative colitis: relation of prognosis to anatomical and clinical varieties. Gastroenterologia 1956;86:549–81.
91. Roth JLA, Valdes-Dapena A, Stein GN, Bockus HL. Toxic megacolon in ulcerative colitis. Gastroenterology 1959;37:239–55.
92. Willard JH. Ulcerative colitis – a review. Int Clinics 1939;4:281–98.
93. Ricketts WE, Palmer WL. Complications of chronic nonspecific ulcerative colitis. Gastroenterology 1946;7:55–66.
94. Kirsner JB, Palmer WL, Maimon JN, Ricketts WE. Clinical course of chronic nonspecific ulcerative colitis. JAMA 1948;137:922–8.
95. Goldgraber MB, Humphreys EM, Kirsner JB, Palmer WL. Carcinoma and ulcerative colitis. A clinical-pathologic study. II. Statistical analysis. Gastroenterology 1958;34:840–6.
96. Rudner HG. Chronic ulcerative colitis. Southern Med J 1935;28:429–34.
97. Monroe CW. Chronic nonspecific ulcerative colitis. Review of 138 cases. Surgery 1937;2:575–80.
98a Mackie TT. Ulcerative colitis due to chronic infection with Flexner Y bacillus. JAMA 1932;98:1706–10.

98b. Mackie TT. The medical management of chronic ulcerative colitis. JAMA 1938; 111:2071–6.
99. Minzer IJ. Pyoderma gangrenosum, onychogryphosis and onycholysis with ulcerative colitis. Arch Dermat Syph 1939;40:541–3.
100. Brust JCM, Bargen JA. Chronic ulcerative colitis among elderly persons. Minnesota Med 1935;18:583–5.
101. Banks BN, Klayman MI. Idiopathic ulcerative colitis beginning after the age of fifty. New Eng J Med 1953;24:91–6.
102. Bercovitz ZT. Ulcerative colitis in older age patients. Gastroenterology 1960; 39:28–33.
103. Bargen JA, Barker NW. Extensive arterial and venous thrombosis complicating ulcerative colitis. Arch Int Med 1936;58:17–31.
104. Comfort MW, Bargen JA, Morlock CG. The association of chronic ulcerative colitis (colitis gravis) with hepatic insufficiency. Med Clin North Am 1938;22: 1089–97.
105. Schlicke CP, Bargen JA. Clubbed fingers and ulcerative colitis. Am J Dig Dis 1940; 7:17–22.
106. Fielding JF, Cooke WT. Finger clubbing and regional enteritis. Gut 1971;12:442–4.
107. Lindahl WW, Bargen JA. Nephrolithiasis complicating chronic ulcerative colitis after ileostomy. A report of six cases. J Urol 1941;46:183–92.
108. Deren JJ, Porush JG, Levitt MF, Rhilrani MT. Nephrolithiasis as a complication of ulcerative colitis and regional enteritis. Ann Int Med 1962;56:843–53.
109. Gelzayd EA, Breuer RI, Kirsner JB. Nephrolithiasis in inflammatory bowel disease. Am J Dig Dis 1968;13:1027–34.
110. Davidson M. Juvenile ulcerative colitis. Arch Int Med 1939;64:1187–95.
111. Benson EE, Bargen JA. Chronic ulcerative colitis as a cause of retarded sexual and somatic development. Gastroenterology 1943;1:147–59.
112. Ricketts WE, Benditt EP, Palmer WL. Chronic ulcerative colitis with infantilism and carcinoma of the colon. Gastroenterology 1945;5:272–80.
113. Welch CS, Adams M, Wakefield EG. Metabolic studies in ulcerative colitis. J Clin Invest 1937;16:161–8.
114. Sappington TS, Bockus HL. Nitrogen metabolism in chronic idiopathic ulcerative colitis and its therapeutic significance. Ann Int Med 1949;31:282–302.
115. Kirsner JB, Sheffner AL, Palmer WL. Studies on amino acid excretion in man. V. Chronic ulcerative colitis and regional enteritis. J Clin Invest 1950;29:874–900.
116. Posey EL, Bargen JA. Metabolic derangements in chronic ulcerative colitis. Gastroenterology 1950;16:39–56.
117. Jankelson IR, McClure CW, Sweetsir FN. Chronic ulcerative colitis. II. Complications outside the digestive tract. Review Gastroenterology 1942;9:99–104.
118. Chisholm TC. Acute fulminating ulcerative colitis with massive perforation and peritonitis – report of a case. Arch Surg 1946;53:462–76.
119. Norland CC, Kirsner JB. Toxic dilatation of colon (toxic megacolon): etiology, treatment and prognosis in 42 patients. Medicine 1969;48:229–50.
120. Jalan KN, Sircus W, Card WI, Falconer CWA, Bruce J, Crean GP, et al. An experience of ulcerative colitis. I. Toxic dilation in 55 cases. Gastroenterology 1969;57:68–82.
121. Ricketts WE, Kirsner JB, Rothman S. Pyoderma gangrenosum in nonspecific ulcerative colitis. Am J Med 1948;5:69–75.
122. Leishman AG. Idiopathic ulcerative colitis with severe ulceration of the skin and peritonitis. Proc Roy Soc Med 1949;42:105–6.
123. Butler EC. Spreading ulceration of the skin associated with idiopathic ulcerative colitis. Proc Roy Soc Med 1948;41:474–6.

124. Maratka Z, Spellberg MA. Observations on the clinical course of nonspecific ulcerative colitis. Gastroenterology 1949;12:79–86.
125. Cuthbertson AM, Hawk WA, Turnbull Jr. RB, Hughes ES. A comparison of primary inflammatory disease of the colon in Australia and in the United States of America. Aust NZ J Surg 1970;39:273–4.
126. Domagk G. Ein beitrag zur chemotherapie der bakteriellen infektione. Dtsch Med Wochschr 1935;61:250–3.
127. Fleming A. The 1928 discovery of penicillin. Br Med Bull 1944;2:4–5.
128. Hench PS, Kendall EC, Slocumb CH, Polley HF. The effect of a hormone of the adrenal cortex (Compound E) and of pituitary adrenocorticotropic hormone on rheumatoid arthritis – preliminary report. Proc Staff Meet Mayo Clinic 1949;24:181–97.
129. Wigley RD, MacLaurin BP. A study of ulcerative colitis in New Zealand showing a low incidence in Maoris. Br Med J 1962;2:228–31.
130. Tandon BN, Mathus AK, Mohapatra LN, Jandon HD, Wig KL. A study of the prevalence and clinical pattern of nonspecific ulcerative colitis in northern India. Gut 1965;6:448–53.
131. Alm T, Ihre B. Colitis ulcerosa. Nord Med 1958;59:572–5.
132. Matsunaga F. Clinical studies in ulcerative colitis and its related increase in Japan. Proc World Congress of Gastroenterology, Washington, Vol. 2. Baltimore: Williams and Wilkins, 1958:955–60.
133. Guangli C. The treatment of chronic ulcerative colitis in Chinese. Analysis of fifty cases. Chinese J Coloproctology 1985;5:9–10.
134. Brooke BN. What is ulcerative colitis? Lancet 1953;1:1220–5.
135. Kirsner JB, Palmer WL. Ulcerative colitis (considerations of its etiology and treatment). JAMA 1954;155:341–6.
136. Kirsner JB, Palmer WL, Klotz AP. Reversibility in ulcerative colitis. Radiology 1951;5:1–14.
137. Kirsner JB, Van Woert M. Irreversibility and reversibility in ulcerative colitis. Med Clinics North Am 1964;48:143–57.
138. Jones JH, Lennard-Jones JE, Young AC. Reversibility of radiological appearances during clinical improvement in colonic Crohn's disease. Gut 1969;10:738–43.
139. Ball PW, Baggenstoss AH, Bargen JA. Pancreatic lesions associated with chronic ulcerative colitis. Arch Pathol 1950;50:347–58.
140. Graef V, Baggenstoss AH, Sauer WG, Spittell Jr. JA. Venous thrombosis occurring in nonspecific ulcerative colitis. Arch Int Med 1966;117:377–82.
141. Kehoe EL, Newcomer KL. Thromboembolic phenomena in ulcerative colitis. Two case reports. Arch Int Med 1964;113:711–5.
142. Pollard HM, Block M. Association of hepatic insufficiency with chronic ulcerative colitis. Arch Int Med 1948;82:159–74.
143. Kleckner, Jr. MS, Stauffer MH, Bargen JA, Dockerty MB. Hepatic lesions in the living patient with chronic ulcerative colitis as demonstrated by needle biopsy. Gastroenterology 1952;22:13–23.
144. Kimmelstiel P, Large, Jr. HJ, Verner HD. Liver damage in ulcerative colitis. Am J Path 1952;28:259–90.
145. Palmer WL, Kirsner JB, Goldgraber M, Fuentes SS. Diseases of the liver in chronic ulcerative colitis. Am J Med 1964;36:856–66.
146. Brooke BN, Slaney G. Portal bacteremia in ulcerative colitis. Lancet 1958;1:1206–7.
147. Rankin JG, Boden RW, Goulston SJM, Morrow W. The liver in ulcerative colitis. Treatment of pericholangitis with Tetracycline. Lancet 1959;2:1110–2.
148. Mistilis SP. Pericholangitis and ulcerative colitis. I. Pathology, etiology and pathogenesis. Ann Int Med 1965;63:1:1–16.

149. Broome V, Lindberg G, Lofberg R. Primary sclerosing cholangitis in ulcerative colitis – a risk factor for the development of dysplasia and DNA aneupoloidy? Gastroenterology 1992;102:1877–80.
150. Wheelock FG, Warren R. Ulcerative colitis – follow up studies. New Engl J Med 1955;252:421–5.
151. Bacon HE, Ouyang LM, Carroll PT, Cates BA, Villalba G, McGregor RA. Nonspecific ulcerative colitis with reference to mortality, morbidity, complications and long-term survivals following colectomy. Am J Surg 1956;92:688–95.
152. Kern, Jr. F, Almy TP, Abbott FK, Bogdonoff MD. The motility of the distal colon in nonspecific ulcerative colitis. Gastroenterology 1951;19:492–503.
153. Chaudhary NA, Truelove SC. Human colon motility. A comparative study of normal subjects, patients with ulcerative colitis and patients with the irritable colon syndrome. I. Resting patterns of motility. Gastroenterology 1961;40:1–17.
154. Chaudhary NA, Truelove SC. Human colon motility. A comparative study of normal subjects, patients with ulcerative colitis and patients with the irritable colon syndrome. II. The effect of prostigmine. Gastroenterology 1961;40:18–26.
155. Chaudhary NA, Truelove SC. Human colon motility. A comparative study of normal subjects, patients with ulcerative colitis and patients with the irritable colon syndrome. III. Effects of emotions. Gastroenterology 1961;40:27–36.
156. Hench PS. Acute and chronic arthritis. Nelson's loose-leaf living surgery. New York: Thomas Nelson and Sons, 1935:104.
157. Bywaters EGL, Ansell B. Arthritis associated with ulcerative colitis – a clinical and pathological study. Ann Rheum Dis 1958;17:169–83.
158. Fernandez-Herlihy J. The articular manifestations of chronic ulcerative colitis. An analysis of 555 cases. New Engl J Med 1959;261:259–63.
159. Wright V, Watkinson G. The arthritis of ulcerative colitis. Medicine 1959;38:243–59.
160. McEwen C, Lingg C, Kirsner JB, Spencer JA. Arthritis accompanying ulcerative colitis. Am J Med 1962;33:923–41.
161. Steinberg VL, Storey G. Ankylosing spondylitis and chronic inflammatory lesions of the intestines. Br Med J 1957;2:1157–9.
162. Romanus R. Intestinal infections and pelvo-spondylitis ossificans. Acta Med Scand Suppl 1953;280:316–23.
163. McBride JA, King MJ, Baikie AG, Crean GP, Sircus W. Ankylosing spondylitis and chronic inflammatory diseases of the intestines. Br Med J 1963;2:483–6.
164. Beal RW, Skyring AP, McRae J, Firkin BG. The anaemia of ulcerative colitis. Gastroenterology 1963;45:589–603.
165. Wasserman F, Krosnick A, Tumen H. Necrotizing angiitis associated with chronic ulcerative colitis. Am J Med 1954;17:736–43.
166. Lehtinen M, Lentinen E, Nikkila E. Microangiopathic hemolytic anemia in ulcerative colitis. Report of a case. Scand J Gastroenterol 1968;3:417–24.
167. McCarthy P, Shklar G. A syndrome of pyostomatitis vegetans and ulcerative colitis. Arch Dermatol 1963;88:913–9.
168. Edwards FC, Truelove SC. The course and prognosis of ulcerative colitis. I. Short-term prognosis and II. Long-term prognosis. Gut 1963;4:299–315. III. Complications and IV. Carcinoma of the colon. Gut 1964;5:1–22.
169. McConnell F, Hanelin J, Robbins LL. Plain film diagnosis of fulminating ulcerative colitis. Radiology 1958;71:674–82.
170. Dawson IMP, Pryse-Davies J. The development of a carcinoma of the large intestine in ulcerative colitis. Br J Surg 1959;47:113–28.
171. Goldgraber MB, Kirsner JB. Carcinoma of the colon in ulcerative colitis. Cancer 1964;17:657–65.

172. Devroede GJ, Taylor WF, Sauer WG, Jackman RJ, Stickler GB. Cancer risk and life expectancy of children with ulcerative colitis. New Engl J Med 1971;285:17–21.
173. MacDougall IPM. Ulcerative colitis and carcinoma of the large intestine. Br Med J 1954;1:852–4.
174. Bargen JA, Sauer WG, Sloan WP, Gage RP. The development of cancer in chronic ulcerative colitis. Gastroenterology 1954;26:32–7.
175. Warren IA, Berk JE. The etiology of chronic nonspecific ulcerative colitis. Gastroenterology 1957;33:395–422.
176. Almy T, Plaut AG. Ulcerative colitis – a report of progress based upon recent literature. Gastroenterology 1965;49:295–314.
177. Rhodes JB, Kirsner JB. Early and late course of patients with ulcerative colitis after ileostomy and colectomy. Surg Gynecol Obstet 1965;121:1303–1314.
178. Wright R. Progress in gastroenterology – ulcerative colitis. Gastroenterology 1970;58:875–97.

Initial Pathology of Ulcerative Colitis and Its Pathogenetic Implications

179. Manson Bahr PH. The differential diagnosis of disease of the colon (dysentery and colitis) and their complications. Trans Med Soc London 1936;59:203 cited by Morson BC. The 1970 Lettsomian Lectures. Trans Med Soc London 1970;86:159–76.
180. Buie LA, Bargen JA. Chronic ulcerative colitis – a disease of systemic origin. JAMA 1933;101:1462–6.
181. Bargen JA, Jackman RJ, Kerr JG. Studies on the life histories of patients with chronic ulcerative colitis (thrombo ulcerative colitis) with some suggestions for treatment. Ann Int Med 1938;12:339–52.
182. Lium R. Etiology of ulcerative colitis. I. The preparation, care and secreting of colonic explants in dogs. Arch Int Med 1939;63:201–9.
183. Lium R. Etiology of ulcerative colitis. II. Effect of induced muscular spasm on colonic explants in dogs with comment on relation of muscular spasm to ulcerative colitis. Arch Int Med 1939;63:210–25.
184. Lium R, Porter JE. Observations on the etiology of ulcerative colitis. III. Distribution of lesions and its possible significance. Am J Pathol 1939;15:73–7.
185. Monaghan JF. Ulcerative colitis. In: Bockus H, ed. Gastroenterology, Vol. 2. Philadelphia: WB Saunders Co., 1944:549–614.
186. Warren S, Sommers SC. Pathogenesis of ulcerative colitis. Am J Pathol 1949;25:657–79.
187. Warren W, Sommers S. Pathology of regional ileitis and ulcerative colitis. JAMA 1954;154:189–93.
188. Dawson B. Discussion of ulcerative colitis. Proc Roy Soc Med 1909;2:94–5.
189. Victor RG, Kirsner JB, Palmer WL. Failure to induce ulcerative colitis experimentally with filtrates of feces and rectal mucosa. Gastroenterology 1950;14:398–400.
190. Stoughton RB. Enzymatic cytolysis of epithelium by filtrates of feces from patients with ulcerative colitis. Science 1952;116:37–9.
191. Fleming WH, Smith EW, Hendrix TR. Acantholytic factor and ulcerative colitis. Bull Johns Hopkins Hosp 1962;111:285–91.
192. Sammons HG. Mucinases in ulcerative colitis. Lancet 1951;261:239–40.
193. Florey HW. The secretion and function of gastrointestinal mucus. Gastroenterology 1962;43:326–9.

194. Greco V, Lauro G, Fabbrini A, Torsoli A. Histochemistry of the colonic epithelial mucins in normal subjects and in patients with ulcerative colitis. A qualitative and histophotometric investigation. Gut 1967;8:491–6.
195. Hellstrom HR, Fisher ER. Estimation of mucosal mucin as an aid in the differentiation of Crohn's disease of the colon and chronic ulcerative colitis. Am J Clin Pathol 1967;48:259–68.
196. Filipe MI, Dawson I. The diagnostic value of mucosubstances in rectal biopsies from patients with ulcerative colitis and Crohn's disease. Gut 1970;11:229–34.
197. Fraser GM, Clamp JR. Changes in human colonic mucus in ulcerative colitis. Gut 1975;16:832–3.
198. Filipe MI. Mucins in the human gastrointestinal epithelium – a review. Invest Cell Pathol 1979;2(3):195–216.
199. Podolsky DK, Isselbacher KJ. Composition of human colonic mucin – selective alteration in inflammatory bowel disease. J Clin Invest 1983;72:142–53.
200. Podolsky DK, Isselbacher KJ. Glycoprotein composition of colonic mucosa. Specific alterations in ulcerative colitis. Gastroenterology 1984;87:991–8.
201. Neutra M, Forstner JF. Gastrointestinal mucus: synthesis, secretion and function. In: Johnson LR, ed. Physiology of the digestive tract. New York: Raven Press, 1987:957–1009.
202. Rhodes JM. Colonic mucus and mucosal glycoproteins: the key to colitis and cancer? Gut 1989;30:1660–6.
203. Brooke BN. Ulcerative colitis and its surgical treatment. London: E&S Livingstone Ltd, 1954.
204. Goldgraber MB, Kirsner JB. Specific diseases simulating "nonspecific" ulcerative colitis (lymphopathia venereum, acute vasculitis, scleroderma and secondary amyloidosis). Ann Int Med 1957;47:939–55.
205. Gallart-Mones F. Concepto radiologico y anatamo patologico de la rectocolite ulcerosa grave. Minerva Chir 1953;9:477–8.
206. Rachet J, Busson A. Etiopathogenesis de la rectocolite hemorragique. Acta Gastroenterol Belg Suppl 1950;11:563–76.
207. Busson A, LeQuintrec Y. Rectocolite mucohemorragique a forme etagee. Arch Med Appar Digest 1954;43:1154–70.
208. McGovern VJ, Archer GT. The pathogenesis of ulcerative colitis. Aust Ann Med 1957;6:68–74.
209. McGovern VJ. The mechanism of inflammation. J Pathol Bacteriol 1957;73:99–106.
210. Mirvish L. The mucosa of the rectosigmoid in ulcerative colitis. S Afr Med J 1960;34:732–4.
211. Sommers SC. Mast cells and paneth cells in ulcerative colitis. Gastroenterology 1966;51:5:841–50.
212. Binder V, Hvidberg E. Histamine content of rectal mucosa in ulcerative colitis. Gut 1967;8:24–8.
213. Lloyd G, Green FH, Fox H, Mani V, Turnberg LA. Mast cells and immunoglobulin E in inflammatory bowel disease. Gut 1975;16:861–6.
214. Balaza M, Illyes G, Vadasz G. Mast cells in ulcerative colitis. Virchow's Arch B Cell Pathol 1989;57:353–60.
215. Stead RH, Dixon MF, Bramwell NH, Riddell RH, Bienenstock J. Mast cells are closely apposed to nerves in the human gastrointestinal mucosa. Gastroenterology 1989;97:575–85.
216. Baum CA, Bhatia P, Miner, Jr P. Increased colonic mucosal mast cells associated with severe watery diarrhea and microscopic colitis. Dig Dis Sci 1989;34:1462–5.
217. Kobayashi HT, Isizuka T, Okayama U. Human mast cells and basophils as sources of cytokines. Clin Exp Allergy 2000;30:1205–12.

218. Raithel M, Winterkamp S, Pacurar A, Ulrich P, Hochberger J, Hahn EG. Release of mast cell tryptase from human colorectal mucosa in inflammatory bowel disease. Scand J Gastroenterol 2001;36:174–9.
219. Sartos J, Yang PC, Soderholm JD, Benjamin M, Perdue MH. Role of mast cells in chronic stress induced colonic epithelial barrier dysfunction in the rat. Gut 2001;48:630–6.
220. Lumb G. The pathology of ulcerative colitis. In: Jones FA, ed. Modern trends in gastroenterology. New York: PB Hoeber Inc., 1958:315–28.
221. Lumb G, Protheroe RHB. Ulcerative colitis. A pathologic study of 152 surgical specimens. Gastroenterology 1958;34:387–407.
222. Morson BC. Pathology of ulcerative colitis. Proc Roy Soc Med 1971;64:976–7.
223. Morson BC. Pathology of ulcerative colitis. In: Kirsner JB, Shorter RG, eds. Inflammatory bowel disease. Philadelphia: Lea and Febiger, 1975:167–81.
224. Riis P, Valdorf-Hansen F, Anthonisen P. Cytology of colonic mucosal secretions from patients with nonspecific haemorrhagic proctocolitis in complete clinical remission. Br Med J 1966;1:712–14.
225. Counsell PB, Dukes CE. The association of chronic ulcerative colitis and carcinoma of the rectum and colon. Br J Surg 1952;39:485–95.
226. Dukes CE. Surgical pathology of ulcerative colitis. Ann Roy Coll Surg 1954;14: 389–400.
227. Morson BC, Pang LS. Rectal biopsy as an aid to cancer control in ulcerative colitis. Gut 1967;8:423–34.
228. Cook MG, Goligher JC. Carcinoma and epithelial dysplasia complicating ulcerative colitis. Gastroenterology 1975;68:1227–36.
229. Riddell RH, Goldman H, Ransohoff DF, Appelman HD, Fenoglio CM, Haggitt RC, et al. Dysplasia in inflammatory bowel disease. Hum Pathol 1983;14:931–68.
230. Blackstone MO, Riddell RH, Rogers BH, Levin B. Dysplasia-associated lesion or mass (DALM) detected by colonoscopy in long-standing ulcerative colitis. An Indication for colectomy. Gastroenterology 1981;80:366–74.
231. Levine MD, Kirsner JB, Klotz AP. A new concept of the pathogenesis of ulcerative colitis. Science 1951;114:552–3.
232. Sommers SC, Anderson LM, Warren S. Basement membranes chronic intestinal diseases. Lab Invest 1953;2:223–6.
233. Streicher MH, Catchpole HB, Pirani CL. Chronic ulcerative colitis – histochemical studies. Illinois Med J 1956;110:172–6.
234. Jacobson MA, Kirsner JB. The basement membranes of the epithelium of the colon and rectum in ulcerative colitis and other diseases. Gastroenterology 1956; 30:279–85.
235. Beeson P. Role of the eosinophil in immunology of the gut. Ciba Foundation Symposium. North Holland, Amsterdam: Elsevier, Excerpta Medica, 1977:203–23.
236. Riis P, Anthonisen P. Eosinophiles in peripheral blood and inflammatory exudate in nonspecific proctocolitis. Acta Med Scand 1964;175:85–9.
237. Walsh RE, Gaginella TS. The eosinophil in inflammatory bowel disease (review). Scand J Gastroenterol 1991;26:1217–24.
238. Desreumaux P, Nutten S, Colombel JF. Activated eosinophils in inflammatory bowel disease: Do they matter? (Editorial) Am J Gastroenterol 1999;94:3396–8.
239. Robertson HE, Kernohan JW. Myenteric plexus in congenital megacolon. Proc Staff Meet Mayo Clinic 1938;13:123–5.
240. Storsteen KA, Kernohan JW, Bargen JA. The myenteric plexus in chronic ulcerative colitis. Surg Gynecol Obstet 1953;997:335–43.
241. Geboes K, Collins SM. Structural changes in the enteric nervous system. Inflammatory Bowel Disease – Neurogastroenterol. Motility 1998;10:189.

242. Kyosola K, Penttila O, Salaspuro M. Rectal mucosal adrenergic innervation and enterochromaffin cells in ulcerative colitis and irritable colon. Scand J Gastroenterol 1977;12:363–7.
243. Collins SM. Altered neuromuscular function in the inflamed bowel. In: Kirsner JB, ed. Inflammatory bowel disease, 5th edn. Philadelphia: WB Saunders Co., 1999:28–86.

Electron Microscopy – Ulcerative Colitis

244. Donnellan WL. The structure of the colonic mucosa, the epithelium and subepithelial reticulohistiocytic complex. Gastroenterology 1965;49:496–544.
245. Donnellan WL. Early histological changes in ulcerative colitis. Gastroenterology 1966;50:519–40.
246. Movat HZ, Ferando NVP. Allergic inflammation. I. The earliest fine structural changes at the blood-tissue barrier during antigen-antibody interaction. Am J Pathol 1963;42:41–59.
247. Dvorak AM. Ultrastructural pathology of Crohn's disease. In: Grobell H, Peskar BM, Malchow H, eds. Inflammatory bowel disease: Basic research and clinical implications. Boston: MJP Press Ltd, 1988:3–41.
248. Kubota Y, Petras RE, Ottaway CA, Tubbs RR, Farmer RG, Fiocchi C. Colonic vasoactive intestinal peptide nerves in inflammatory bowel disease. Gastroenterology 1992;102:1242–51.
249. Gonzales-Licea A, Yardley JH. A comparative ultrastructural study of the mucosa in idiopathic ulcerative colitis, shigellosis and other human colonic diseases. Johns Hopkins Hosp Bull 1966;118:444–61.
250. Gonzalez-Licea A, Yardley JH. Nature of the tissue reaction in ulcerative colitis: Light and electron microscopic findings. Gastroenterology 1966;51:5:825–40.
251. Prescott SM, McIntyre TM, Zimmerman GA. Events at the vascular wall – the molecular basis of inflammation. J Invest Med 2001;49:104–11.

"Natural" and Experimental Ulcerative Colitis

252. Ginsberg R, Ivy AC. The etiology of ulcerative colitis: An analytical review of the literature. Gastroenterology 1946;7:67–90.
253. Stewart HL, Jones BF. Pathologic anatomy of chronic ulcerative colitis: A spontaneous disease of the rat. Arch Pathol 1941;31:37–54.
254. Berkhoff GA, Campbell SG. Etiology and pathogenesis of ulcerative enteritis (Quail disease). The experimental disease. Avian Dis 1974;18:205–12.
255. Scott GB, Keymer IF. Ulcerative colitis in apes: A comparison with the human disease. J Pathol 1975;115:241–4.
256. Cave DR, Kirsner JB. Animal models of inflammatory bowel disease. Ztschr Gastroenterol 1979;17(Suppl):125–35.
257. Strober W. Animal models of inflammatory bowel disease. Am J Dig Dis 1985;30 (Suppl):3S–10S.
258. Chalifoux LV, Bronson RT, Escajadillo A, McKenna S. An analysis of the association of gastroenteric lesions with chronic wasting syndrome of marmosets. Vet Pathol 1982;19:(Suppl 7):141–62.
259. Lushbaugh CC, Humason GL, Swartzendruber DC, Richter CB, Gengozian N. Spontaneous colonic adenocarcinoma in marmosets. Primate Med 1978;10:119–34.

260. Tilden EB, Miller EG Jr. The response of the monkey (maccacus rhesus) to withdrawal of vitamin A from the diet. J Nutr 1930;3:121–40.
261. Wintrobe MM, Follis RH Jr, Alcayaga P, Paulson M, Humphreys S. Pantothenic acid deficiency in swine. Bull Johns Hopkins Hosp 1943;73:313–41.
262. Rinehart JF, Greenberg LD. Colitis in the folic acid deficient monkey with notes on similarities to ulcerative colitis in man. Am J Pathol 1948;24:710 (Abstract).
263. Penner A, Bernheim AI. Experimental production of digestive tract ulcerations. J Exp Med 1939;70:453–63.
264. MacPherson BR, Pfeiffer CJ. Experimental colitis. Digestion 1976;14:424–52.
265. Freeman HJ. Animal models of inflammatory bowel diseases and colon cancer. Inflammatory bowel disease, Vol. 1. Boca Raton, FL: CRC Press, 1989:141–53.
266. Melnyk CS. Experimental enteritis and colitis. In: Kirsner JB, Shorter RG, eds. Inflammatory bowel disease, 2nd edn. Philadelphia: Lea and Febiger, 1980:25–43.
267. Portis SA, Block L, Necheles H. Studies on chronic ulcerative colitis and some biological effects of detergents. Gastroenterology 1944;3:106–13.
268. Ivy JH, Clark BG. Is bile and pancreatic juice a factor in the genesis of ulcerative colitis. Gastroenterology 1945;5:416–17.
269. Lake M, Nickel Jr. WF, Dew Andrus W. Possible role of pancreatic enzymes in the etiology of ulcerative colitis. Gastroenterology 1951;17:409–13.
270. Marcus R, Watt J. Seaweeds and ulcerative colitis in laboratory animals. Lancet 1969;2:489–90.
271. Watt J, Marcus R. Experimental ulcerative disease of the colon in animals. Gut 1973;14:506–10.
272. Onderdonk AB, Hermos JA, Dzink JL, Bartlett JB. Protective effect of metronidazole in experimental ulcerative colitis. Gastroenterology 1978;74:521–6.
273. Roediger WE. The colonic epithelium in ulcerative colitis: An energy-deficiency disease? Lancet 1980;2:712–15.
274. Roediger WE, Nance S. Metabolic induction of experimental ulcerative colitis by inhibition of fatty acid oxidation. Br J Exp Path 1986;67:773–82.
275. Gibson PR, van de Pol E, Barratt PJ, Doe WF. Ulcerative colitis – a disease characterized by the abnormal colonic epithelial cell? Gut 1988;29:516–21.
276. Fedorak RN, Madsen KL. Naturally occurring and experimental models of inflammatory bowel disease. In: Kirsner JB, ed. Inflammatory bowel disease, 5th edn. Philadelphia: WB Saunders Co., 1999:113–43.
277. Arsenau KO, Pizarro TT, Cominelli F. Discovering the cause of inflammatory bowel disease. Curr Opin Gastroenterol 2000;16:310–17.
278. Strober W, Fuss IJ, Ehrhardt RO, Neurata M, Boirivant M, Ludviksson BR. Mucosal immunoregulation and inflammatory bowel disease: New insights from murine models of inflammation. Scand J Immunol 1998;48:5:453–8.

Part II

Crohn's disease

ORIGINS

Inflammatory bowel disease descriptively consistent with Crohn's disease apparently was observed three hundred years ago, possibly earlier in Carson's "Iliac Passion."[279] Wilhelm Fabry[280] (Guilhelmus Fabricius Hildanus) of Hilden-Cologne, Germany (1560–1629), had noted at autopsy in a boy who had experienced persistent "subhepatic pain" that "the cecum (was) contracted and invaginated into the ileum ... such that it was not possible for anything to pass from the proximal intestine into the colon." On extracting the cecum, it was ulcerated and fibrous. J.H. Baron,[281] in a review of early instances of possible Crohn's disease, cites J.J. Bernier et al.[282] on La Maladie de Louis XIII. Baron writes "... Louis XIII is known to have been prone to attacks of diarrhea for decades, associated with fever and a rectal abscess that discharged spontaneously. In 1642, he experienced bloody diarrhea, fever, abdominal pain and a perianal abscess or fistula. He died the following year, at age 42. Autopsy revealed ulcerations of small and large bowel, with abscesses and fistulas, compatible with ileocecal tuberculosis or regional enteritis." The noted pathologist G.B. Morgagni[283] of Forli, Italy (1682–1771) in his "De Sedibus et Causis Morborum" in 1761, described ulcerations and perforation of an inflamed, narrowed distal ileum and enlarged mesenteric lymph nodes in a young man of 20 with a history of diarrhea and fever culminating in death after 14 days.

C. Combe and W. Saunders[284] (1813) of England, reporting a patient who had experienced abdominal cramps and diarrhea, wrote: "The lower part of the ileum as far as the colon was ulcerated and contracted for three feet to the size of a turkey quill." J. Abercrombie[285] (1828) of England observed an inflamed, ulcerated and thickened ileal segment in a 13-year-old girl who had suffered from diarrhea.

As reported by J. Fielding,[286,287] Abraham Colles[288] of Dublin, Ireland, as early as 1830, had described an apparent Crohn's disease among children, including perianal, rectovaginal, and rectovesical fistulas,

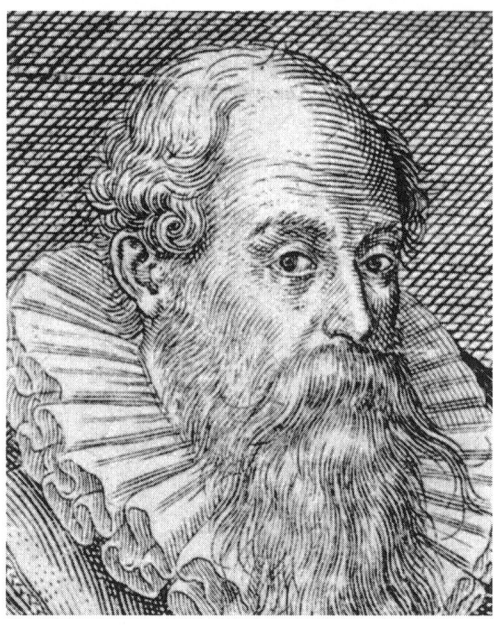

Wilhelm Fabricus Hildanus

attributed initially to tuberculosis. Corrigan[289] of Ireland in 1853 reported a patient with a thickened ileum and "snail track ulceration." Fielding,[287] noting that the disease had appeared at least since the middle of the 19th century, summarized the features in 31 patients seen in London from 1850 to 1899. The group included 11 males and 20 females, with ages from 5 to 59 years. The disease involved the large bowel in 15, the small and large bowel in 12 and the small intestine only in 4. Findings included enlarged mesenteric lymph nodes, toxic dilatation of the bowel, free perforation of the intestine and liver disease (fatty infiltration, hepatitis). Fielding also tabulated the findings in 25 additional patients considered as "possible Crohn's disease." A review of the Transactions of the Pathological Society of London for the same period included: N. Moore's[290] (1882) first microscopic description of Crohn's disease and case reports by S.J. Sharkey (1884), R.E. Carrington (1886), and C. Ogle (1895). "It is of interest that the large majority of cases involved the large bowel." J.F. Walker and J. Fielding[291] compiled 29 additional 19th century instances of apparent Crohn's disease from Dublin hospitals during the same period. The Dublin series included 19 males and 10 females, ages 16 to 68. The large bowel was affected in 8, large and small bowel 15 and small intestine in 6.

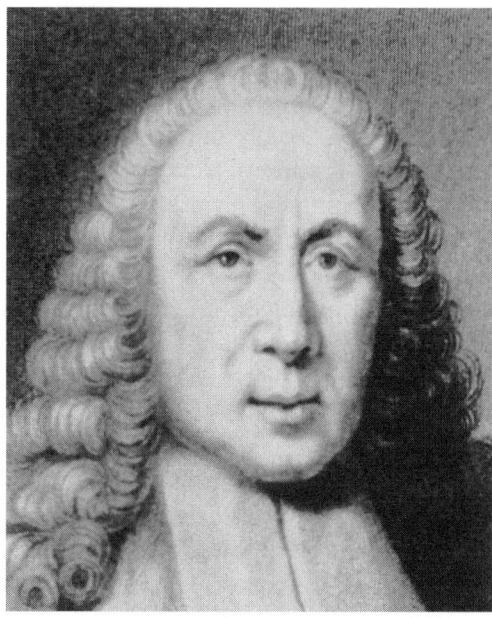

G.B. Morgagni

Interesting features included extracutaneous fistulas, entero-vesical fistula, intra-abdominal abscesses, one instance of toxic dilatation of the colon, free bowel perforations, and perianal suppurative disease. In a 25-year-old male patient, "the contraction (in the colon) was so great that a common crow quill could scarcely be passed through it."

J.S. Bristowe[292] (1853) of London found at autopsy in a 32-year-old woman with a history of persistent diarrhea narrowing and ulceration of the mid jejunum and ileum; the ileum was thickened, the lumen narrowed, a fistula involved several segments of the ileum and the colon was ulcerated and perforated. As noted earlier, the transmural "ulcerative colitis" described by Samuel Wilks[19] in 1859 (patient Isabella Bankes) was re-classified in 1970 by J. Fielding[293] as Crohn's disease of the colon. In 1889 Samuel Fenwick[294] of London, in a 27-year-old woman with a history of diarrhea and weight loss, wrote: "Many of the coils of intestine were adherent and a communication existed between the cecum and a portion of the small intestine adherent to it. Whilst the sigmoid flexure was adherent to the rectum and a communication also existed between them, the lower end of the ileum was much dilated and hypertrophied and the ileocecal valve was contracted to the size of a swan's quill."

H.I. Goldstein[295] of Camden, New Jersey (USA), in a paper entitled the History of Regional Enteritis, begins: "In the American Medical and Philosophical Register or Annals of Medicine, Natural History, Agriculture and the Arts conducted by a Society of Gentlemen, New York (Volume I, July 1870), John Wakefield Francis of New York reports a case of enteritis accompanied with a 'preternatural formation of the ileum,' suggestive of Crohn's disease." G. Hellers[296] of Stockholm in his monograph (Crohn's disease in Stockholm County 1955–1974) states: "Between 1870 and 1900, case histories of all inpatients in the Surgical Department at the Serafimer Hospital (Stockholm) included a case described by John Berg (1898) possibly due to Crohn's disease. The patient, a 20-year-old man, was admitted after a three weeks' illness, in very poor condition and with a mass in the right iliac fossa. At operation, a thickened ileum was found with several mesenteric abscesses. A normal appendix was removed. The patient died on the second day. Postmortem examination revealed perforation of the bowel and peritonitis." Heller adds that a 1932 thesis by Strombeck[297] entitled Mesenteric Lymphadenitis included 349 patients. "Most of these cases were probably due to acute terminal ileitis but some may well have been due to Crohn's disease." While conclusive diagnoses were not possible several centuries earlier, these early reports similar in clinical and anatomic features represented the emergence of an inflammatory intestinal disorder later designated as Crohn's disease.

EARLY CLINICAL RECOGNITION

The early years of the 20th century were characterized by increasing recognition of patients with "regional enteritis," descriptions of associated clinical problems and by limited attempts to clarify the nature of this entity. The first important observation was by A.J. Lartigau,[298] pathologist at Columbia University (New York). In a 1901 detailed study of "a form of tuberculosis of the small intestine," characterized by pronounced thickening of the wall of the intestine, he reviewed the already substantial German and French literature on the subject, noted the first such case recognized by Hartman and Pilliet[299] in 1891 and astutely described in detail the unique case of Simon S., age 49, who in 1895 succumbed after three years of symptoms, including weight loss, abdominal cramping pain, alternating diarrhea and constipation and darkening of skin color. Autopsy demonstrated no evidence of pulmonary tuberculosis. The liver and gallbladder were normal. The major finding was thickening of the distal two thirds of the intestine, involving the cecum and a thickened and rigid ileocecal valve. Although the initial "diagnosis" was hyperplastic tuberculosis of the small and large intestine, Lartigau noted several critical differences: many "tubercles" were mere aggregations of lymphoid cells with occasional giant cells, without epithelioid cells and, in contrast to tuberculosis, "with little or no tendency to necrotic change." The typical histologic features of tuberculosis were absent. These histologic findings in modern times are consistent with Crohn's disease and Lartigau probably was the first to recognize the histologic difference from tuberculosis and define an important feature of Crohn's disease. The long-time significant involvement with pulmonary and intestinal tuberculosis clearly had influenced physicians, unaware of the "new" entity of "Crohn's disease," to overlook this diagnosis.

The early case reports by Braun[300] (1901), J. Koch[301] (1903), Wilmanns[302] (1905), H. Senn (1905) and H. Lilienthal (1906) of the United States, Moynihan[303] (1907), R. Proust[304] (1907) and Lejars[305] (1908) of France, Monsarrat[306] (1907) of Liverpool, England and von Bergmann[307] (1911) of Germany, (cited by Shapiro[308]) were noteworthy for their presentation as abdominal (inflammatory) masses, clinically resembling tumors, assumed erroneously to be "malignant" and, at a time of limited abdominal surgery, were assessed by clinicians, unaware of IBD, as "untreatable." R. Shapiro's[308] 1939 review (289 references) identified many instances of apparent Crohn's disease masquerading as "tumors." Two hundred and sixty one of the 413 cases collected from the literature in this report involved the terminal ileum and 22 the right colon. E.G. Janeway[309] of New York had presented a similar paper ("Inflammatory Abdominal Masses Simulating Malignant Growths") at the 1907 annual meeting of the Association of American Physicians in New York and N.M. Jones and A.A. Eisenberg[310] (1918) of Cleveland, Ohio reported a similar patient; neither paper attracted attention. E. Schmidt[311] (1911), (Dresden, Germany), S. Goto[312] (1912) (Fukuoka, Japan) each described patients misdiagnosed initially as "intestinal cancer," with pathologic features resembling Crohn's disease. Since these publications antedated the recognition of Crohn's disease, the central issue at the time was the masquerading of intestinal inflammatory "masses" as abdominal tumors.

The landmark 1913 paper by T. Kennedy Dalziel,[313] a Glasgow surgeon, antedating Crohn's paper by nearly 20 years, included 13 patients and was the second important clinical development, a model of accurate clinical description. The first case, a physician, since 1901 had experienced episodes of cramping abdominal pain and diarrhea progressing to intestinal obstruction. At autopsy, the entire small intestine was

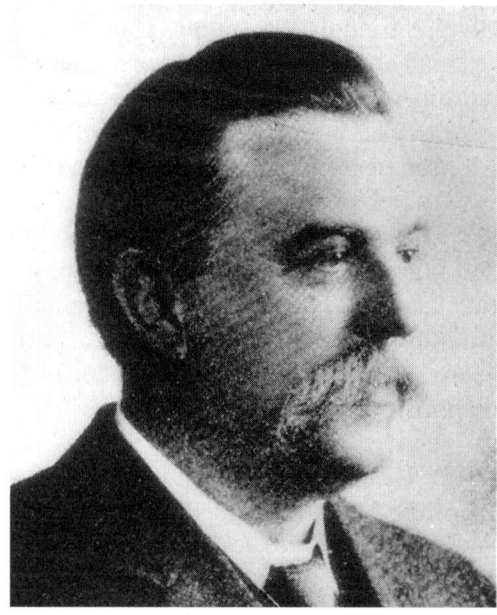

Sir T. Kennedy Dalziel

chronically inflamed and narrowed and the mesenteric lymph nodes were enlarged. In another patient, "The affected bowel gives the consistence and smoothness of an eel in rigor mortis, and the mesenteric glands, though enlarged, are evidently not caseous." In other patients, the process involved the jejunum, midportion of the ileum, and the transverse and sigmoid colon. Histologic examination demonstrated vascular congestion, submucosal edema, acute and chronic transmural inflammation, increased numbers of eosinophils and scattered giant cells. Dalziel distinguished the process from tuberculosis and related his "chronic intestinal ileitis" to Johne's disease of cattle (M. paratuberculosis) described first in 1895 and publicized by McFadyean in 1907.[314] Crohn's disease recently has been differentiated from Johne's disease by Van Kruiningen.[315] Although Dalziel had presented his paper at the 81st annual meeting of the British Medical Association, it was unnoticed for many years.

In 1914 A. Läwen[316] of Leipzig, Germany in a 20 page report described an "appendicitis fibroplastica," simulating a tumor. Twenty four years later from Königsberg, Läwen, now aware of the paper by Crohn, Ginzburg, and Oppenheimer, reported the identical patient, re-evaluated as a "chronic stenosing terminal ileitis,"[317] illustrating the impact of new information in physician recognition of previously overlooked clinical and pathologic entities (Goethe: "was man weiss, man sieht"). By 1920 Tietze[318] of Breslau, Germany had reviewed 281 cases from the medical literature. Korte[319] of Berlin (1921) and Bundschuh and Wolff[320] (1925) Wurzburg, Germany each described groups of patients with similar findings, reviewed the considerable early German literature (Korte – between 1908–1920) (Bundschuh and Wolff – between 1895–1924) respectively and concluded in 1925 that "chronic ileitis" was more common than had been appreciated.

By 1925, American physicians began to increasingly report instances of "nonspecific" hyperplastic and granulomatous lesions of the intestinal tract, previously labelled "intestinal tuberculosis." T.H. Coffen[321] of Portland, Oregon in 1925 described a clinical situation familiar today. A 20-year-old man with abdominal cramping pain since 1915 underwent surgery in 1916 because of small bowel obstruction, with resection of six inches of thickened inflamed bowel. Five months later, 24 inches of bowel were removed for recurrent obstruction. Eight months later, 24 inches of bowel were removed for recurrent obstruction. Eight months later, a fourth bowel resection was necessary for obstruction, emphasizing not only the cicatrizing nature of Crohn's disease but also the individually consistent recurrence of the same complication.

The 1932 paper by Crohn, Ginzburg and Oppenheimer,[322] the third significant event, dramatically increased clinical recognition of regional ileitis (Crohn's disease); approximately 500 cases were reported in the medical literature during the four year period 1932 to 1937! H.W.L. Molesworth[323] of England in 1933, in a 33-year-old woman with the history of an appendectomy in 1921, found at surgery for intestinal obstruction, hypertrophy of the small intestine, thickening of the terminal ileum and adjacent mesentery and stenosis of the ileocecal valve. The mimicry of intestinal neoplasm by "chronic cicatrizing enteritis" (Crohn's disease) was re-emphasized by Donchess and Warren[324] of Boston in a 1934 case report: a 62-year-old woman, with involvement of the cecum and the ascending colon. Twenty-four similar instances, often with appendiceal involvement, recorded in the literature during the 1920s and 1930s were reviewed.

Many reports expanded the clinical spectrum of regional enteritis.[325–331] Brown, Bargen and Weber[332] in 1934 and Pemberton and Brown[333] in 1937 reviewed their considerable experience with regional enteritis at the Mayo Clinic dating back to the 1920s. The clinical and pathologic features in all patients were similar, regardless of geography, age (children, teen-

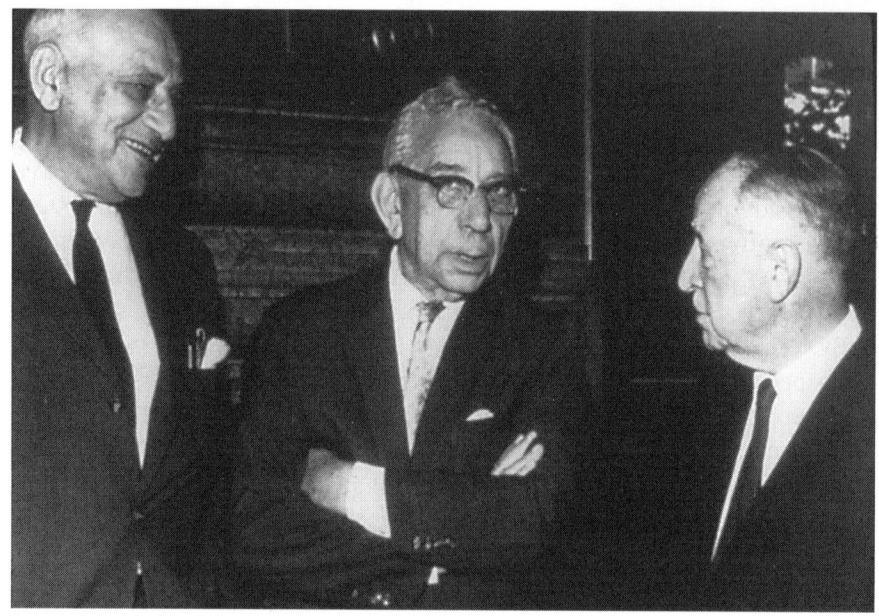

G. Oppenheimer, B. Crohn and L. Ginzburg

agers, and young adults), symptoms of abdominal cramps, diarrhea, low grade fever, and weight loss, often presenting as acute "appendicitis" and treated by appendectomy. In 1933, Harris et al.[334] recorded involvement of the jejunum and the colon. Also in 1933, American surgeons Homans and Hass[335] described regional ileitis as "a clinical not a pathological entity." Anal disease and fistula formation had been noted in the 1932 paper by Crohn et al. and these findings were emphasized in 1934 by A.D. Bisell,[336] R.J. Jackman[337] (1943) and later (1965) by Gray, Lockhart-Mummery and Morson.[338] In 1934 G. Anschutz[339] of Kiel, Germany, apparently unaware of the 1913 Dalziel and 1932 Crohn papers on regional enteritis, described in detail a series of patients with chronic inflammation of the small intestine clinically resembling malignant abdominal tumors. Gastroenterologist J.L. Kantor[340] of New York in 1934 reported observations identifiable today as late roentgen findings in six private patients with regional enteritis (rigid, narrowed terminal ileum). Dyer et al.[341] (St. Bartholomew hospital, London), also emphasized contraction and rigidity as two signs with low observer variation. The expert IBD radiologist R. Marshak[342] of Mt. Sinai Hospital, New York, based upon his extensive experience with regional enteritis as the radiologist for B. Crohn et al., described the roentgen findings in meticulous detail and Crohn's 1949 monograph on regional ileitis included this authoritative information.[343]

ANIMAL AND EXPERIMENTAL CROHN'S DISEASE

In 1934 H.G. Bell[344] of California reported (without details) that experiments "interfering with the blood supply of the intestinal tract" had failed to produce a cicatrizing enteritis, ulceration of the mucosa or any lesion resembling regional enteritis. The early concept of a possible endolymphangitis (subcutaneous lymphatic dilatation and lymphoid prominence) as observed in resected bowel from three patients with cicatrizing regional enteritis (thickening of bowel wall, engorged lymphatics) resembling chronic lymphedema of the extremities, was the rationale for the 1936 experiments of Reichert and Mathes of Stanford University.[345] Adopting the method of Homans, Drinker and Field[346] of the Massachusetts General Hospital, Boston, Massachusetts, at intervals of weeks to months, they repeatedly injected fine sand (crystalline silica (200 mesh) or sodium morrhuate) and a sclerosing solution of 26% bismuth oxychloride, rose aniline dye (indelible lead) with and without E. coli into the cannulated mesenteric lymphatics of dogs. Chronic edema of the ileocecal area developed; mucosal inflammation, ulceration or granulomas were not observed. In 1941 J.K. Poppe[347] of Yale University, New Haven, Connecticut, seeking to reproduce an "ulcerative colitis," similarly injected a 26% aqueous solution of bismuth oxychloride with and without bacteria (B. coli, Streptococcus viridans, Staphylococcus aureus and Streptococcus hemolyticus) into the intestinal lymphatics, made prominent by a prior fat meal in 15 dogs. Lymph nodes draining the injected segments of intestine were inflamed and ulcerations of the small and large bowel developed but neither ulcerative colitis nor Crohn's disease was duplicated. Sinaiko and Necheles[348] of Michael Reese Hospital, Chicago, in 1946 injected seven dogs with bismuth oxychloride solution and sodium morrhuate (without bacteria) producing only partial obstruction of intestinal lymphatics; they attributed Poppe's findings to vascular thromboses rather than to lymphatic obstruction. Emphasizing inflammation of intestinal lymphatics or an etiologic possibility, Chess et al.[349] of the University of Illinois (Chicago) in 1950 instilled suspensions of 200 and 400 mesh sand or talc powder into Thiry-Vella fistulas of an isolated loop of terminal ileum and also fed dogs finely ground silica and talc. A mixture of S. aureus, Streptococcus and E. coli organisms was injected intravenously in one dog. Gross findings included bowel thickening, friable mucosa and hemorrhagic areas.

Histologic changes included lymphoid hyperplasia, enlarged mesenteric lymph nodes and granulomatous lesions on the liver. Talc was thought to be more pathogenic than finely divided sand. The authors compared the pathologic changes to those of regional enteritis. Kalima et al.[350] (1976) of Finland injected dilute formalin solution into the mesenteric lymphatics of the terminal ileum in 21 pigs ("chosen because spontaneous ileitis is common in pigs"). Endolymphangitis developed with congestion and edematous thickening of the distal small bowel and ileocecal area and mucosal ulceration. Histologic examination demonstrated inflammation of the subserosa with occasional foreign body giant cells, not Crohn's disease. Transmural inflammation developed after three weeks. Kalima et al.[350] stated: "The early phase of Crohn's disease includes mucosal aphthoid ulcerations, hyperplasia of intestinal lymphoid tissue with superficial ulcerations, crypt abscesses and obstructive lymphedema. The advanced phase of Crohn's disease is characterized by: (a) a transmural inflammatory process, (b) mucosal ulcerations and entero-enteric or enterocutaneous fistulas, (c) fibrosis and (d) inflammation in the serosa and mesentery." Kalima's conclusion: "Changes caused by lymphatic obstruction do not enlighten the etiology of Crohn's disease." Kalima, Saloniemi and Rahko[351] also described a "lymphostatic enteropathy," characterized by partial or total lymphatic obstruction of intestinal lymph vessels ... "closely related to many clinical diseases." Warren and Sommers in 1948 considered the possibility of an endolymphangitis in Crohn's disease, attributable to the intestinal absorption of an (unidentified) lipid but this possibility was not pursued.

Van Patter and Bargen et al.[352] in a 1954 review of 600 patients with Crohn's disease, suggested, as had earlier observers, that "the causative agent may be found in the fecal stream and ... appears initially in the proximal part of the small intestine. If this agent resides in the fecal stream, it may exert its influence on the normal epithelial cell. The further course of the agent appears to be by way of the lymphatic vessels where it causes focal intralymphatic endothelial hyperplasia, lymphatic obstruction, and dilatation, lymphoid hyperplasia and lymphatic endothelial proliferation." Bargen,[353] in a 1955 reprise of the Van Patter article, rejected bacterial, viral, and protozoan agents, sarcoid and abdominal trauma as causes, but accepted "intestinal allergy" as a possibility.

Early Crohn's disease, in its gross and histologic features, to some observers resembled the porcine terminal ileitis described from Copenhagen in 1951.[354,355] Emsbo of the Royal Veterinary and Agricultural College, Copenhagen, in a comprehensive article on porcine terminal ileitis,[354] wrote: "In a couple of cases I too have encountered familial occurrences of ileitis in several pigs of the same litter." As evidence of the predisposition of the porcine ileum to pathological changes, he noted: the frequent occurrence of uncomplicated hypertrophy of the bowel, the often pronounced hyperplasia of Peyer's patches, the presence of epithelial changes, local fibrosis and foreign-body giant cells in the lymph follicles. However, the histologic findings were not comparable to those of Crohn's disease, including an absence of granulomatous changes. No specific organism was identified in the Danish porcine ileitis. Emsbo was convinced that porcine ileitis and human ileitis "fundamentally are identical." A campylobacter-type organism was isolated in Scottish and Swedish pigs[356] and a corona virus-like particle was associated with diarrhea in Belgian swine.[357] Strande, Sommers and Petrak[358] (Angell Memorial Animal Hospital, Boston – 500 autopsies annually) described morphologic features consistent with regional enteritis in two cocker spaniel dogs and raised the question of an infection transmitted by animals. As described by N.K. Mottet,[17] in one instance, lesions involved the colon and rectum and the terminal 6 cm of ileum with skip areas. The microscopic features included chronic inflammation with cicatrization of the intestinal wall producing an obliterative lymphangitis. Similar changes were present in the mesenteric and regional lymph nodes. Geil, Davis and Thompson,[359] Fitzsimmons General Hospital, Denver, Colorado, described a spontaneous ileitis in albino rats histologically different from human regional ileitis and the regional ileitis of swine. Cross et al.[360] of the Ohio Agricultural Research Center in 1973 described a terminal ileitis involving the distal 50 to 75 cm in 7 lambs ranging in age from 4 to 6 months. Intestinal nematodes were not found, bacterial cultures were negative. The predilection for the terminal ileum in animals, as in humans, is intriguing and deserves further study (?increased microbial adhesion sites).

Investigating staphylococcus related pseudomembranous enterocolitis, J. Prohaska[361] (University of Chicago) produced an enterocolitis in (a) chinchillas given multiple antibiotics, preparatory to the oral administration of S. aureus and (b) in mongrel dogs given single infusions of Staphylococci purified enterotoxin. Van Kruiningen[362] and Kennedy and Cello[363] reported histologic abnormalities resembling regional enteritis in Boxer dogs and favored a microbial-viral etiology for Crohn's disease. Limited microbiological studies and attempts to transmit the disease experimentally were unsuccessful. Cimprich[364] of the University of Pennsylvania Veterinary Medical School, in 1974 described a "granulomatous enteritis" in 10 malnourished horses. Bacterial, fungal and acid fast stains were negative in nine animals, acid-fast organisms (avian tuberculosis) were identified in one horse. In 1991 Roediger[365] of Woodsville, Australia, noting that "the stimulus for the immune response in Crohn's disease is unknown," proposed an unusual "updated lipid theory." In each of 19 cases of Crohn's disease evaluated by electron microscopy, he had observed that epithelial cells of the ileum contained phagolysosomes with lamellar layers of lipid. These structures, termed R or reactant bodies, he suggested were the proffered antigenic stimulus, as an amalgam of lipid (cholesterol esters, or phospholipids) and bacterial fragments (mycoplasma, mycobacteria or streptococci), presumed to induce a powerful immunological adjuvant response. For disease expression to occur, lipids and specific bacterial populations were required in the bowel lumen.

As noted by Pizarro et al.,[366] "the more recent availability of genetically engineered mouse models of CD provided an exceptional opportunity to identify the complex mechanisms involved in the pathogenesis of human IBD" (e.g. interleukin-10 deficient mice). Elson, Sartor, Tennyson and Riddell[367] commented in 1995: "no animal model exactly reproduced these human diseases ... However, multiple models are available to study the major components involved in IBD and today these serve as an important complement to the studies of IBD in humans."[368–370] The animal studies already have suggested multiple pathogenic pathways to IBD.[371] Indeed, Kosiewicz et al.[372] recently described a new murine model of spontaneous gastrointestinal inflammation that, according to W. Strober et al.,[373] "bears remarkable similarity to human Crohn's disease," the Samp1/yit mouse. The development of the disease is dependent upon a "benign intestinal microflora."

ABDOMINAL TRAUMA

In 1932 G. Pupini[374] of Italy described a post abdominal traumatic narrowing of the small bowel resembling Crohn's disease. A.W. Fischer and H. Lürmann[375] of Germany in 1933 and Blumenthal and Berman[376] of the USA in 1939 reported similar cases. After operating on a 22-year-old motorcyclist who developed a severe jejunitis of the proximal jejunum following a severe blow to the abdomen[377] when he ran into the rear end of a truck, abdominal trauma was investigated by M. Spellberg and A. Ochsner[378] of New Orleans as a possible cause of regional ileitis. Experimental constriction of the small bowel of dogs by steel clamps produced gross lesions of the intestine but not regional ileitis. Two instances of "regional enteritis" following external trauma were reported from the Mayo Clinic.[379] Crohn and Yarnis[380] added 11 patients with a history of abdominal trauma but, as noted by Kyle et al.,[381] this possibility was invalidated by the vast majority of CD patients without any history of abdominal trauma.

THE EARLY MT. SINAI (NEW YORK) EXPERIENCE

Antedating the 1932 "CGO" paper, A.H. Aufses Jr.[382] cited patients admitted to the Mt. Sinai (NY) Hospital in 1855, 1889, 1899 and 1919, with clinical findings suggestive of Crohn's disease (fistula in ano, abdominal abscess with enterovesical fistula, "hyperplastic colitis," right lower quadrant mass in 23-year-old male). Aufses also described the pivotal surgical approaches to the disease throughout the years by Mt. Sinai (NY) surgeons. Immediately preceding the paper by Crohn, Ginzburg, and Oppenheimer[322] in 1932, F.J. Nuboer[383] of Holland had described two male patients with "chronic phlegmonous ileitis" and implicated an "abnormal intestinal microflora" secondary to an "achylia gastrica." M. Golob[384] of New York (1932) had reported a "chronic infectious granuloma" of the ileocecal region in a 44-year-old man who had bled per rectum.

The New York Mt. Sinai experience actually began with E. Moschowitz and A.O. Wilensky, who in 1923[385] and 1927[386] described patients with "nonspecific" granulomas of the intestine, reflecting the long-time interest of that institution in intestinal granulomas and its early commitment to medical-surgical gastroenterology. The 1923 paper described four young patients, each with a history of appendicitis and an appendectomy. The colon was involved in three and the small intestine and colon in the fourth. The 1927 paper described an 18-year-old male with an apparent acute appendicitis, perforation and abscess formation. One week after operation a fecal fistula developed necessitating a second operation. Mock[387] of Northwestern University, Chicago, aware of the 1923 Moschowitz/Wilensky paper, in 1931 described 10 patients with "infective granulomas" involving various parts of the gastrointestinal tract, including the small intestine and the colon. The lesions were evaluated in the context of chronic inflammatory masses simulating tumor and not in relation to Crohn's disease.

The decisive 1932 Mt. Sinai events appeared to be as follows: Leon Ginzburg,[388] associated with the noted surgeon A.A. Berg, who had operated on all the Mt. Sinai patients, first as Berg's resident and then his

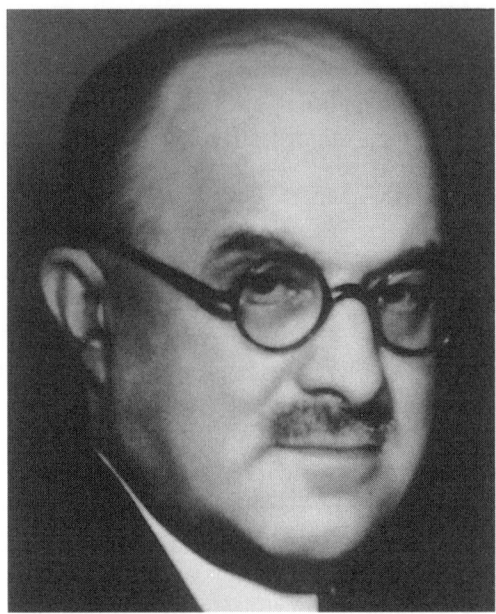

Eli Moschcowitz

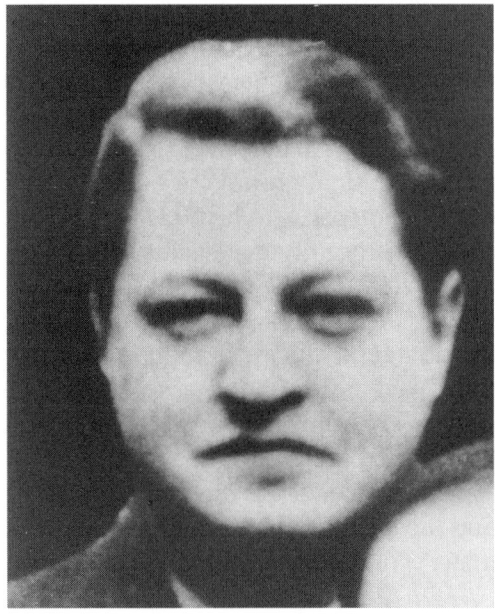

A.O. Wilensky

colleague, and Gordon Oppenheimer, then resident in surgical pathology, in studies beginning in 1925, had collected a group of 12 patients dating back to 1920, characterized by an hypertrophic and ulcerative stenosis of the distal two or three feet of the terminal ileum, "ending rather abruptly at the ileocecal valve." Ginzburg's early involvement in the study of the intestinal granulomas was acknowledged by Crohn in 1945.[389] Amebiasis, syphilis and actinomycosis, Hodgkin's disease or lymphosarcoma were eliminated as possible causes by histologic examination. Intestinal tuberculosis, the chief differential diagnostic problem of the time, was excluded by negative chest X-rays and negative Von Pirquet and intradermal tuberculin tests and by the absence of acid-fast bacilli histologically. In cooperation with pathologist William Antopol, the granulomas were evaluated as incidental findings. Fistula formation was a constant feature. However, as discovered by J.H. Baron[281] of England in his account of the Mt. Sinai (NY) terminal ileitis story and the L. Ginzburg–B. Crohn relationship (and brought to my attention by Dr. Henry Janowitz – November 2000), it is historically important to note that L. Ginzburg[390] presented a paper entitled "Nonspecific Granulomata of the Intestines (Inflammatory Tumors and Strictures of the Bowel)" "in conjunction with Burrill B. Crohn," at the May 2–3, 1932 meeting of the American Gastroenterological Association (Transactions Thirty-Fifth Annual Meeting of American Gastroenterological Association, Hotel Traymore, Atlantic City, N.J.), a publication with limited circulation. The paper was published later in the 1933 Annals of Surgery[391] and is noteworthy for its accurate description of terminal ileitis, chronologically antedating by one month the June 1932 paper by Crohn et al. The fifty-two cases comprising the Ginzburg study previously had been diagnosed as "malignancy" or "localized hypertrophic tuberculosis." An abdominal mass was palpable in every subacute and chronic case. Approximately half of the group had previous appendectomies. Chronic, incomplete small intestinal obstruction was the most common clinical manifestation.

Clinically, the patients were divided into 6 groups, some overlapping: (1) Pericolonic or peri-intestinal granulomata due to sealed-off perforation, (2) intestinal stenosis due to known vascular lesions of the bowel, (3) localized hypertrophic ulcerative ileitis, (4) localized hypertrophic colitis, (5) penetrating ulcers of the colon, and (6) granulomata secondary to inflammation of appendages or diverticula of the bowel.

All patients were operated upon by Dr. A.A. Berg. In Group 3, the terminal ileum was the exclusive site of the process. The end stage, the one most frequently observed, was conversion of the terminal ileum into a thickened hose-like tube. The mucosal folds were partially destroyed with polypoid excrescences. Linear or oval ulceration along the mesenteric border was a constant finding. The submucosa was "enormously thickened and the bowel lumen was greatly narrowed." Microscopic examination disclosed acute and chronic inflammation; numerous non-caseating giant cells, pronounced fibrous proliferation, many lymphocytes, monocytes, plasma cells, occasional polymorphonuclear cells and areas of lymphoid hyperplasia.

In the ensuing discussion, H. Bockus raised the question of "undue ptosis rotating the ascending branch of the ileocolic artery supplying the terminal ileum, causing vascular insufficiency." W. Alvarez stated he had seen instances of terminal ileitis but had not appreciated their significance. He suggested as a possible mechanism, "reversal of the intestinal gradient in the terminal ileum." B.B. Crohn, showing four slides, indicated he had been interested in the problem "for some time." He noted the fourteen cases with which he was familiar (two, his patients, 12 from Ginzburg and Oppenheimer), the tendency to intestinal stenosis and obstruction and to fistula formation. He added that three, four or five cases were seen each year at Mt. Sinai Hospital and that the condition was more common than had been appreciated. Ginzburg dismissed the etiologic possibilities of amebic infection, syphilis or vascular insufficiency and concluded that the etiology was yet to be determined.[392]

As an intern at New York's Mt. Sinai Hospital (1907–8) Burrill Crohn (1884–1983) had participated "in all autopsies, to cut and to take dictation on all surgical sections." In 1930 Burrill Crohn (now Dr. Berg's gastroenterology consultant) had under his care two young patients with a similar process. Crohn's first case seen in 1930 was a 17-year-old young man with diarrhea, fever, a mass in the right lower abdominal quadrant, and pain, requiring ileocecal resection. The patient's sister also was operated upon for regional ileitis several years later.[393] As related to me by Henry Janowitz of Mt. Sinai Hospital, the two groups united at the recommendation of surgeon Dr. A.A. Berg and chief pathologist Dr. Paul Klemperer, providing the 14 cases published in the 1932 JAMA article as "terminal ileitis." The article was credited to the surgical service of Dr. A.A. Berg and had Berg accepted the invitation to join the alphabetically arranged authorship of the paper, we might today be writing about Berg's disease! At the time the paper was presented in New Orleans (May 13, 1932), J.A. Bargen of Rochester, Minnesota, wisely anticipating the more extensive involvement of the small intestine, suggested the term regional enteritis. As noted earlier, Ginzburg, with G. Oppenheimer, "had been studying the pathology and clinical features of patients with intestinal granulomas of various origins and instances of distal ileal stenosis for many years; and his claim for eponym co-designation (Crohn–Ginzburg–Oppenheimer or "CGO" disease) seems justified.

R. Lewisohn,[394] on the Surgical Service of Mt. Sinai, New York in 1938, aware of regional enteritis in other areas of the small bowel and also in the colon, preferred the term "segmental enteritis." Lewisohn wrote further: "... As our views on ileitis and ileocolitis stabilize with accumulated experience during the next few years, this lesion may turn out simply to represent a milder form of ulcerative colitis." Although reports of regional ileitis were increasing, clinical and investigative interest in the new entity remained low. Crohn,[395] reviewing his Mt. Sinai experience later, queried: "Are these new diseases the product of our modern civilization in the nature of psychosomatic disease or the end product of the industrial revolution?" The significant contributions of Mt. Sinai Hospital (New York) physicians to the knowledge of regional ileitis have been collected by D. Sachar.[396] Kovalcik of Eastern Virginia Medical School[397] in 1982 provided an "outside" perspective on the Mt. Sinai story.

MORE EARLY 20TH CENTURY REPORTS (CD)

Emphasizing the frequent need for surgery, in 1933 A.W. Fischer and H. Lürmann[375] of Frankfurt am Main, Germany described 3 patients with regional enteritis; each had presented with tumor-simulating inflammatory abdominal masses, in one instance associated with perforation of bowel. In the same year, J.F. Erdmann and C.V. Burt[398] of the New York Postgraduate Medical School, apparently unaware of the 1932 paper on regional ileitis, added 5 similar cases. In 1934 Brown, Bargen and Weber[332] describing involvement of the entire ileum and jejunum, validated the term "regional enteritis." In 1934 A.S. Bisell[336] (University of Chicago) described two male patients, ages 28 and 39, with ileocecal masses and a fistula requiring resection. Corr and Boeck[399] (Los Angeles, California) almost simultaneously contributed additional instances of the disease. Harold Edwards[400] of London in 1936 characterized the resected bowel from a 23-year-old woman, who had been treated for abdominal tuberculosis, as having the "consistency of a hose pipe." He added: "Recurrences sometimes occurred at the anastomotic site ... it was well to remember that Crohn's disease was a rather fatal condition, about half the cases dying." In his 1968 Bradshaw lecture on Crohn's disease before the Royal College of Surgeons of England, Edwards[401] agreed with Meadows

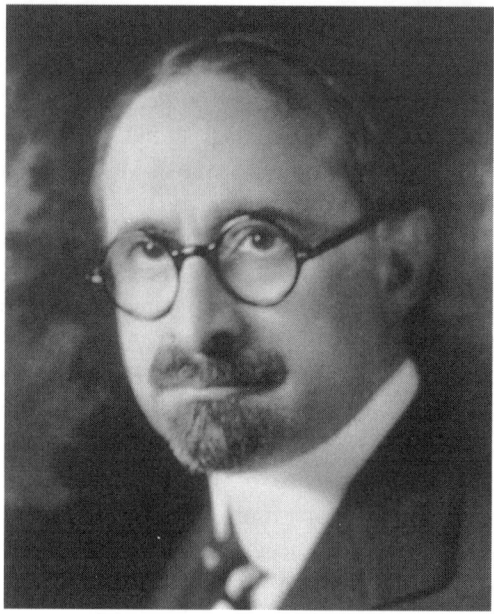

A.A. Berg

and Batsakis[402] (1963) of Ann Arbor, Michigan "that the main early feature ... of Crohn's disease is a pronounced edema of the entire bowel wall, most marked in the submucosa and accompanied by a hyperemia and lymphangiectasis." Appendicitis was the initial diagnosis in one-third of 240 patients. The 1936 series of Koster, Kasman, and Sheinfeld[403] of Brooklyn, New York included "17 instances of peculiar inflammatory lesions localized in the terminal portion of the ileum." The preoperative diagnosis had been appendicitis in 13 of the 17 patients. In 1936 Crohn and Rosenak[404] reported 9 instances of combined ileitis and colitis, another early indication of Crohn's disease of the colon. Also in 1936 A.A. Berg[405] (Mt. Sinai Hospital, New York) had described an operative procedure for "right-sided ulcerative ileocolitis" ("ulcerative colo-ileitis") "to put the diseased colon at rest," provide "an outlet" for the discharge of blood and pus and "cleansing of the diseased colon by irrigating fluids."

R.A. Leonardo[406] of Rochester, New York in 1937 described the interesting course of a 33-year-old white male hospitalized in 1935 for abdominal cramps and diarrhea, diagnosed as "early appendicitis." One year earlier, a lesion on his face had been resected, described histologically as "lymphoid tissue with many characteristic tubercles" and diagnosed as tuberculous lymphadenitis. An appendectomy (retrocecal appendix) was performed with "more than the usual amount of trauma to the ileocecal region." Within days the patient was re-hospitalized with abdominal cramps and diarrhea. Laboratory studies were unremarkable. X-rays indicated small bowel dilatation. At operation, a large inflammatory mass involved the last 8 inches of terminal ileum, the cecum and 4 inches of the ascending colon. The mesentery of the terminal ileum was greatly thickened and the terminal ileum was adherent to the peritoneum. No tubercles were identified histologically. The differential diagnosis included: operative trauma (preceding operation), tuberculosis of the cecum (negative chest X-ray) or carcinoma. A simple ileostomy was performed. Within days, all symptoms disappeared and the patient apparently had no further difficulty. The author, aware of the 1932 paper on regional ileitis, diagnosed combined "regional ileitis" and colitis. The favorable course after the "simple ileostomy" was an early indication of the benefits of diversion of the fecal stream. In retrospect, the facial lesion probably was "metastatic Crohn's disease!"

I. Snapper and A. Pompen[407] of Amsterdam, Holland (1936), describing five patients, implicated "intestinal stagnation" proximal to the ileocecal valve, recognized the clinical similarity to acute appendicitis, and the tendency to fistula formation and suggested its higher frequency among Jewish individuals. T.G.I. James[408] of England in 1937, describing an inflammatory mass with histologic features of Crohn's disease involving the transverse colon in a 19-year-old male, was an early advocate of the entity of Crohn's disease of the colon. In 1937 Jellen[409] of Los Angeles, California (formerly radiologist at Mt. Sinai) reviewed the clinical features in fifty patients with regional ileitis ("nonspecific ulcerative granuloma") with emphasis upon the roentgen findings. I.S. Ravdin and C.G. Johnston[410] University of Pennsylvania, in 1939 suggested twelve possible etiologic factors: (1) bacteria, (2) bacterial toxins, (3) viruses, (4) protozoa, (5) metazoa, (6) achylia gastrica, (7) allergy, (8) foreign bodies, (9) nonspecific inflammation of appendix, (10), impairment of blood supply, (11) interference with lymphatic supply and (12) trauma.

By the latter 1930s, Crohn's disease was global in distribution, with reports from Italy,[411,412] Sweden,[413] Germany,[414] Holland,[415] Australia[125] and later among Chinese in Hong Kong[416] and among Chinese immigrants to Vancouver, British Columbia, Canada.[417] In 1937 C. Gottlieb and S. Alpert[418] (Lincoln Hospital, New York) described the roentgen appearance of regional jejunitis in a 44-year-old Greek man; the diagnosis, suspected on X-ray, was confirmed at abdominal operation. In

1940 Sherrill and Hall[419] of Nashville, Kentucky, reported two interesting cases of regional ileitis. In one, a 17-year-old male presented with intestinal obstruction caused by a thickened adherent distal ileum necessitating operation. In the second instance, a 16-year-old male presented with abdominal pain and fever, found at operation to be caused by a Meckel's diverticulitis enveloped in the ileitis. The ileum was thickened and adherent with pronounced fibrosis of the distal ileum necessitating bowel resection. In 1943 A. Tallroth[420] of Gothenberg, Sweden impressed by the large numbers of eosinophils in the inflammatory reaction, considered "intestinal allergy" as the underlying mechanism.

A detailed clinical report by E. Schiff[421] of Basel, Switzerland in 1945 documented the increasing frequency of the disease in young patients and cited numerous European references to Crohn's disease. F.N. Silverman[422] of Cincinnati (1966) reviewing 14 children with Crohn's disease (8 male, 6 female) emphasized the alerting clinical features: "children with atypical appendicitis, pyrexia of undetermined origin, growth failure, recurrent abdominal pain and anorexia nervosa." Koop et al.[423] of the United States in 1947 reported a cicatrizing enterocolitis in a newborn involving the entire small intestine and colon. Walter and Chaffin[424] (University of Southern California, Los Angeles) in 1957 reported two cases of apparent segmental enteritis in infancy: one in a newborn female who was operated upon ten hours after birth, disclosing acute inflammation of the distal ileum and the second, in a baby whose symptom of gastrointestinal bleeding began at the age of one month and who was operated upon at the age of three months. A second operation disclosed segmental inflammation of the mid-ileum, fistula formation, skip areas of disease, and "typical" histologic findings.

As with ulcerative colitis, the clinical spectrum of Crohn's disease steadily expanded. In 1948 Kirsner, Owens and Humphreys[425] described regional enteritis in father and son with exactly the same disease in the terminal ileum. Ginzburg and Oppenheimer[426] directed attention to the urological complications in regional ileitis, expanded later by F. Gross of Stuttgart, Germany[427] (1959). J.R. Ross[428] (1949) of the Lahey Clinic, Boston described in sequence cicatrizing ulcerative enteritis, colitis and gastritis in a 21-year-old white female, undergoing multiple operations including: resections of terminal ileum (38 inches of terminal ileum), an abdominoperineal resection and partial (50%) gastric resection. Another instance of Crohn's disease of the stomach was reported by Martin and Carr of London.[429] In 1950, Franklin and Taylor[430] of London described Crohn's disease involvement of the esophagus. The 1951 review of 40 patients with regional enteritis by G.F. Dashiell, J.B. Kirsner et al.[431] (Chicago) emphasized the pathophysiology of the disease. Of the four deaths, two resulted from complications of the disease, one patient died of coronary occlusion, and the fourth death was a suicide. In 1954 Crohn and Janowitz,[432] reflecting on the status of regional enteritis after 20 years, emphasized the vulnerability of the entire small intestine. One year later, Janowitz,[433] reviewing current problems of regional enteritis, implicated "materials in the intestinal content in the recurrences gaining access via the ileal lymphatics." This aspect was reviewed comprehensively in 1998.[434]

In 1956 Zetzel[435] of Boston, in a survey of 69 publications, updated the clinical status of regional enteritis and current etiologic concepts. Chapin, Scudamore, Baggenstoss, and Bargen[436] in 1956 enumerated the complications of regional enteritis at autopsy in 39 patients, including peritonitis (49%), fatty liver (51%), glomerulitis (33%) and vascular thrombosis (21%). Ford and Vallis[437] described the clinical course of the arthritis associated with ulcerative colitis and with regional ileitis. Other complications reported during this time included perforation of the bowel,[438] the only case of generalized amyloidosis[439] in a 33-year-old female with regional enteritis of the terminal ileum seen at Mt. Sinai Hospital. The recognition of carcinoma of the jejunum in a patient with regional ileitis[440] was followed by the comprehensive study of carcinoma complicating Crohn's disease by Weedon et al., comprising 440 patients with an impressive 92% followup.[441] L. Falla-Alvarez (a former student of H.L. Bockus in Philadelphia) and R. Albacete[442] in 1958 recorded their experience with 20 patients with regional enteritis in Cuba, observed between 1950 and 1957, illustrating the importance of physician awareness acquired at a major medical center in facilitating recognition of the disease in their home countries yet unaware of the problem. A second report of regional enteritis in Cuba appeared in 1966.[443] Seeking a reliable laboratory index of disease activity in IBD, W.T. Cooke et al.[444] of Birmingham, England, in 1958 proposed the measurement of seromucoids as an index of disease activity in regional enteritis, but this test was not adopted generally.

General Eisenhower's intestinal obstruction secondary to an old regional enteritis (thickened, narrowed terminal ileum), managed successfully by an intestinal bypass operation (ileotransverse colostomy without bowel resection) in 1956,[445,446] stimulated interest in Crohn's disease, particularly in the United States, and encouraged a onetime modest ($100,000) multiple center outlay of research funds from the National Institutes of

Health. Eisenhower died in 1969 and autopsy demonstrated a thick-walled, fibrotic "burned-out" regional enteritis, unchanged since the bypass procedure 13 years earlier. The prevailing surgical operation for Crohn's disease for many years had been extensive intestinal resection (guided by multiple intestinal biopsies to ensure the absence of any histologic evidence of visible Crohn's disease at the resection margins) and intestinal re-anastomosis, in a futile effort to eliminate disease, with serious physiologic consequences (short bowel syndrome). The frequent recurrence of disease after bowel resection and re-anastomosis as noted by D.J. Fone,[447] among many others, and the favorable outcome of Eisenhower's intestinal bypass operation encouraged a short trial of the intestinal bypass procedure, soon discontinued because of concern with the associated bacterial (anaerobic) overgrowth in the isolated bypassed segment and the associated hazard of intestinal carcinoma.

In time, Crohn's disease was identified in virtually all areas of the gastrointestinal tract from mouth to anus and elsewhere in the body. Crohn's-type lesions were observed in the mouth,[448] skin,[449] the umbilicus,[450] bone,[451] muscles, and lungs.[452] Involvement of the mouth in Crohn's disease attracted considerable attention in the 1970s. Basu, Asquith, Thompson and Cooke[453] of Birmingham, England found decreased production of salivary IgA in Crohn's patients with active Crohn's disease. T. Lehner[454] of Guy's Hospital, London, extensively reviewed the problem of oral ulceration, comparing Crohn's disease with Behçet's syndrome; a viral infection with clinical similarities to Crohn's disease. In a letter to the editor, Matthews et al.,[455] (England) utilizing buccal biopsies, noted that "some patients with Crohn's disease produced antibodies to perinuclear components in buccal mucosal epithelial cells." In 1969, Present, Rabinowitz, Banks and Janowitz[456] described the occasionally unrecognized complication of obstructive hydronephrosis resulting from envelopment of the lower end of the ureters in the intestinal inflammation. Heaton and Rich[457] of Bristol, England (1969) described the altered bile salt metabolism and the pathophysiology underlying the frequency of gallstones in patients with regional ileitis. Smith, Fromm and Hoffman[458] in 1972 reviewed the pathophysiology of acquired hyperoxaluria and nephrolithiasis in small intestinal disease.

In 1963, J. Kyle et al.[381] of Aberdeen, Scotland investigated possible causes of regional enteritis in a study of 54 patients. In 15% of cases, the disease did not begin until after the age of 50. None of the patients was Jewish. Kyle already had noticed a rising incidence of the disease during the latter years of his study. The series included one instance of familial incidence (mother and daughter) and one patient in whom abdominal trauma preceded the occurrence of Crohn's disease. In 30 patients, intestinal tissue cultures and serum antibody studies for adenovirus and Coxsackie B were indecisive. Intestinal autoantibodies (immunofluorescent and double diffusion in agar techniques) were not found.

In 1966 Gjone, Orning and Myren of Oslo, Norway[459] soon noted the increasing prevalence of Crohn's disease in Norway, a trend soon evident in other Scandinavian countries and continuing today. Clinical reports from Norway[460] and Northern Ireland,[461] added to the increasing interest in IBD. A workshop (Leiden, Holland), focusing solely on Crohn's disease therapy,[462] included 300 references published during the 1960s and 1970s. A major United States Cooperative Crohn's Disease Study during the 1970s examined various clinical parameters of the disease and developed a Crohn's disease activity index (CDAI), often utilized today in the evaluation of drug therapy.[463–465]

CROHN'S DISEASE OF THE COLON – DELAYED RECOGNITION

Despite early accounts of Crohn's-like inflammatory lesions in the colon, the reports of Dalziel in 1913, Moschowitz and Wilensky in 1923 and 1927 describing "non-specific granulomatous lesions" in both the small and large intestine, a right-sided colitis by Bargen and Weber[466] (1930) and case reports from Mt. Sinai Hospital, New York by R. Colp,[467)] and by Crohn and A.A. Berg[468] (1938) for reasons still unclear, the concept of a "Crohn's colitis" was difficult to accept in the United States. The 1930 Bargen-Weber paper described 23 patients with "regional migrating colitis." The sole available method of diagnosis was the single contrast barium examination of the colon. Review of that report revealed (understandably) poor quality X-ray views, identifying only the most pronounced changes in the colon; identifiable today as advanced Crohn's disease (not ulcerative colitis).

Charles Wells[469] of Liverpool in 1952 differentiated ulcerative colitis from Crohn's colitis and recognized "segmental colitis" as a variant of Crohn's disease. W.T. Cooke and B. Brooke[470] of Birmingham, England (1955), described 11 patients, teenagers and young adults with a "non-infective disorder," "non-specific enterocolitis" affecting the small bowel initially and spreading to the colon. Diarrhea was the predominant symptom. Pathologically, the lesion in the small intestine was confined to the mucosa (multiple small ulcers "differing from Crohn's disease" and "backwash ileitis." In the colon the disease was evident initially in the

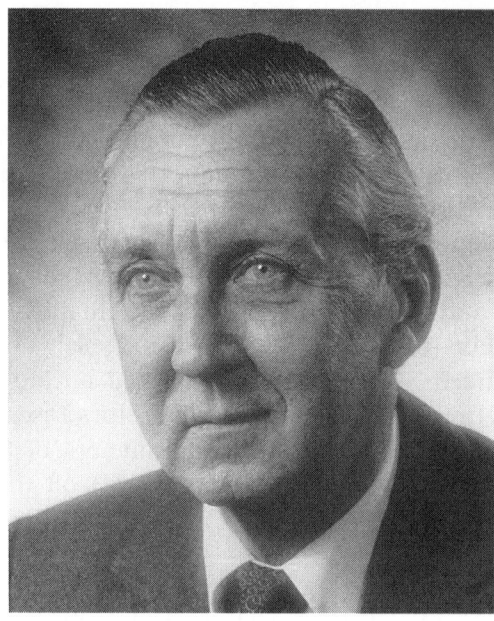

H.E. Lockhart-Mummery

right colon and resembled ulcerative colitis except for the right-sided involvement ... "it is different ... from ulcerative colitis and from cicatrizing regional enteritis or colitis."

Brooke[471] conclusively identified "right-sided colitis" as Crohn's disease in 1959. But not until the reports of Morson and H.E. Lockhart-Mummery[472] in 1959 and Cornes and Stecher[473] (1961) was Crohn's colitis finally accepted as a distinct entity in the United States, Great Britain and in Europe. (See also review by R.W. Nevin[493a].) Despite the long-term familiarity with granulomatous intestinal disease at Mt. Sinai Hospital (NY), physicians and surgeons at that institution refused for many years to recognize that regional enteritis could involve the colon. Resected specimens of inflammatory disease of both ileum and colon were consistently reported as regional enteritis of the small bowel and ulcerative colitis respectively.

As early as 1951, radiologist R. Marshak (New York) had noted changes in the colon resembling regional ileitis in some patients with so-called ulcerative colitis. Also, other patients with definite regional ileitis presented radiologically-identical disease in the colon, observations he reported at a meeting of the Inter-American Association of Radiologists

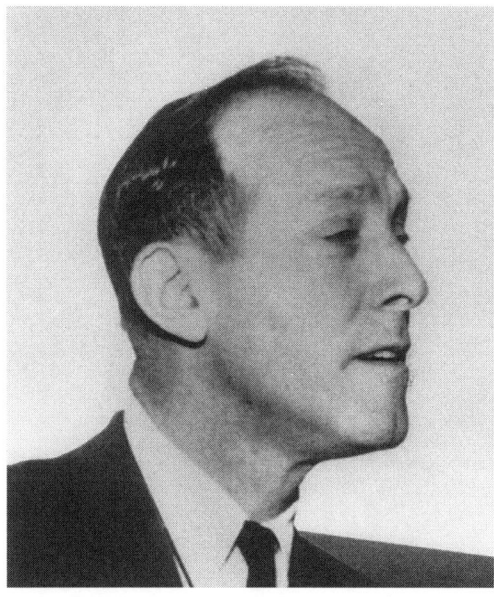

R. Marshak

in 1951. At the 1955 meeting of the American Gastroenterological Association, he described the roentgen differences between ulcerative and granulomatous colitis. The discussants of the paper, however, took the erroneous position that granulomatous colitis was a form of chronic ulcerative colitis. In 1959, Marshak[474] published his findings on granulomatous colitis in a paper entitled "Segmental Colitis" but he too suggested that most of the cases of segmental colonic disease probably were instances of ulcerative colitis. However, in 1962 Marshak,[475] in a major presentation to the Radiological Society of North America, entitled "Granulomatous Disease of the Intestinal Tract (Crohn's Disease)", reviewed his remarkable experience with approximately 8000 cases of regional enteritis and 4000 of granulomatous colitis. The paper included his "10 principles of Crohn's disease." He concluded in part: "The main purpose of this talk is to present an overall perspective of granulomatous disease and provide a stimulus, especially to the younger men, for further study of a disease in which there are so many unsolved problems." Numerous papers in the 1960s and subsequently, dealing with the overlapping findings in ulcerative colitis and Crohn's disease of the colon, outlined differentiating features of ulcerative colitis and Crohn's disease of the colon.[476–479] McGovern and Goulston[480] in 1968 re-emphasized the

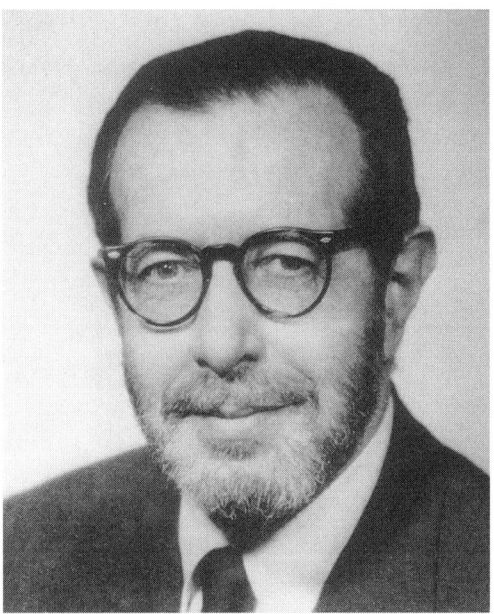

Henry D. Janowitz

characteristic histologic features of submucosal fibrosis and prominent lymphoid aggregates.

In addressing the question, Why was the recognition of Crohn's colitis so slow?, Janowitz[481] remarked: "The reasons at the home of the American pioneers I believe I can account for. From the 1920s on, Pathology was king, not only at Mt. Sinai but especially there, where Paul Klemperer, who had just arrived from Vienna was to start his long, distinguished career, and under whom Moschowitz and Wilensky and later Ginzburg and Oppenheimer were to work. The central dogma firmly held by the pathologist Dr. Otani of Klemperer's department was that the ileocecal valve was more than a landmark of separation. It was a virtual Mason–Dixon line. In the north, from the duodenum to the ileum occurred regional enteritis. To the south occurred ulcerative colitis and never the twain were to meet or mingle. This perspective determined the attitude through which inflammatory bowel disease was viewed at that time. So fixed was this widely held point of view that these were two geographically as well as nosologically different diseases, that the idea that Crohn's ileitis could occur in the colon was hard to accept by the original Mt. Sinai workers, especially Crohn himself. The tidiness of the original separation also played its part in the stereotyping of clinical perception. If the hold was so strong at the home of Crohn, Ginzburg and Oppenheimer, it is not difficult to see why others on the American side of the Atlantic failed to accept what had been under their eyes for at least a generation." Following the acceptance of Crohn's disease of the colon as a valid entity, its differentiation from nonspecific ulcerative colitis became an important clinical challenge in 10 to 15% with IBD of the colon. In 1975 Price and Morson of St. Marks Hospital[482] and Kirsner[483] each published helpful differentiating features of Crohn's colitis and ulcerative colitis.

EARLY PATHOLOGY OF CROHN'S DISEASE

In 1938 Coffey[484] (Mayo Clinic) emphasized the early principal anatomic features of Crohn's disease as: subacute or chronic granulomatous inflammation, the tendency to stenosis of the bowel, the fistula formation and the absence of tuberculosis. In 1939 G. Hadfield[485] of St. Bartholomew Hospital, London, in a study of 20 cases of regional ileitis, noting "obstructive lymphedema" and lymphoid hyperplasia in the intestinal submucosa, had suggested "lymphadenoid hyperplasia with the formation of non-caseating giant cell systems in the submucosa" and also in the regional lymph nodes as the earliest and possibly the "specific" histological lesion of regional enteritis. Hadfield et al. concluded: "From the purely histological point of view ... the appearance, evolution and retrogression of the giant cell systems of regional ileitis more closely resemble the tissue reaction of Boeck's sarcoidosis than of tuberculosis infection."[486] Testing this hypothesis, Kveim skin tests for sarcoidosis later were negative in patients with regional enteritis.

The production of granulomas by antigen-antibody complexes[487,488] in 1966 and 1969 stimulated interest in possible contributory immune mechanisms. In the 1970s the etiologic significance of the granuloma in Crohn's disease was unclear, although the microgranuloma was considered an early indication of Crohn's disease.[489] Chambers and Morson[490] in 1979 stated, "It (the granuloma) is generally assumed to represent a response to the aetiological agent (for example, a 'poorly soluble antigenic agent') ... It is conceivable that it follows mucosal ulceration with resulting penetration of bowel contents into tissues ..." although "granulomas are often seen in non-ulcerated bowel wall and no luminal debris can be identified." The early emphasis upon the possible etiologic importance of the intestinal granulomas generated modest interest in the nature of the granuloma and in conditions associated with granuloma formation.

Though differing in some features, as originally noted by Lartigau in 1901, the association of granulomas with tuberculosis, actinomycosis, schistosomiasis, sarcoid, and histoplasmosis, as well as foreign body granulomas (talc, lipid, silica, mercury and beryllium) actually diminished their diagnostic usefulness in Crohn's disease. Furthermore, Whitehead[491] of Australia demonstrated microgranulomas and giant cell reactions also in ulcerative colitis. Kirsner also had observed granulomas in experimental injury of the bowel. In 1973 Aaronson and Spiro[492] (Yale University) speculated on a possible role for mercury in inflammatory bowel disease and in 1987 P.O. Ganrot[493] (Orebro, Sweden) proposed aluminum as a "possible etiologic agent" in Crohn's disease, but neither suggestion attracted attention. In 1992 J.V. Weinstock,[494] University of Iowa, Iowa City, authoritatively reviewed the subject of the granuloma and Crohn's disease.

The 1948 study of 120 cases and the comprehensive literature review by S. Warren and S.C. Sommers[495] of the New England Deaconess Hospital, Boston had emphasized the cicatrizing nature of the tissue reaction, in addition to the "granulomatous response in the intestine." Giant cell systems, including giant cell inclusions, were present in lymph nodes even when not present in the intestine. As stated by Warren and Sommers: "A progressive sclerosing granulomatous lymphangitis, probably as a reaction to an irritative lipid substance," is of interest in relation to the later implication of lipids in Crohn's disease.[496]

H. Rappaport et al.,[497] at the U.S. Armed Forces Institute of Pathology in Washington D.C., in 1951 reviewed 100 cases, including 85 bowel resections and 15 autopsies. In 72 instances, sections from mesenteric lymph nodes and in 35, appendices were available for study. The "tubercle-like granuloma observed in about half of the group, differed from foreign body granulomas and from the sarcoid lesion. Lymphedema and lymphangiectasis were common." Ulceration was not the primary lesion in regional enteritis but was preceded by lymphoid hyperplasia. Rappaport et al. were able to histologically differentiate regional enteritis from chronic ulcerative colitis. S. Otani[498] of Mt. Sinai Hospital (1955) and R. Whitehead of Australia[499] (1980) each provided detailed reviews of the pathology of regional enteritis and regional enterocolitis. Otani concluded "since the pathological picture of the colonic lesions is so identical with that of regional enteritis, it is logical to assume that the simultaneous association of regional ileitis and colitis should not be interpreted as a mere coincidence, since they may have a common etiological factor."

In 1954 Warren and Sommers,[187] comparing the pathology of ulcerative colitis and regional ileitis, reaffirmed: "The histopathology of regional ileitis would suggest a reaction to irritative lipid substances. It appears possibly to represent a by-product of some biochemical abnormality of lipid absorption in the intestine," but this possibility was not pursued.

In 1955 Davis, Dockerty and Mayo[500] examined the myenteric plexus of the ileum in 24 patients with regional enteritis (with allowance for thickening and shrinkage of tissue) and, as in ulcerative colitis, found a threefold increase in the number of ganglion cells, compared to controls. The increased ganglion cells were present in adjacent, apparently normal bowel as well as in diseased areas. The only explanation offered, as in the ulcerative colitis study, was "the stimulus of ulceration and increased function to the growth of small undeveloped nerve cells."

Binney[501] observed endarteritis obliterans and perivascular infiltration of plasma cells in the small intestine but made no etiologic inferences. Interestingly, Warren and Sommers[187] had observed "inflammatory necrosis" of arteries and veins also in ulcerative colitis. B.C. Morson[502] for many years had identified foci of vasculitis (arteritis) in surgically resected and in biopsy tissue of Crohn's disease and "I often wondered about the importance of this lesion." Recent interest in a possible focal "granulomatous" mesenteric vasculitis involving mucosal and submucosal vessels, inducing focal ischemic damage, and mini-infarctions of the intestine related to the measles virus as an explanation for the focal distribution of Crohn's disease[503] has not received strong support. Also, the specificity of "focal lesions" (CD) may be in question if "multifocal colitis" also characterizes colitis of infectious origin[504] and allergic proctocolitis in infants.

In 1961, R.W. Ammann (Zurich, Switzerland) and H.L. Bockus[505] (Graduate Hospital, Philadelphia), emphasizing "immunologically-induced edema" as the earliest histologic lesion, re-examined surgical specimens from 40 patients with regional enteritis. In the proximal pre-ulcerous segments, the changes (edema, mucosal distortion, inflammatory reaction of the lamina propria with PAS-positive macrocytes and 'Brunner's glands') were attributed to an obstructive lymphedema, similar to the changes observed in experimental chylous obstruction. Granulomatous changes within or around lymph vessels were noted frequently. Similar alterations had been recorded by Schepers[506] in 1945. In 1964 T.K. Shnitka[507] of Edmonton, Alberta, Canada, like others, emphasized lymphangiectasis, lymphedema, lymphoid hyperplasia and granulomatous inflammation of the submucosal and subserosal layers of the intestine. Chronic ulcerative colitis, on the other hand, began in the mucosa with "crypt abscesses" and progressed transmurally only in its later stages.

In the absence of acceptable endoscopic biopsy technology, the "early" pathologic studies of Crohn's disease had dealt with advanced stages of the disease.[508] In 1972 B.C. Morson[509] of London identified the "earliest macroscopic lesion of Crohn's disease as the tiny aphthoid ulceration (micro-erosion)," as had been noted by B. Brooke in 1953.[134] Poulsen et al.[510] of Copenhagen, Denmark identified microerosions often associated with granulomas in rectal biopsies in patients with Crohn's disease. In 1980 the aphthoid ulcer was located by Rickert and Carter of Livingston, New Jersey precisely over the special membranous M cell[511] situated in the epithelium overlying lymphoid follicles in Peyer's patches, a finding of considerable, as yet incompletely evaluated pathogenetic importance. The M cell, a membranous cell type that allows molecules and microorganisms to reach the organized mucosa-associated lymphoid tissue, only now is attracting increased scientific attention. (See later.)

Morson[502] in the 1960s and 1970s had summarized the gross pathological features of Crohn's disease, including thickened adherent mesentery, thickened small bowel, enteric fistulas, intestinal narrowing, aphthous ulcers, and linear serpiginous ulcers, cobblestone appearing mucosa, and the asymmetrical focal distribution of the disease. Distinctive histologic findings included focal lesions, transmural inflammation, dilated submucosal lymphatics, prominent lymphoid aggregates, knife-like fissuring ulcerations, granulomas, hypertrophy of the muscular layer and neural hyperplasia. The diagnostic emphasis histopathologically was upon a collection of features, rather than a single abnormality (focal submucosal involvement, dilated lymphatics, lymphoid prominence, non-tuberculous granuloma, vertical fissures). None of these features, in fact, was an early manifestation of a disease that probably also involves the intestinal mucosa.

The development of gastrointestinal endoscopy,[512] including the fiber-optic colonoscope and the associated improvements in biopsy technology during the 1950s provided access to intestinal tissue at earlier stages of IBD. Increased knowledge of intestinal epithelial function and the response to injury provided new insights into the nature of the IBD tissue reaction.[513]

ELECTRON MICROSCOPY – CROHN'S DISEASE

In a 1971 electron microscopic study, Aluwihare,[514,515] St. Marks Hospital, London, examined colon tissue obtained at operation or biopsy specimens from the colon and rectum of patients with Crohn's disease, fixed in 1% osmium tetroxide. Where the bowel was not ulcerated, the epithelial cells appeared normal, as did their microvilli. In contrast to ulcerative colitis, the epithelial cells, initially intact, appeared smaller, with stunted microvilli. There was mild edema between the cells but the underlying basement membrane and collagen were intact. Numerous plasma cells and lymphocytes were present in the broadened lamina propria. The lymphocytes contained prominent nucleoli, as seen in immunologically-stimulated lymphocytes. Most of the nerve and muscle cells and the blood vessels appeared normal. The epithelioid cells in the granulomas contained large nuclei with finely dispersed chromatin and a clear-cut nucleolus. The margins between the epithelioid cells were undulating and interdigitating, without a true basement membrane. Towards the periphery of a granuloma, the endoplasmic reticulum of the epithelioid cells appeared coarse in texture. Nearer the center, they contained vacuoles, representing metabolic activity. Electron microscopic histochemistry demonstrated acid phosphatase, an important lysosomal enzyme in the clear vesicles present in the epithelioid cells. Clusters of bacteria were seen in the deep layers of the colon. Organisms were not seen in similar sites of normal colon. Aluwihare regarded the changes in the lymphocytes, plasma cells and epithelioid cells as compatible with "some immunological reaction," but secondary manifestations were not excluded.

Ranlov, Nielsen and Wanstrup[516] (Copenhagen) in 1972 reported electron microscopic findings in surgical tissues from two patients with "advanced Crohn's disease of the ileum" (one male 26, one female 24) and were impressed with the many small and large lymphocytes, plasma cells, epithelioid cell granulomas and unusually large number of mast cells, "attributable to cell-mediated immune mechanisms." Microorganisms were not seen. In 1974 Siemers and Dobbins[517] of San Diego, California published a light and electron microscopy study of the Meissner submucosal plexus in normal colon and the colon of patients with Crohn's disease. Ganglion cells of the plexus in Crohn's disease appeared normal. Minor changes included axon dilatation, increased numbers of neurofilaments and penetration of nerve fibers by plasma cells and mast cells. There was no hypertrophy of ganglion cells but centrioles in ganglion cells were prominent. The authors speculated on a process of "mitotic division of otherwise normal neurons." Although the emphasis in Crohn's disease traditionally has been upon submucosal and transmural disease, Dourmashkin et al.[518] (England) in 1981 on electron microscopy noted "early epithelial lesions."

The axonal necrosis of autonomic nerve fibers and ganglion cells in Crohn's disease, observed at electron microscopy by A. Dvorak (Beth Israel Hospital, Boston),[519–521] and the earlier observation of mast cell hyperplasia in the ileum of Crohn's disease,[522] presumably consequences of the inflammatory reaction (or perhaps "the ultrastructural correlate of an autonomic neuropathy") remain unexplained. Additional findings such as mast cell degranulation, release of basic protein-containing eosinophilic granules[523] (primarily affecting autonomic nervous system axons), myofibroblast proliferation, increased numbers of polymorphonuclear leukocytes, lymphocytes, eosinophils, macrophages, basophils, and Paneth's granular cells and alterations in epithelial cells reflected the complexity of the CD tissue reaction.

In 1981, Otto (Hamburg, Germany) and Gebbers (Lucerne, Switzerland)[524] described immunohisto- and ultracytochemical studies on surgical and biopsy specimens from 27 patients with Crohn's disease of the ileum or colon. Control specimens were obtained from 16 patients with nonspecific proctitis or neoplastic disorders of the cecum or rectum. The initial lesions in Crohn's disease were associated with a "typical humoral immune response." In non-ulcerated mucosa a uniform increase of IgA-, IgG- and IgM-cells was found, whereas disproportional increases of IgG- and IgE-cells were observed in ulcerated mucosa. The IgE-cell multiplication in ulcerated areas suggested a local hypersensitivity reaction. Macrophages and granulocytes contained IgG, also present in multinucleated giant cells. The granulomas contained extracellular IgG, acid phosphatase and peroxidase. The finding of "potentially harmful" extracellular lysosomal enzymes was attributed to "autoimmune phenomena." Micro-ulcerations of the dome epithelium of hyperplastic Peyer's patches were an early lesion through which luminal antigens gained uncontrolled access to Peyer's patches. C1q or C3 bound to epithelial or vascular basement membranes were not detected and no electron dense deposits were found. Viral particles or bacteria were not demonstrated by electron microscopy.

Later studies by Marin et al.[525] of New York, utilizing freeze fracture electron microscopy, demonstrated a variety of changes in the ileal mucosa of Crohn's disease, including large lysosomal inclusions in epithelial cells, alterations in villi, dilated goblet cells and pinpoint aphthoid ulcers and in the involved colonic mucosa, loss of the normal mucosal architecture, changes thought to represent secondary tissue reactions. Marin et al.[526] were intrigued by the fusion of "limiting and inclusion granule membranes" within the epithelial cells in CD and considered their pathogenetic significance. In 1995 Nagel et al.[527] of Hannover, Germany, in a scanning-electron-microscopic study of surgically-resected bowel from 29 patients with Crohn's disease and 11 control subjects, correlated a triad of early lesions: mucosal architectural alteration, epithelial bridge formation and goblet cell hyperplasia with the frequent recurrences of CD. These observations extended the 1976 findings of Goodman, Skinner and Truelove,[528] who, with light microscopy, had noted more diffuse involvement of the small intestine than was apparent visually. In considering the "early" vs. late pathologic studies of IBD, the 1972 comments by James Kyle are relevant 30 years later. "Probably too much attention has been paid in the past to the end-product (and I would include the granuloma). All routine and most research pathology studies tend to concentrate on the worst affected part of the intestine ... but this type of examination is most unlikely to throw much new light on the early stages of the disease when aetiological clues are more likely to be discerned," (as in early colonoscopic biopsies). The issue of "early" and "late" Crohn's disease continues to be debated by physicians, surgeons and pathologists; in part because of the difficulty in assigning "time-related labels" (early, late) to the complex biologic phenomena characterizing CD.

ORIGIN OF EPONYM OF CROHN'S DISEASE

Many terms have been applied to the disorder originally labelled terminal ileitis: regional enteritis, chronic cicatrizing enteritis, nonspecific granuloma of the intestine, hyperplastic ileitis, chronic ulcerative ileitis, enteritis phlegmonosa, ileocolitis, inflammatory pseudo-tumor of the intestine, regional ileitis of the colon and Crohn's colitis. British reports of "granulomatous inflammation" of the small bowel in Great Britain in the 1930s occasionally were referred to as Crohn's disease.[529,530] In the United States, the term Crohn's disease probably was first employed as an eponym by F.I. Harris[334] (1933) in the article "Chronic cicatrizing enteritis of the ileum: Regional ileitis (Crohn)." B.C. Cushway[531] of Chicago in a 1934 case report used the title "Chronic Cicatrizing Enteritis, Regional Ileitis (Crohn)." R.F. Barbour and A.B. Stokes[532] of the Maudsley Hospital, London wrote in 1936: "To this localized condition the name of regional

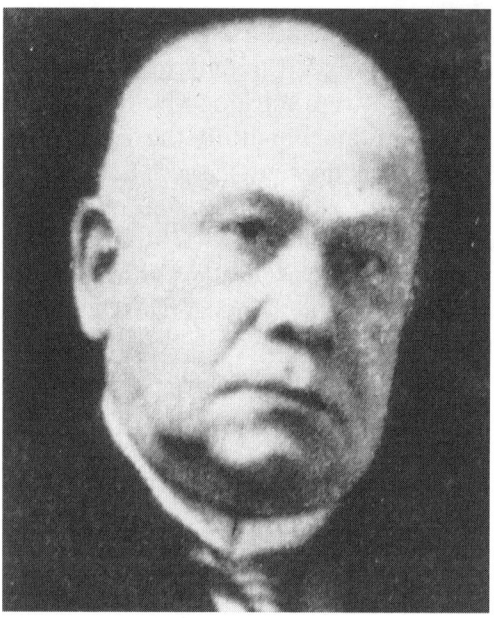

Antoni Lesniowski

enteritis was given, although in America it also became known as Crohn's disease. A.F. Hurst and G.A.M. Lintott[533] (London) in 1937 also referred to Crohn's disease. Physicians in other countries likewise claimed publication priority. Thus, in Poland, this entity was called "Lesniowski–Crohn's disease."[534] (Antoni Lesniowski and his contribution to Regional enteritis [Crohn's Disease]). H.I. Goldstein[295] utilized the term: "Saunders–Abercrombie–Crohn's ileitis," to recognize early British describers of the entity.

To American observers, this entity might justifiably have been designated "CGO disease" to reflect the important contributions of not only B. Crohn but also L. Ginzburg and G. Oppenheimer who provided 12 of the 14 cases in the 1932 JAMA paper. Also Ginzburg was acknowledged by Crohn himself as having studied intestinal granulomas and intestinal inflammatory pseudotumors long before Crohn, justifying Ginzburg's claim for co-designation. The term Crohn–Dalziel disease as suggested by M. Harmer[535] appealed to many, in recognition of Dalziel's significant 1913 paper, including J.F. Fielding[536] and J. Kyle.[537,538] The term "cicatrizing enteritis" proposed by Warren and Sommers, according to Armitage and Wilson,[539] "though a fair term is far from euphonious." "The name Crohn's disease has been adhered to in most cases at this hospital (Leeds). It avoids confusion, makes no pretense of pathological exactitude, conveys an exact meaning, is easily remembered by students, and pays a well deserved tribute." Apparently unaware of the precise chronological events, the designation of Crohn's disease was endorsed at the 8th International Congress of Gastroenterology in Prague, Czechoslovakia in 1968. Whatever the "labeling" circumstances, the entity today carries the eponym Crohn's disease as the most convenient designation, now sanctioned by worldwide, long-term usage, for an unique inflammatory process involving any part of the gastrointestinal tract, characterized by chronicity, recurrences, and numerous complications.

To the credit of Crohn, Ginzburg, and Oppenheimer is the globally-acknowledged fact that their timely clinical description and subsequent numerous, important contributions, although initially focussed on the terminal ileum, stimulated interest in an emerging worldwide disease. As Brooke, Morson, Truelove, Heller and other IBD observers had suggested in personal communications, "the time (1932) was right" for the description of this disorder and, had the Mt. Sinai group not assembled their paper, others soon would have done so (see also A.H. Aufses[540]).

On the matter of eponyms, the comment of Thomas Lewis[541] in 1944 remains pertinent today: "Diagnosis is a system of more or less accurate guessing, in which the end point achieved is a name. These names applied to disease come to assume the importance of specific entities ... whereas they are, for the most part, no more than insecure and therefore temporary conceptions." Presumably, the Crohn's designation will yield to the etiology of the disease when it is discovered!

EDITORIAL NOTE

With the conclusion of this overview of origins, early discovery and increasing clinical recognition of ulcerative colitis and Crohn's disease, the remainder of this publication is focused on the nature and etiopathogenesis of ulcerative colitis and Crohn's disease. The following sections include: early epidemiology, psychogenic aspects, microbiological possibilities, immune mechanisms, including M cell, epithelial permeability and inflammation, genetic possibilities and a concluding commentary. The early treatment of inflammatory bowel disease is reviewed in the appendix, together with a listing of earlier IBD publications.

REFERENCES

Crohn's Disease – Origins

279. Carson HW. The iliac passion. Ann Med Hist 1931;3:638–94.
280. Fabry W. Ex scirrho et ulcere cancioso in intestino cocco exorta iliaca passio. In Opera, Observatio LXI, Centuriae I. Frankfort:31. J.L. Dufour, 1682: 49 cited by J.F. Fielding (286).
281. Baron JH. Inflammatory bowel disease up to 1932. Mt. Sinai J Med (New York) 2000;67:174–89.
282. Bernier JJ, Chevauer P, Teysseire D, Andre J. La maladie de Louis XIII: Tuberculose intestinale ou maladie de Crohn? (Louis XIII's disease: Intestinal tuberculosis or Crohn's disease?). Nouv Presse Med 1981;10(27):2243, 2247–50.
283. Morgagni GB. The seats and causes of disease investigated by anatomy. In: Johnson, Payne, eds. Five books containing a great variety of dissections with remarks (Translated from the Latin of G.B. Morgagni by Benjamin Alexander.) In three volumes. Vol. 2 Letter XXXi: Flores of the belly with and without blood. London: A Millar and T Cadell, 1769.
284. Combe C, Saunders W. A singular case of stricture and thickening of ileum. Med Tran Roy Coll Physicians London 1813;4:16–18.
285. Abercrombie J. Pathological and practical researches of the stomach, the intestinal tract, and other viscera of the abdomen. Edinburgh: Waugh and Innes, 1828:238.
286. Fielding JF. Dalziel's (Crohn's) disease. Hist Med 1973;4:20–3.
287. Fielding JF. Crohn's disease and Dalziel's syndrome. J Clin Gastroenterol 1988;10: 279–85.
288. Colles A. Practical observations upon certain diseases of intestines, colon and rectum. Dublin Hosp Reports 1830;5:131–57.
289. Corrigan D. Ulceration of the intestines. Proc Pathol Soc Dublin 1853;1:245.
290. Moore N. Stricture of intestine at the ileocecal valve. Trans Pathol Soc London 1882;34:112. In: Kyle J, Crohn's disease. New York: Appleton–Century–Crofts, 1972.
291. Walker JF, Fielding JF. Crohn's disease in Dublin in the latter half of the nineteenth century. Irish J Med Sci 1988;157:235–7.
292. Bristowe JS. Ulceration, stricture, perforation of the small intestines. Trans Pathol Soc London 1853;4:152–3.
293. Fielding JF. Crohn's disease in London in the latter half of the nineteenth century. Irish J Med Sci 1984;153:214–20.
294. Fenwick S. Clinical lectures on some obscure diseases of the abdomen. London: Churchill, 1889:37–55.
295a. Goldstein HI. The history of regional enteritis. Schweiz Med Wochschr 1950;38: 1035–6.
295b. Goldstein HI. The history of regional enteritis (Saunders – Abercrombie – Crohn ileitis). In: Kagan S, ed. Victor Robinson memorial essays on history medicine. New York: Froben Press, 1948:99–104.
296. Hellers G. Crohn's disease in Stockholm County 1955–1974. A study of epidemiology, results of surgical treatment and long-term prognosis. Acta Chir Scand Suppl 1979;490:1–84.
297. Strombeck JP. Mesenteric lymphadenitis. Acta Chir Scand Suppl 1932;20:1–254.

Early 20th Century – Clinical Recognition of Crohn's Disease

298. Lartigau AJ. A study of chronic hyperplastic tuberculosis of the intestine with report of a case. J Exp Med 1901;6:23–51. Cited by Kyle J, Crohn's disease. New York: Appleton–Century–Crofts, 1972.
299. Hartman H, Pilliet AH. Notes sur une variete de typhlite tuberculose simulant les cancers de la region. Bull Soc Anat Paris 1891;5:471–503.
300. Braun H. Uber entzundliche geschwulste es netzes. Arch Klin Chir 1901;63:378–81.
301. Koch J. Ueber einfach entzundliche stricturen des dickdarms. Arch Klin Chir 1903;70:876–96. Cited by Kyle J, Crohn's disease. New York: Appleton–Century–Crofts, 1972.
302. Wilmanns R. Ein fall von darmstenose infolge cronisch etzundlicher vrdickung der ieocacal kappe. Beit z Klin Chir 1905;46:221–32.
303. Moynihan BGA. The mimicry of malignant disease in the large bowel. Edinburgh Med J 1907;21:203–28.
304. Proust R. Tumeur paraintestinale. Bull Mem Soc Chir Paris 1907;33:1158–60.
305. Lejars F. Des tumeurs inflammatoires paraintestinal. Bull Mem Soc Chir Paris 1908;34:9–11.
306. Monsarrat KW. A clinical lecture on the simulation of malignant disease by chronic inflammatory affections of the sigmoid flexure. Br Med J (Clin Res) 1907;2:65–7.
307. von Bergmann A. Tumorbildung bei appendicitis und ihre radikale behandlung. St. Petersburger Med Wochschr 1911;36:512–23.
308. Shapiro S. Regional ileitis – A summary of the literature. Am J Med Sci 1939;198:269–92.
309. Janeway EG. (1907) Inflammatory abdominal masses simulating malignant growths. Cited by McGeehee Harvey A, The Association of American Physicians (1886–1986). Baltimore, MD: Waverly Press 1986:155.
310. Jones NM, Eisenberg AA. Inflammatory neoplasms of the intestine simulating malignancy. Surg Gynecol Obstet 1918;20:420–3.
311. Schmidt E. Ueber dickdarmgeschwultse. Bruns Beitrage Klin Chir 1911;74:401–24.
312. Goto S. Ueber die einfache Chronische entzundliche strictur des darmes. Arch Klin Chir 1912;97:190–206.
313. Dalziel TK. Chronic interstitial enteritis. Br Med J (Clin Res) 1913;2:1068–70.
314. McFadyean J. Johne's disease: A chronic bacterial enteritis of cattle. J Comp Pathol Therapeut 1907;20:48–60.
315. Van Kruiningen HJ. Lack of support for a common etiology in Johne's disease of animals and Crohn's disease in humans. Inflamm Bowel Dis 1999;5:183–91.
316. Lawen A. Uber appendicitis fibroplastica. Dtsch Ztschr Chir 1914;129:221–41.
317. Lawen A. Appendicitis fibroplastica Chronische stenosierende ileitis terminalis und unspezifische entzundliche ileo-coecal tumoren. Zentrlbl f Chir 1938;65:911–15.
318. Tietze A. Die entzundliche geschwulste die dickdarms. Ergebn Chir Orth 1920;12:211. Cited by Warren S, Sommers SC, Cicatrizing enteritis (regional ileitis) as a pathologic entity. Am J Pathol 1948;24:475–501.
319. Korte W. Ueber enzundliche geschwultse am darm. Arch Klin Chir 1921;118:138–63.
320. Bundschuh E, Wolff EP. ZurKenntnis der darmphlegmone. Arch Klin Chir 1925;136:438–48.
321. Coffen TH. Nonspecific granuloma of the intestine causing intestinal obstruction. JAMA 1925;35:1303–4.

322. Crohn BB, Ginzburg L, Oppenheimer J. Regional ileitis. JAMA 1932;99:1323–9.
323. Molesworth HWL. Granuloma of intestine – stenosis of ileocecal valve. Br J Surgery 1933;21:370–2.
324. Donchess JC, Warren S. Chronic cicatrizing enteritis. Arch Pathol 1934;18:22–9.
325. Ralphs FG. On chronic inflammatory "tumours" of the gastrointestinal tract. Br J Surg 1937–38;25:524–9.
326. Dudley GS, Miscall I. Inflammatory tumors of the gastrointestinal tract. Ann Surg 1938;107:55–73.
327. Erb IH, Farmer AW. Ileocolitis – its relation to "regional ileitis" or chronic cicatrizing enteritis. Surg Gynecol Obstet 1935;61:6–14.
328. Bockus HL, Lee WE. Regional (terminal) ileitis. Ann Surg 1935;102:412–21.
329. Galambos A, Mittelmann W. Typical and atypical terminal ileitis. Am J Dig Dis Nutr 1935;2:442–7.
330. Meyer KA, Rosi PA. Regional enteritis (nonspecific). Surg Gynecol Obstet 1936;62:927–88.
331. Cutler EC. A neglected entity in abdominal pain and a common disease – cicatrizing enteritis. NY State J Med 1939;39:328–37.
332. Brown PW, Bargen JA, Weber HM. Inflammatory lesions of the small intestine (regional enteritis). Am J Dig Dis Nutr 1934;1:426–31.
333. de J. Pemberton J, Brown PW. Regional ileitis. Ann Surg 1937;105:855–70.
334. Harris F, Bell G, Brunn H. Chronic cicatrizing enteritis: regional ileitis (Crohn). Surg Gynecol Obstet 1933;57:637–45.
335. Homans J, Hass GM. Regional ileitis. A clinical not a pathological entity. N Engl J Med 1933;209:1315–24.
336. Bisell AD. Localized chronic ulcerative colitis. Ann Surg 1934;99:956–66.
337. Jackman RJ. Anal abscess and anal fistula in association with regional ileitis. Proc Staff Meet Mayo Clinic 1943;18:154–5.
338. Gray BK, Lockhart-Mummery HE, Morson BC. Crohn's disease of the anal region. Gut 1965;6:515–24.
339. Anschutz G. Uber unspezifische entzundliche geschwulste des dickdarmes. Dtsch Zschr Chir 1934;243:377–99.
340. Kantor JL. Regional ileitis – its roentgen diagnosis. JAMA 1934;103:2016–21.
341. Dyer NH, Rutherford C, Visick JH, Dawson AM. The incidence and reliability of individual radiographic signs in the small intestine in Crohn's disease. Br J Radiol 1970;43:401–8.
342. Marshak RH. Granulomatous disease of the intestinal tract (Crohn's disease). Radiology 1975;114:3–22.
343. Maklansky D. Pioneer gastroenterological radiologic studies. Mt Sinai J Med 2000;67:204–7.

Crohn's Disease – Animal and Experimental Observations

344. Bell HG. Chronic cicatrizing enteritis. California West Med 1934;41:239–41.
345. Reichert FL, Mathes ME. Experimental lymphoderma of the intestinal tract and its relation to regional cicatrizing enteritis. Ann Surg 1936;104:601–14.
346. Homans J, Drinker CK, Field ME. Elephantiasis and clinical implications of its experimental reproduction in animals. Ann Surg 1934;100:812–32.
347. Poppe JK. Reproduction of ulcerative colitis in dogs. Arch Surg 1941;43:551–8.
348. Sinaiko ES, Necheles H. Experiments in ulcerative enteritis. Surgery 1946;20:395–7.

Part II – Crohn's Disease

349. Chess S, Chess D, Olander G, Benner W, Cole WH. Production of chronic enteritis and other systemic lesions by ingestion of finely divided foreign materials. Surgery 1950;27:221–34.
350. Kalima TV, Saloniemi H, Rahko T. Experimental regional enteritis in pigs. Scand J Gastroenterol 1976;11:353–62.
351. Kalima TV, Saloniemi H, Rahko T. Lymphostatic enteropathy. In: Foldi M, ed. Ergebnisse der angiologie. Stuttgart: FK Schahauer, 1976:199–218.
352. Van Patter WN, Bargen JA, Dockerty MB, Feldman WH, Mayo CW, Waugh JM. Regional enteritis. Gastroenterology 1954;26:347–450.
353. Bargen JA. Regional enteritis. Wisconsin Med J 1955;54:367–74.
354. Emsbo P. Terminal or regional ileitis in swine. Nord Vet Med 1951;3:1–28.
355. Jonsson L, Martinsson K. Regional ileitis in pigs: Morphological and pathogenetical aspects. Acta Vet Scand 1976;17:223–32.
356. Gunnarsson A, Hurvell B, Jonsson L. Regional ileitis in pigs – isolation of campylobacter from affected ileal mucosa. Acta Vet Scand 1976;17:267–9.
357. Pensaert MB, DeBouck P. A new corona virus-like particle associated with diarrhea in swine. Arch Virol 1978;58:243–7.
358. Strande A, Sommers M, Petrak M. Regional enterocolitis in cocker spaniel dogs. Arch Pathol 1954;57:357–62.
359. Geil RG, Davis CL, Thompson SW. Spontaneous ileitis in rats – a report of 64 cases. Am J Vet Res 1961;22:932–6.
360. Cross RF, Smith CK, Parker CF. Terminal ileitis in lambs. J Am Vet Med Assoc 1973;162:564–6.
361. Prohaska J. Development and fate of experimentally induced enteritis. Gastroenterology 1966;51:913–25.
362. Van Kruiningen HJ. Granulomatous colitis of boxer dogs. Comparative aspects. Gastroenterology 1967;53:114–22.
363. Kennedy PC, Cello RM. Colitis of boxer dogs. Gastroenterology 1966;51:926–31.
364. Cimprich RE. Equine granulomatous enteritis. Vet Pathol 1974;11:535–47.
365. Roediger WE. A new hypothesis for the aetiology of Crohn's disease – evidence for lipid metabolism and intestinal tuberculosis. Postgrad Med J 1991;67:666–71.
366. Pizarro TT, Arseneau KO, Cominelli F. Lessons from genetically engineered animal models. XI. Novel mouse models to study pathogenic mechanisms of Crohn's disease. Am J Physiol-Gastrointest Liver Physiol 2000;278:G665–9.
367. Elson CO, Sartor RB, Tennyson GS, Riddell RH. Experimental models of inflammatory bowel disease. Gastroenterology 1995;109:1344–67.
368. Sartor RB, Cromartie WJ, Powell DW, Schwab JH. Granulomatous enterocolitis induced in rats by purified bacterial cell wall fragments. Gastroenterology 1985;89:587–95.
369. Elson CO, Cong Y, Brandwein S, Weaver ET, Mahler M, Sandberg I. Experimental models of IBD: Old hypotheses confirmed and new paradigms generated. In: Emmrich J, Liebe S, Stange EF, eds. Innovative concepts in inflammatory bowel disease. Dordrecht, Netherlands: Kluwer Academic Publishers, 1999:35–42.
370. Rath HC. Spontaneous colitis and gastritis in HLA-B27/B2 microglobulin transgenic rats and its association with normal luminal bacteria. In: Emmrich J, Liebe S, Stange EF, eds. Innovative concepts in inflammatory bowel disease. Dordrecht, Netherlands: Kluwer Academic Publishers, 1999:52–60.
371. Elson CO. Workshop X – Experimental models of IBD – lesions from mice – summary. In: Tytgat GNJ, Bartelsman JFWM, Huan Deventer SJ, eds. Inflammatory bowel disease. Dordrecht, Holland: Kluwer Academic Publishers, (Falk Symposium 85), 1995:395–400.

372. Kosiewicz MM, Nast CC, Krishnan A, Rivera-Nieves J, Moskaluk CA, Matsumoto S, et al. Th1-type responses mediate spontaneous ileitis in a novel murine model of Crohn's disease. J Clin Invest 2001;107:695–702.
373. Strober W, Nakamura K, Kitani A. The Sampl/yit mouse: Another step closer to modeling human inflammatory bowel disease. J Clin Invest 2001;107:667–9.

Abdominal Trauma

374. Pupini G. Considerazioni su di un caso di stenosi del tenue postraumatica. Policlinico Sez Prat 1932;39:847–53.
375. Fischer AW, Lurmann H. Uber eine tumorbildende ulcerose stenoosierende und perforierende entzundung des unteren ileum. Arch Klin Chir 1933;177:638–50.
376. Blumenthal JS, Berman R. Terminal ileitis with extension into the cecum following non-perforating abdominal trauma. Minnesota Med 1939;22:406–8.
377. Spellberg MA, Gray LW. Regional enteritis of proximal jejunum following trauma. Surgery 1945;17:343–50.
378. Spellberg MA, Ochsner A. Role of traumas as possible etiologic factor in regional enteritis: Effect of non-penetrating trauma in small intestine of dogs. Am J Med Sci 1947;213:579–84.
379. Morlock CG, Bargen JA, de J. Pemberton J. Regional enteritis following severe external violence. Proc Staff Meet Mayo Clinic 1939;14:631–5.
380. Crohn BB, Yarnis H. Regional ileitis. New York: Grune and Stratton, 1958.
381. Kyle J, Bell TM, Porteous LB, Blair DW. Factors in the aetiology of regional enteritis. Bull Soc Int Chir 1963;22:575–84.

The Mt. Sinai (New York) Experience

382. Aufses Jr. AH. The history of surgery for Crohn's disease at The Mt. Sinai Hospital. Mt Sinai J Med 2000;67:198–203.
383. Nuboer FJ. Chronische phlegmone van het ileum. Med J Geneesk 1932;76:2989. Cited by Weterman I. Course and long term prognosis of Crohn's isease. Delft, Holland: WD Meinema BV, 1976:9.
384. Golob M. Infectious granuloma of the intestines. Med J Rec 1932;135:390–3.
385. Moschowitz E, Wilensky AO. Nonspecific granulomata of the intestines. Am J Med 1923;166:48–65.
386. Wilensky AO, Moschowitz E. Nonspecific granulomata of the intestine. Am J Med Sci 1927;173:374–80.
387. Mock HE. Infective granuloma. Nonspecific chronic tumor-like productive inflammations of the gastrointestinal tract. Surg Gynecol Obstet 1931;52:672–89.
388. Ginzburg L. The road to regional enteritis. J Mt Sinai Hospital 1961;41:272–5.
389. Crohn BB. Gastroenterology at the Mt. Sinai Hospital. J Mt. Sinai Hosp 1945;12:129–36.
390. Ginzburg L, Oppenheimer GD. Nonspecific granulomata of the intestines (inflammatory tumors and strictures of the bowel). Trans Am Gastroenterol Assoc 1932;35:241–83.
391. Ginzburg L, Oppenheimer GD. Non-specific granulomata of the intestines, inflammatory tumors and strictures of the bowel. Ann Surg 1933;98:1046–62.
392. Janowitz H. Inflammatory bowel disease after 1932. Mt Sinai J Med 2000;67:190–7.

393. Crohn BB. The early days of regional ileitis at Mount Sinai Hospital. Reminiscences. J Mt Sinai Hospital 1955;22:143–6.
394. Lewisohn R. Segmental enteritis. Surg Gynecol Obstet 1938;66:215–22.
395. Crohn BB. Granulomatous diseases of the small and large bowel. A historical survey. Gastroenterology 1967;52:767–72.
396. Sachar DB. Planting seeds of knowledge about inflammatory bowel disease (half a century of science, prescience and prophecy in the pages of Mt. Sinai Journal). J Mt Sinai Hosp, 2001 – To be published.
397. Kovalcik PJ. Early history of regional enteritis. Curr Surg 1982;39:395–400.

More Early 20th Century Reports (CD)

398. Erdmann JF, Burt CV. Nonspecific granuloma of the gastrointestinal tract. Surg Gynecol Obstet 1933;57:71–80.
399. Coor P, Boeck WC. Chronic ulcerative enteritis. Am J Dig Dis Nutr 1934–35;1:161–3.
400. Edwards H. Specimen of Crohn's disease. The Medical Society's Transactions 1936;59:87–8. Cited by Hawkins C. Historical review. In: Allan RN, Keighley MRB, Alexander-Williams J, Hawkins C, eds. Inflammatory bowel diseases. London: Churchill Livingstone, 1983:1–7.
401. Edwards H. Crohn's disease. An inquiry into its nature and consequences. Ann Roy Coll Surg Engl 1969;44:121–39.
402. Meadows TR, Batsakis JB. Histopathological spectrum of regional enteritis. Arch Surg 1963;87:976–81.
403. Koster H, Kasman LP, Sheinfeld W. Regional ileitis. Arch Surg 1936;32:789–809.
404. Crohn BB, Rosenak BD. A combined form of ileitis and colitis. JAMA 1936;106:1–7.
405. Berg AA. An operating procedure for rightsided ulcerative ileocolitis. Ann Surg 1936;104:1019–23.
406. Leonardo RA. Intestinal obstruction due to nonspecific ileocecal granuloma (combined "regional ileitis" and colitis). Am J Surg 1937;35:607–8.
407. Snapper I, Pompen AWM. Ileite regionale. Ann Med Interne (Paris) 1936;29:5–23.
408. James TGI. Chronic regional colitis. Br J Surg 1937;25:511–16.
409. Jellen J. Regional ileitis. A review of fifty cases. Am J Roentg Radium 1937;37:190–201.
410. Ravdin IS, Johnston CG. Regional ileitis: A summary of the literature. Am J Med Sci 1939;198:269–92.
411. Razzaboni G. Di una rara lesione della parete intestinale ad infiltrato plasmacellulare. Arch Ital di Chir 1927;19:615–32. Cited by Shapiro R (Reference 308).
412. Ragnotti E. Regional enteritis with two cases. Arch Ital di Chir 1939;56:237–71.
413. Strombeck JP. Ileitis terminalis. Acta Chir Scand 1937;80(Suppl 50):1–59.
414. Landois F. Uber ileitis ulcerosa. Zentr Chir 1937;64:1690–2.
415. Tenkate J. Two cases of terminal ileitis. Nederl Tijdschr v. Geneesk 1936;80:5660–4.
416. Chan CW, Lam KC, Ho JCI, Lai CL. Crohn's syndrome in Chinese (Hong Kong). Am J Proctology, Gastroenterol Colon Rectal Surg 1984;35:3:8–17.
417. Chaun H, Freeman HJ. Crohn's disease in Chinese people in Vancouver, British Columbia. Can J Gastroenterol 1993;7:28–32.
418. Gottlieb C, Alpert S. Regional jejunitis. Am J Roentg Radium Ther 1937;38:861–83.
419. Sherrill JG, Hall DP. Regional ileitis. Am J Surg 1940;48:669–74.

420. Tallroth A. Regional enteritis with special reference to its etiology and pathogenesis. Acta Chir Scand 1943;88:407–32.
421. Schiff E. Die regionale enteritis (terminal ileitis, Crohn's disease). Ann Paediatr (International) 1945;165:281–311.
422. Silverman FN. Regional enteritis in children. Aust Paediatr J 1966;2:207–10.
423. Koop CE, Perlingiero JG, Weiss W. Cicatrizing enterocolitis in a newborn infant. Am J Med Sci 1947;214:27–32.
424. Walter LE, Chaffin L. Regional ileitis in infancy. West J Surg Obstet Gynecol 1957;65:354–7.
425. Kirsner JB, Owens FM, Humphreys EM. Regional enteritis in father and son. Gastroenterology 1948;10:883–91.
426. Ginzburg L, Oppenheimer GD. Urological complications in regional ileitis. J Urol 1948;59:948–52.
427. Gross F. Urologische komplikationen bei der ileitis regionalis. Med Klin 1959;54:1453–9.
428. Ross JR. Cicatrizing enterits, colitis and gastritis – a case report. Gastroenterology 1949;13:344–50.
429. Martin FRR, Carr RK. Crohn's disease involving the stomach. Br Med J 1953;1:700–2.
430. Franklin RH, Taylor S. Nonspecific granulomatous (regional) esophagitis. J Thorac Surg 1950;19:292–7.
431. Dashiell GF, Kirsner JB, Klotz AP, Palmer WL. Regional enteritis. A followup study of forty cases. Med Clin North Am 1951;35:227–41.
432. Crohn BB, Janowitz HD. Reflections on regional ileitis, twenty years later. JAMA 1954;156:1221–5.
433. Janowitz HD. Problems of regional enteritis. J Mt. Sinai Hospital (NY) 1955;22:223–8.
434. Janowitz HD, Croen EC, Sachar DB. The role of the fecal stream in Crohn's disease: An historical and analytic review. Inflamm Bowel Dis 1998;4:29–39.
435. Zetzel L. Regional enteritis. N Engl J Med 1956;254:990–5, 1029–32.
436. Chapin LE, Scudamore HH, Baggenstoss AH, Bargen JA. Regional enteritis: Associated visceral changes. Gastroenterology 1956;30:404–15.
437. Ford DK, Vallis DG. The clinical course of arthritis associated with ulcerative colitis and regional ileitis. Arthritis Rheum 1959;2:526–36.
438. Neeley JC. Perforation in regional enteritis. JAMA 1960;174:86–8.
439. Cohen H, Fishman AP. Regional enteritis and amyloidosis. Gastroenterology 1949;12:502–8.
440. Ginzburg L, Schneider KM, Dreizin DH, Levinson C. Carcinoma of the jejunum occurring in a case of regional enteritis. Surgery 1956;39:347–51.
441. Weedon DD, Shorter RG, Ilstrup DM, Huizenga KA, Taylor WF. Crohn's disease and cancer. N Engl J Med 1973;289:1099–102.
442. Falla-Alvarez L, Albacete R. Further experience with chronic regional enteritis in Cuba. Southern Med J 1958;51:1556–61.
443. Chacon CEA. Regional enteritis in Cuba. Revista Cubana de Cirug 1966;5:221–7.
444. Cooke WT, Fowler DI, Cox EV, Gaddie R, Meyrell MJ. The clinical significance of seromucoids in regional ileitis and ulcerative colitis. Gastroenterology 1958;34:910–19.
445. Heaton LD, Ravdin IS, Blades B, Whelan TJ. President Eisenhower's operation for regional enteritis. A footnote to history. Ann Surg 1964;159:661–6.
446. Hughes CW, Baugh JH, Mologne LA, Heaton LD. A review of the late General Eisenhower's operations: Epilog to a footnote to history. Ann Surg 1971;173:793–9.
447. Fone DJ. Regional enteritis (Crohn's disease). Med J Aust 1966;1:865–7.

448. Sircus W, Church R, Kelleher J. Recurrent aphthous ulceration of the mouth. Q J Med 1957;26:235–49.
449. McCallum DI, Gray WM. Metastatic Crohn's disease. Br J Dermatol 1976;95:551–4.
450. Nugent FW, Glaser D, Fernandez-Herlihy L. Crohn's colitis associated with granulomatous bone disease. N Engl J Med 1976;294:262–3.
451. Shah SM, Texter, Jr. EC, White HJ. Inflammatory bone disease associated with granulomatous lung disease. Gastrointest Endosc 1976;23:98–9.
452. Veloso FT, Cardosa V, Fraga J, Carvalho J, Dias LM. Spontaneous umbilical fistula in Crohn's disease. J Clin Gastroenterol 1989;11:197–200.
453. Basu MK, Asquith P, Thompson RA, Cooke WT. Oral manifestations of Crohn's disease. Gut 1975;16:249–54.
454. Lehner T. Oral ulceration and Behcet's syndrome. Gut 1977;18:491–511.
455. Matthews N, Tapper-Jones L, Mayberry JF, Rhodes J. Buccal biopsy in diagnosis of Crohn's disease (Letter to Editor). Lancet 1979;1:500–1.
456. Present DH, Rabinowitz JG, Banks PH, Janowitz HO. Obstructive hydronephrosis – a frequent but seldom recognized complication of granulomatous disease of the bowel. N Engl J Med 1969;280:523–8.
457. Heaton KW, Rich AE. Gallstones in patients with disorders of the terminal ileum and disturbed bile salt metabolism. Br Med J 1969;3:494–6.
458. Smith LH, Fromm H, Hoffman AF. Acquired hyperoxaluria, nephrolithiasis and intestinal disease. Description of a syndrome. N Engl J Med 1972;286:1371–5.
459. Gjone E, Orning OM, Myren J. Crohn's disease in Norway 1956–63. Gut 1966;7:372–4.
460. Myren J, Gjone E, Hertzberg JN, Rygvold O, Semb LS, Fretheim B. Epidemiology of ulcerative colitis and regional enterocolitis (Crohn's disease) in Norway. Scand J Gastroenterol 1971;6:511–14.
461. Humphreys WG, Parks TG. Crohn's disease in northern Ireland – a retrospective survey of 159 cases. Irish J Med Sci 1975;144:437–46.
462. Weterman IT, Pena AS, Booth CC, eds. The management of Crohn's disease. Amsterdam: Excerpta Medica, 1976.
463. Best WR, Becktal JM, Singleton JW, Kern, Jr. F. Development of a Crohn's disease activity index. Gastroenterology 1976;70:439–44.
464. Winship DH, Summers RW, Singleton JW, Best WR, Becktel JM, Lenk LF, et al. National Cooperative Crohn's Disease Study: Study design and conduct of the study. Gastroenterology 1979;77:829–42.
465. Summers RW, Switz DM, Sessions, Jr. JT, Becktel JM, Best WR, Kern Jr. F, et al. National Cooperative Crohn's Disease Study: Results of drug treatment. Gastroenterology 1979;77:847–69.

Crohn's Disease of the Colon

466. Bargen JA, Weber HM. Regional migratory chronic ulcerative colitis. Surg Gynecol Obstet 1930;50:964–72.
467. Colp R. Case of nonspecific granuloma of terminal ileum and cecum. Surg Clin North Am 1934;14:443–9.
468. Crohn BB, Berg AA. Right-side (regional) colitis. JAMA 1938;110:32–8.
469. Wells C. Ulcerative colitis and Crohn's disease. Ann Roy Coll Surg Engl 1952;11:105–20.
470. Cooke WT, Brooke BN. Nonspecific enterocolitis. Q J Med 1955;24:1–22.
471. Brooke BN. Granulomatous disease of the intestine. Lancet 1959;2:745–9.

472. Morson BC, Lockhart-Mummery HE. Crohn's disease of the colon. Gastroenterologia 1959;92:168-72.
473. Cornes J, Stecher M. Primary Crohn's disease of the colon and rectum. Gut 1961; 2:189-201.
473a. Nevin RW. A review of granulomata of the large intestine. Proc Roy Soc Med 1961;54:137-42.
474. Marshak RH, Wolf BS, Eliasoph J. Segmental colitis. Radiology 1959;73:706-16.
475. Wolf BS, Marshak RH. Granulomatous colitis (Crohn's disease of the colon). Am J Roentg 1962;88:662-70.
476. Korelitz BI. Prognosis of granulomatous colitis with onset in childhood. J Mt Sinai Hosp 1968;35:1-13.
477. Lennard-Jones JE, Lockhart-Mummery HE, Morson BC. Clinical and pathological differentiation of Crohn's disease and proctocolitis. Gastroenterology 1968;54: 1162-70.
478. Capek V, Maratka Z, Kubernatova D, Kudmann J. Roentgenology of regional colitis. (Crohn's disease of the colon and rectum). Cs Gastroenterologie 1968;22: 254-62.
479. Price AB. Overlap in the spectrum of nonspecific inflammatory bowel disease – 'colitis indeterminate'. J Clin Pathol 1978;31:567-77.
480. McGovern VJ, Goulston SJ. Crohn's disease of the colon. Gut 1968;9:164-76.
481. Janowitz HD. Editorial: Why was the recognition of Crohn's colitis so slow? J Clin Gastroenterol 1989;11:125-6.
482. Price AB, Morson BC. Inflammatory bowel disease – the surgical pathology of Crohn's disease and ulcerative colitis. Hum Pathol 1975;6:7-29.
483. Kirsner JB. Problems in the differentiation of ulcerative colitis and Crohn's disease of the colon – the need for repeated diagnostic evaluation. Gastroenterology 1975;68:187-91.

Pathology of Crohn's Disease – Etiologic Implications

484. Coffey RJ. Pathologic manifestations of regional enteritis. Mayo Clin Proc 1938; 13:541-4.
485. Hadfield G. The primary histological lesion of regional ileitis. Lancet 1939;2:773-5.
486. Blackburn G, Hadfield G, Hunt AH. Regional Ileitis. St Bart's Hosp Reports 1939; 72:181-224.
487. Spector WG, Lykke AWJ. The cellular evolution of inflammatory granulomata. J Pathol Bacteriol 1966;92:163-77.
488. Spector WG, Heesom N. The production of granulomata by antibody-antigen complexes. J Pathol 1969;98:31-9.
489. Rotterdam H, Korelitz BI, Sommers SC. Microgranulomas in grossly normal rectal mucosa in Crohn's disease. Am J Clin Pathol 1977;67:550-4.
490. Chambers TJ, Morson BC. The granuloma in Crohn's disease. Gut 1979;20:269-74.
491. Whitehead R. Mucosal biopsy of the gastrointestinal tract. In: Major problems in pathology, Vol. 3. Philadelphia: WB Saunders Co., 1973.
492. Aaronson RM, Spiro HM. Mercury and the gut. Am J Dig Dis 1973;18:583-94.
493. Ganrot PO. Aluminum: Possible etiologic agent in Crohn's disease. In: Jarnerot G, ed. Inflammatory bowel disease. New York: Raven Press, 1987:119-28.
494. Weinstock JV. The granuloma and Crohn's disease. In: MacDermott RP, Stenson WF, eds. Inflammatory bowel disease. New York: Elsevier Science Publishing Co., 1992:163-76.

495. Warren S, Sommers SC. Cicatrizing enteritis (regional ileitis) as a pathologic entity: Analysis of 120 cases. Am J Patholo 1948;24:475–501.
496. Guthy E. Aetiologie des morbus Crohn. Dtsch Med Wochenschr 1983;45:1729–33.
497. Rappaport H, Burgoyne FH, Smetana HF. The pathology of regional enteritis. Military Surg 1951;109:463–502.
498. Otani S. Pathology of regional enteritis and regional enterocolitis. J Mt Sinai Hosp 1955;22:147–58.
499. Whitehead R. Pathology of Crohn's disease. In: Kirsner JB, Shorter RG, eds. Inflammatory bowel disease, 2nd edn. Philadelphia: Lea and Febiger, 1980:296–307.
500. Davis DR, Dockerty MB, Mayo CW. The myenteric plexus in regional enteritis: A study of the number of ganglion cells in the ileum in 24 cases. Surg Gynecol Obstet 1955;101:208–16.
501. Binney H. Discussion of paper by C.G. Mixter – regional ileitis. Ann Surg 1935;102:689–90. Cited by Crohn and Yarnis (380).
502. Morson BC. Histopathology of Crohn's disease. Scand J Gastroenterol 1971;6:573–5.
503. Wakefield AJ, Sawyer AM, Dhillon AP, Pittilo RM, Rowles PM, Lewis AA, et al. Pathogenesis of Crohn's disease. Multifocal gastrointestinal infarction. Lancet 1989;2:1057–62.
504. Janda RC, Conklin JL, Mitros FA, Parsonnet J. Multifocal colitis associated with an epidemic of chronic diarrhea. Gastroenterology 1991;100:458–64.
505. Ammann RW, Bockus HL. Pathogenesis of regional enteritis. Arch Int Med 1961;107:504–13.
506. Schepers GWH. The pathology of regional ileitis. Am J Dig Dis 1945;12:97–116.
507. Shnitka TK. Current concepts of the pathogenesis and pathology of inflammatory lesions of the intestine. Can Med Assoc J 1964;97:7–22.
508. Whitehead R. Pathology of Crohn's disease. In: Kirsner JB, Shorter RG, eds. Inflammatory bowel disease. Philadelphia: Lea and Febiger, 1975:182–98.
509. Morson BC. The early histological lesion of Crohn's disease. Proc Royal Soc Med 1972;65:71–2.
510. Poulsen SS, Pederson NT, Jarnum S. Microerosions in rectal biopsies in Crohn's disease. Scand J Gastroenterol 1984;19:607–12.
511. Rickert RR, Carter HW. The "early" ulcerative lesion of Crohn's disease: Correlative light and scanning electron microscopic studies. J Clin Gastroenterol 1980;2:11–19.
512. Haubrich WS. Gastrointestinal endoscopy. In: Kirsner JB, ed. The growth of gastroenterologic knowledge during the twentieth century. Philadelphia: Lea and Febiger, 1994:474–90.
513. Chang EB. Intestinal epithelial function and response to mucosal injury. In: Kirsner JB, editor. Inflammatory bowel disease, 5th edn. Philadelphia: WB Saunders Co., 1999:1–19.

Electron Microscopy – Crohn's Disease

514. Aluwihare APR. Electron microscopy in Crohn's disease. Gut 1971;12:509–18.
515. Aluwihare APR. The electron microscope and Crohn's disease. In: Brooke BN, ed. Clinics in gastroenterology – Crohn's disease. London: WB Saunders Co., Ltd., 1972:279–94.
516. Ranlov P, Nielsen MH, Wanstrup J. Ultrastructure of the ileum in Crohn's disease. Scand J Gastroenterol 1972;7:471–6.

100 *Origins and Directions of Inflammatory Bowel Disease*

517. Siemers PT, Dobbins III WO. The Meissner plexus in Crohn's disease of the colon. Surg Gynecol Obstet 1974;138:39–42.
518. Dourmashkin RR, Davies H, Wells C, Shah D, Price A, O'Morain C, et al. Early epithelial lesions in Crohn's disease revealed by electron microscopy. In: Pena AS, Weterman IT, Booth CC, Strober W, eds. Recent advances in Crohn's disease. Boston: Martinus Nijhoff, 1981;117–23.
519. Dvorak AM, Connell AB, Dickersin GR. Crohn's disease: a scanning electron microscopic study. Hum Pathol 1970;10:165–77.
520. Dvorak AM. Axonal necrosis in Crohn's disease. In: Watanabe S, Wolff M, Sommers SC, eds. Digestive disease pathology, Vol. 2. Philadelphia: Field and Wood Inc., 1988.
521. Dvorak AM, Monahan RA, Osage JE, Dickersin GR. Mast cell degranulation in Crohn's disease (Letter to Editor). Lancet 1978;1:498.
522. Dvorak AM. Mast cell hyperplasia and degranulation in Crohn's disease. In: Pepys J, Edwards AM, eds. The mast cell: Its role in health and disease. Kent: Pitman Publishing Co., (Ltd), 1979:657–62.
523. Dvorak AM. Ultrastructural evidence for release of major basic protein-containing crystalline cores of eosinophil granules in vivo: Cytotoxic potential in Crohn's disease. J Immunol 1980;125:460–2.
524. Otto HF, Gebbers JO. Electron microscopic, ultracytochemical and immunohistological observations in Crohn's disease of the ileum and colon. Virchow's Arch 1981;391:189–205.
525. Marin ML, Geller SA, Greenstein AJ, Marin RH, Gordon RE, Aufses Jr. AH. Ultrastructural pathology of Crohn's disease: Correlated transmission electron microscopy, scanning electron microscopy and freeze fracture studies. Am J Gastroenterol 1983;78:355–64.
526. Marin ML, Greenstein AJ, Geller SA, Gordon RE, Aufses Jr. AH. Freeze fracture analysis of epithelial cell lysosomal inclusions in Crohn's disease. Ultrastruct Pathol 1984;6:39–44.
527. Nagel E, Bartels M, Pichlmayr R. Scanning electron microscopic lesions in Crohn's disease – relevance for the interpretation of postoperative recurrence. Gastroenterology 1995;108:376–82.
528. Goodman MJ, Skinner JM, Truelove SC. Abnormalities in the apparently normal bowel mucosa in Crohn's disease. Lancet 1976;1:275–8.

Eponym of Crohn's Disease

529. Barrington-Ward L, Norrish RE. Crohn's disease or regional ileitis. Br J Surg 1938–39;25:530–7.
530. Hodgson JC. Regional ileitis – Crohn's disease. Lancet 1937;1:926–7.
531. Cushway BC. Chronic cicatrizing enteritis – regional ileitis (Crohn). Illinois Med J 1934;66:525–33.
532. Barbour RF, Stokes AB. Chronic cicatrizing enteritis. Lancet 1936;1:299–303.
533. Hurst AF, Lintott GAM. Crohn's disease. Br Encyclopedia Med Pract 1937;3:508–13.
534. Lesniowski A. Przczynck do chirurgii kiszek. Granulomatous inflammation of intestine (probable title). Medyeyna 1903;31:21:460–518. Cited by Licharowicz AM, Mayberry JF. J R Soc Med 1988;81:468–70. Also: Towarzystwa Lekarskiego Warszawskiego 1904;100:630–1, 1905;101:669–71.
535. Harmer M. Crohn's disease – a misnomer? Bristol Medico-Chirurgical J 1988; 103:9–10.

536. Fielding JF. An enquiry into certain aspects of regional enteritis (MD Thesis). Cork: National University of Ireland, 1970.
537. Kyle J. Dalziel's disease – 66 years on. Br Med J 1979;1:876–7.
538. Kyle J. Dalziel's disease. Hist Med 1973;4:20–3.
539. Armitage G, Wilson M. Crohn's disease – a survey of the literature and a report on 34 cases. Br J Surg 1950;38:182–93.
540. Aufses Jr. AH. The history of Crohn's disease. Surg Clin North Am 2001;81:1–11.
541. Lewis T. Reflections upon reform in medical education. I. Present state and needs. Lancet 1944;1:619–21.

Part III

Etiology and Pathogenesis of IBD – Origins and Directions

EPIDEMIOLOGY

The concept embodied in epidemiology involving study of the distribution and the determinants of disease in human populations originated with Hippocrates (370–460 BC) and his "Airs, Waters and Places" (Epidemics I and III) but did not emerge as a distinct discipline until mid 19th century. Organization of the Statistical Society of London in 1834 and the Epidemiological Society of London in 1850,[542] together with the seminal descriptions of John Snow[543] (1813–1858) (cholera) in 1849 and by W. Budd[544] (1811–1880) (London) (typhoid fever) in 1873 had established epidemiology as an important approach to the understanding of human illness but its application to inflammatory bowel disease was not possible for many years. Instances of "nonspecific" inflammatory bowel disease appeared during the nineteenth century, concurrently with a "substantial decline in mortality from intestinal infections,"[545] but initial attempts to estimate the incidence, prevalence and demography of inflammatory bowel disease were impractical because of the small number of identified patients, diagnostic uncertainty and limited clinical understanding. J.L. Kantor,[546] in a 1929 review of 2500 private patients with digestive complaints in New York, had suggested the proportion of ulcerative colitis admissions as nine in a thousand, contrasting with such estimates as constipation 500 per 1000 and irritable colon 200 per 1000. E.I. Spriggs,[547] in a 1934 analysis of 35 patients in the Oxford area, had estimated the occurrence of ulcerative colitis as "5 in a thousand." Sedlack et al.[548] of Rochester, Minnesota reported the average annual incidence rate of ulcerative colitis in Olmsted County, Minnesota, USA as 3.4 per 10^5 for the period 1935–1964. For Crohn's disease, Sedlack et al.[549] estimated the mean annual incidence for the period 1935–1975 as 1.9 per 10^5. Rose et al.[550] (Cardiff, Wales) for the period 1935–1985 reported a large increase from 0.18 cases/10^5 in the 1930s to current values of 8.3/10^5 per year. The incidence continues to rise with an increasing proportion of patients with colorectal disease. A.G. Melrose[551] of Glasgow in 1955 obtained information on idiopathic ulcerative colitis from thirty British teaching hospitals for the years 1946 to 1950 (1426 cases). The overall incidence of the disease per 10,000 general admissions was 10.9%. The overall case mortality was 12%. The incidence rate per 10,000 general admissions was 6.9% for the five Scottish towns in contrast to 15.5% for the London hospitals, an early indication of the urban:rural differential in IBD incidence.

Houghton and Naish[552] of Bristol, England in 1958 had identified 170 patients with ulcerative colitis and 32 with ileitis from the records of the three main hospitals in Bristol, England (population 800,000) for the years 1953, 1954 and 1955. The estimated annual incidence of 0.85 per 1000 for ulcerative colitis and 0.14 per 1000 for regional ileitis were similar to those of E.I. Spriggs (1934) and A.G. Melrose (1955). H.J. Ustvedt[553] (1958), reviewing hospital admission rates on all cases discharged from Norwegian hospitals during the ten year period 1945–55, noted a mean annual rate of 1.2 per 100,000 population.

Acheson[554] in 1960 examined the data for all 2320 male veterans discharged from the 174 hospitals of the U.S. Veterans Administration with diagnoses of regional ileitis, ulcerative colitis, or enteritis not specified as ulcerative, and noted a fourfold increase of Jewish patients, regardless of geographic origin of birth within the USA or orthodoxy, over a sample of all discharges for general medical and surgical conditions, as had been noted in 1950 by Sloan, Bargen and Gage of the Mayo Clinic and by J.W. Paulley[555] of London. The Jewish preponderance was re-emphasized by Acheson and Nefzger[556] in a follow-up of 525 patients who had been diagnosed as ulcerative colitis for the first time in the U.S. Army in 1944 and by Weiner and Lewis (V.A. Hospital, East Orange, New Jersey)[557] in a 1960 review of 88 male veterans with ulcerative colitis. In Israel, IBD, Crohn's disease in particular, was more frequent among Ashkenazi (European) Jews than among those of North African and Asiatic origin (Sephardic).[558,559] An epidemiological study of ulcerative colitis in the Jewish population of Tel-Aviv, Israel from 1968 to 1970[560] indicated an average annual incidence of 3.66 per 10^5 population and prevalence of 37.4 per 10^5; figures considerably lower than those reported for Oxford, England, Rochester, Minnesota and Copenhagen, Denmark. A 1989 review by Odes and Fraser[561] (Ben-Gurion University of the Negev, Beer Sheva, Israel) indicated that "ulcerative colitis was twice as common as

Crohn's disease and had increased in all ethnic sections of the Jewish population since 1960." The disease was more prevalent among European and American-born Jews than Asian, African and Israeli-born Jews. The disease also increased in the Arab population. A similar review of Crohn's disease in Israel by Odes, Fraser and Hollander[562] in 1989–90 indicated that it also had increased in frequency during the past 20 years, although less common than ulcerative colitis and uncommon in the Arab population. In the United States, IBD apparently was more frequent among Jews of middle European ancestry[563] (Germany, Austria, Poland, Czechoslovakia and Russia). Surveys from Basel, Switzerland[564] (1971), Nottingham, England[565] (1976) and from Aberdeen, Scotland did not indicate a higher incidence of IBD among Jewish individuals.

Inflammatory bowel disease actually occurs among ethnic groups worldwide, including Arabs,[566] Iranians,[567] Africans,[568] and Chinese populations.[133,416,417] The Kuwait 1984[569] series included 91 Arab patients with ulcerative colitis and 17 with Crohn's disease. Reportedly rare in South African blacks,[570,571] a 1969 survey reported 5 instances of Crohn's disease among the Transvaal Bantu.[572] A 1979 report[573] from the West Indies included 34 patients with ulcerative colitis and 14 with Crohn's disease; 26 Negroes, 18 Indians, three mixed, and one Caucasian. In the United States, the number of black individuals developing IBD continues to rise.[574,575] H. Fahrländer[576] of Basel, in a 1967 clinical review of 172 patients, observed: "Apparently ulcerative colitis at present is relatively milder in Switzerland than in the Anglo-American region and in Scandinavia." Acheson also noted a 20-fold increase in the incidence of ankylosing spondylitis among the 2320 U.S. veterans with IBD. J.G. Evans and E.D. Acheson,[577] in a 1965 study of ulcerative colitis and regional ileitis in Oxford, England for the 1951–1960 period, confirmed the rising incidence of ulcerative colitis and also demonstrated a bimodal age-related incidence pattern. A seasonal trend in the onset or recurrence of symptoms was not observed.

In the first published population study of IBD, Iversen, Bonnevie, Anthonisen and Riis[578] in a 1968 survey of ulcerative colitis in Copenhagen county (Gentofte municipality, Denmark) for the period 1961–1966, reviewed 310 patients (excluding proctitis). The prevalence rate was 44.1 per 100,000 inhabitants. Considering the 231 patients only in whom ulcerative colitis was diagnosed for the first time, the incidence of the disease averaged 7.3 per 100,000 per year. The prevalence of diagnosed cases was 109 per 100,000. The mortality rate was threefold higher than the general mortality. Subsequent population-based studies from this

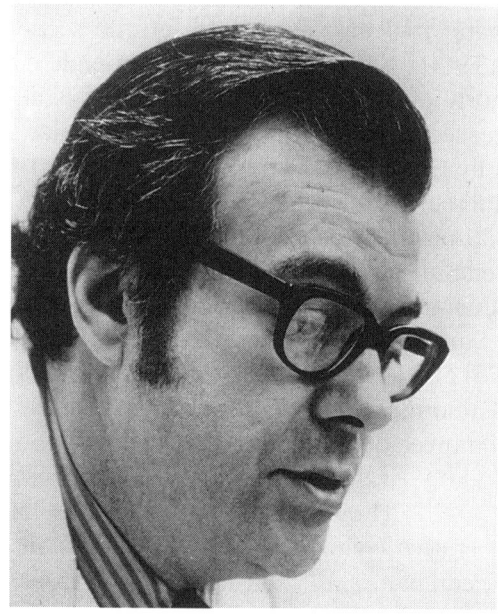

A.I. Mendeloff

center under the leadership of P. Riis and then V. Binder[579] (1982) contributed important epidemiological information on IBD in the Danish population over time. In the 1982 study, 909 patients were diagnosed in the county of Copenhagen (approximately 500,000 inhabitants). The mean incidence of ulcerative colitis was 8.1 per 10^5 inhabitants. The incidence of Crohn's disease was 2.7 per 10^5 inhabitants, noting "a remarkable rise in the incidence of Crohn's disease, similar to results from other industrial countries." A population study of two counties in central Sweden for the period 1956–1967 by Norlen, Krause and Bergman[580] for Crohn's disease indicated a mean incidence of 2.5/100,000 for the first six years of the 12 year span and 5.0 during the second six year period; as noted also in other Scandinavian countries; data from Stockholm (urban) and from Gotland (rural) did not differ.

A series of major epidemiologic studies by Mendeloff et al.[581,582] of Johns Hopkins University, Baltimore, MD in the well-defined Baltimore area documented the rising incidence of ulcerative colitis during the first half of the 20th century, exceeding Crohn's disease in a proportion of 4 to 5:1, similar to the early University of Chicago experience. The incidence of ulcerative colitis stabilized during the latter half of the 20th century, concurrently with the rising incidence of Crohn's disease, a trend observed in many geographic areas. In 1981 Garland, Mendeloff et al.,[583] in a report on incidence rates of ulcerative colitis and Crohn's disease in fifteen areas of the United States, estimated between 20 and 25,000 new patients with IBD would be admitted to community hospitals in 1980. The incidence rates for ulcerative colitis were the same in both sexes and among whites and blacks. For regional enteritis, the incidence rates in whites were the same in both sexes. The white/non-white ratio of IBD for males was 1.85:1. In other data, average annual age and sex-adjusted rates for ulcerative colitis ranged from 2.8 in Baltimore (whites) to 5.9 in Malmo and 6.0 in Oxford, England. For Crohn's disease, rates varied from 0.8 in Oxford and 1.2 in Baltimore to 4.8 in Stockholm and 5.95 in Cardiff, Wales. Rogers et al.[584] of the University of Chicago in 1971 provided extensive demographic data on a cohort of 1400 patients with inflammatory bowel disease, including 844 patients with ulcerative colitis and 556 with Crohn's disease. J. Kyle's[585] (1972) epidemiologic survey of Crohn's disease during the same time period emphasized the role of environmental influences (industrialization). Kyle identified in the early literature instances of Crohn's disease from Australia, Asia, Africa as well as Europe and the Americas.

Summarizing their detailed studies between 1960 and 1979 in the Baltimore area, B.M. Calkins and A.I. Mendeloff[586,587] noted an increase in the age adjusted rate for Crohn's disease over ulcerative colitis for whites of both sexes and for non-white females from the first to the second analysis. Mendeloff also confirmed the bimodality of the age related incidence of both Crohn's disease and ulcerative colitis. The fivefold increase of Crohn's disease among white women of childbearing age (1965 to 1975 period) suggested thrombogenic birth control medication as a factor in this age group, a relationship not confirmed in subsequent studies. Mendeloff et al.[582] in 1975 had described the IBD population in the United States as follows:

(a) Males and females nearly equally affected
(b) Patients more commonly western than oriental, especially of northern European origin
(c) More often urban than rural dwellers
(d) More often caucasian than colored
(e) IBD more common among Jews living in northern Europe and North America than among non-Jews, but not as common among Israelis

(f) An increasing frequency of Crohn's disease over ulcerative colitis
(g) A higher familial distribution than expected.

According to Kyle,[585] Crohn's disease was "most common in northwest Europe and in the northeastern part of North America." "Caucasians in the southern hemisphere were less liable to develop Crohn's disease." F. Brahme et al.,[588] surveying a defined urban population in (Malmo) Sweden, reached a similar conclusion. Later studies from Italy did not indicate a "north-south gradient" for that country (Milan to Palermo).[589]

The early clinical reports on ulcerative colitis and later Crohn's disease had originated more often in "northern" (colder) geographic areas (Great Britain, Europe, and the United States) and less often in southern geographic areas (South America, Africa, Asia), perhaps reflecting in part a lesser tendency to publication. Subsequent regional epidemiologic surveys[590] documented the worldwide distribution of IBD, the now apparently stabilized incidence of ulcerative colitis (excluding proctitis) and the rising incidence of Crohn's disease. Crohn's disease was identified now in formerly "lagging" countries[591] Baragwanath, Africa,[592] Brazil,[593] Egypt,[594] India,[595] and South Korea, and also in Japan[596] and among Chinese immigrants to Vancouver, Canada.

The higher incidence and prevalence of inflammatory bowel disease in the North Tees Health District of England[597] (especially colonic Crohn's disease and anal lesions [35%]), in the Nord-Pas de Calais region and Somme Departments of France,[598] in Basel (Switzerland),[564] and in Manitoba, Canada, consistent with etiologically significant environmental circumstances (?microbial, industrial) are of particular interest as promising areas for etiological investigation. A retrospective epidemiological study of ulcerative colitis[599] and proctitis from 1972–1980 in Leicestershire, England, with a large population of South Asian immigrants, revealed a twofold higher risk of UC among the immigrants than among British. The risk was greatest among Hindus and Sikhs "in whom the incidence is one of the highest in the world."

According to G. Whalen (1990) of Melbourne, Australia,[600] population factors ideally required for feasible epidemiologic studies and not often met include (a) a relatively stable population of adequate size, (b) a geographically well-defined area, (c) demographically heterogeneous and (d) uniform access to health care services. "The annual incidence for inflammatory bowel disease ranges from 3 to 20 new cases per 100,000 population in most countries where it has been measured." At the University of Chicago and, in general, the incidence of Crohn's disease now exceeds that of ulcerative colitis, undoubtedly reflecting a referral bias rather than an epidemiological increase. Time-space clustering of IBD, indicative of an infectious etiology, was not demonstrated early in the 20th century, but several instances of IBD clustering have been reported recently by H.J. Van Kruiningen and his colleagues.

McKeown[545] points out that "Most non-communicable diseases have arisen from exposure to conditions of life for which we are genetically ill-equipped, but some, such as accidents and industrial diseases, are caused by hazards to which genetic adaptation is hardly conceivable. The diseases can therefore be said to be due to maladaptation and to certain hazards which have emerged in the industrial period."

Smoking and IBD

The relationship between ulcerative colitis and non-smoking, especially the occurrence of ulcerative colitis among former smokers, first mentioned by R. Boller[601] of Vienna in a 1956 review of 89 patients with ulcerative colitis, has been an intriguing issue. It was documented by S.M. Samuelsson[602] in a 1976 thesis (University of Uppsala, Sweden) and expanded by J. Rhodes of Wales. In response to my inquiry as to the origin of his interest in IBD and tobacco, Professor John Rhodes of Cardiff, Wales (personal communication October 1991) related the following: "Between 1980 and '81 I had working with me a research registrar, Dr Tony Harries, now Chair of Tropical Medicine in Blantyre, Malawi. Dr Harries was doing his research into nutritional problems in Crohn's disease and was particularly assessing the value of anthropometric measurements, relating them to other nutritional parameters. The mid-arm circumference was one of the simple measurements and assessment involved taking into account several variables – age, sex, dominant arm and smoking status. The rule of thumb we had at the time was that smokers on average were 10% lighter in weight than non-smokers and it was, therefore, important to take this factor into consideration when making comparison with controls.

The group of patients with Crohn's disease under study was to be compared with controls (taken from a normal population attending an Orthopaedic Clinic) but we also wanted to include a patient group and what better group than ulcerative colitis. At first we had 100 patients with colitis, taken at random and the results which related to smoking status were 'irritating'. This was because hardly any of them were smokers, which made it difficult to get meaningful statistics from the comparison. After musing over the figures, however, we wondered whether it might just be a possibility that patients with colitis were largely non-smokers. This prompted us to carry out a larger survey of both patients with colitis and Crohn's disease with matched controls. Unfortunately, the original matching with controls was between colitis and normal controls. The patients with Crohn's disease did not have any tight matching with controls and results looked similar to the control population at that time (only subsequently did the story develop showing that those with Crohn's tended to be smokers compared with the general population). Because the 'non-smoking' status with UC was new, we determined to do no further work on it for a time – but would await data from other groups to see whether or not they confirmed our observations.

I often relate the story because it is curious and fascinating. The observation was made during the course of a piece of research where we allowed ourselves the liberty of looking at data and rather than discarding useless statistics, raised another possibility to account for them ..."

Harries, Baird and Rhodes[603] of Cardiff, Wales, utilizing a 1982 mail questionnaire, reported the infrequency of cigarette smoking in patients with ulcerative colitis and an excess of cigarette smoking in Crohn's disease or controls: 8% of the ulcerative colitis series were current cigarette smokers compared with 42% of the group with Crohn's disease and 44% of controls. 48% of the ulcerative colitis group had never smoked compared with 30% for Crohn's disease and 36% for controls. This finding was rapidly confirmed by Bures et al.[604] of Czechoslovakia in a study of 50 patients with ulcerative colitis and 31 with Crohn's disease. de Castella[605] in the same year described a young woman whose ulcerative colitis began when she stopped smoking cigarettes – subsided on resumption of smoking, and returned when she again discontinued the use of tobacco. Roberts and Diggle[606] described the course of a woman with severe ulcerative colitis who recovered after three years of symptoms when she began to smoke cigarettes. After seven "smoking" years of well-being, she stopped smoking with prompt return of the ulcerative colitis. Nicotine chewing gum containing 40 mg nicotine subsequently maintained remission of the disease.

The negative association between ulcerative colitis and cigarette smoking was reaffirmed by Jick and Walker[607] in a survey of patients in the Boston Collaboration Drug Surveillance program and since then by observers from many geographic areas. Unaccountably, the risk of ulcerative colitis was greater among ex-smokers than in those who had never smoked.[608] Benowitz[609] estimated that the simultaneous ingestion of 10 unchewed pieces of 4 mg nicotine gum results in peak blood concentrations of nicotine of less than 10 mg per milliliter, of interest in relation to the benefit obtained by the patient of Roberts and Diggle from this amount of nicotine.

The negative association of cigarette smoking with ulcerative colitis and the positive association with Crohn's disease, after 20 years of scrutiny, remain unexplained. Therapeutic speculation has included nicotine-induced immunosuppression, decreased production of proinflammatory leukotreine B4, increased mucus secretion by the colon, an undefined "effect on blood circulation in the colon," cholinergic inhibition and reduction in circular muscle activity through the release of nitric oxide.[610] Nicotine is a tertiary amine composed of a pyridine and a pyrolidine ring with profound pharmacological, biochemical and metabolic actions affecting the central nervous system (acetylcholine receptors), cardiovascular, endocrine and gastrointestinal systems, neurohumoral pathways and tissue oxygenation. The possible effects of nicotine upon intestinal blood flow, intestinal inflammation, intestinal neurotransmitter activity, tissue cytokine profiles and a possible genetic basis for nicotine-association are under investigation. The ulcerative colitis-tobacco connection is not exclusive to inflammatory bowel disease. A similar negative relationship characterizes patients with Parkinson's disease[611] and possibly adult celiac disease.

Epidemiologic Comment

Significant clinical information emerged from the early epidemiologic surveys: the role of the environment in the pathogenesis of IBD, especially Crohn's disease, the increased incidence of IBD, especially Crohn's disease,[550] in the industrialized, (northern) colder climates of the world, the development of Crohn's disease among previously healthy persons who move from rural areas to urban locations, and the similar clinical manifestations, radiologic and pathologic features of ulcerative colitis and Crohn's disease everywhere, despite differing ethnic populations, climatic conditions, dietary habits and socio-cultural customs over long periods of time. Because of limited clinical knowledge and diagnostic resources and because of the many mild to moderate cases revealed only by endoscopy in population-based surveys (e.g. proctitis) or not recognized at all, the overall numbers of patients with ulcerative colitis and with Crohn's disease worldwide undoubtedly exceed published figures.

The early epidemiologic studies also revealed the increased familial incidence, especially for Crohn's disease, the elevated colorectal cancer risk, for both ulcerative colitis and Crohn's colitis, the association of ulcerative colitis with immune disorders (e.g. autoimmune hemolytic anemia, systemic lupus erythematosus, Hashimoto's thyroiditis), the genetically-influenced association of ulcerative colitis with ankylosing spondylitis, and the association of Crohn's disease with genetic disorders (Hermansky–Pudlak, Chediak–Hidashi and Wiskott–Aldrich syndromes).

The 1988 agenda suggested by Mendeloff and Calkins[612] for continuing epidemiologic investigation remains relevant today: (a) verification of incidence trends in various populations (diseases that change incidence over a few decades, as noted for Crohn's disease, reflect environmental causes), (b) study of the incidence trends in age-specific categories and in birth cohorts (a higher incidence in a particular birth cohort over time would suggest a common environmental exposure involved in etiology), (c) further study of racial, religious, ethnic and social characteristics ... including studies of Hispanic and Asian groups and of Amish, Mormon, and Seventh-day Adventist populations (socio-cultural and dietary clues to IBD vulnerability or to IBD protection), and (d) the more detailed study of families, accounting also for adopted children, the association of IBD with other diseases, and distinctive individual dietary customs prior to disease onset. I would add multiple case families, particularly with regard to geographic and sociocultural epidemiology. Other risk factors requiring investigation include childhood hygiene and the suspected role of the appendix and the tonsils for ulcerative colitis. Expanding epidemiologic studies, especially population-based studies, including genetic epidemiology,[613] socio-cultural epidemiology, geographic and environmental epidemiology[614] (local agriculture, food and water supplies) and nutritional epidemiology[615] should provide important clues to the causation of IBD. Epidemiologist R.S. Sandler in 1999 similarly stated: "researchers must now move beyond descriptive studies to more focused analytic ones; perhaps to include more completely correlative environmental (agriculture, sanitation) and psychosocial descriptions of IBD populations."

PSYCHOGENIC ASPECTS (UC, CD)

The relationship between mind and body has interested mankind from earliest times and was recognized in the ancient Babylonian, Chinese and Greek civilizations.[616,617] Plato (400 BC) observed: "For this is the great error of our day, in the treatment of the human body, that physicians separate the soul from the body." As noted by S. Wolf,[618] P.J.G. Cabanis[619] (1757–1808) of Paris in 1796 had proposed that thoughts and emotions, as well as general somatic and visceral behavior, are shaped, not only by new experiences perceived through the senses, but also by remote and long-forgotten experiences stored somewhere in the brain, in fact, describing the unconscious – a fundamental tenet of psychoanalysis. Scientific awareness of the physiologic responses of the body to emotional stress probably originated with the classic observations of C. Darwin[620] (1872), I.P. Pavlov,[621] and W.B. Cannon.[622] According to H. Sprinz,[623] Julius Cohnheim[624] as early as 1882 had postulated a connection between diarrhea and the nervous system, presumably on the basis of an earlier experiment by A. Moreau,[625] who produced a "paralytic hypersecretion of the succus entericus" by denervating a segment of intestines. In the 1965 experiment of H. Sprinz[623] wherein massive "propulsive watery diarrhea developed in the 'reserpinized' guinea pig challenged with bacterial endotoxin, autopsy demonstrated degenerative changes in both the intramural plexus and extramural abdominal sympathetic ganglia." "Direct injection of endotoxin into the abdominal sympathetic ganglia did not result in diarrhea, suggesting that the peripheral network, distributed within the gut wall, is relatively independent of the central portions or even of the extramural ganglia." Charles Richet of Paris, Adolph Meyer of Baltimore, Stanley Cobb of Boston, and Hans Selye of Montreal, among others, and animal researchers, Victor Horsley of England, H. Gantt and Curt Richter of Baltimore, and Howard Lidell of Ithaca, N.Y. early in the 20th century contributed substantially to concepts associating somatic illness with neuro-psychogenic disturbances. A.J. Sullivan[626] and G.F. Solomon[627] also contributed to the subject. Mohr[628] expressed the psychogenic relationship thusly: "There is no such thing as a purely psychic illness or a purely physical one, but only a living event taking place in a living organism which is itself alive only by virtue of the fact that in it psychic and somatic are united in a unity."

Psychogenic factors were "formally" implicated in ulcerative colitis following the reports of C. Murray[629] (1930) (first observed in a patient at the Presbyterian Hospital, New York) and A.J. Sullivan and C.A. Chandler[630] of Yale University, New Haven, Conn. (1932). Murray later studied four and then 12 patients with ulcerative colitis at Yale. In each he was impressed with a chronological relationship between an emotional disturbance and the onset of bowel symptoms. None of the seven men in the series had been married or had ever been away from his mother. The five women each had emotional difficulties involving their marriage or home life. Murray previously had worked in the "constitutional" clinic of George Draper at Columbia University (New York), himself interested in psychosomatic origins of disease. This experience developed Murray's

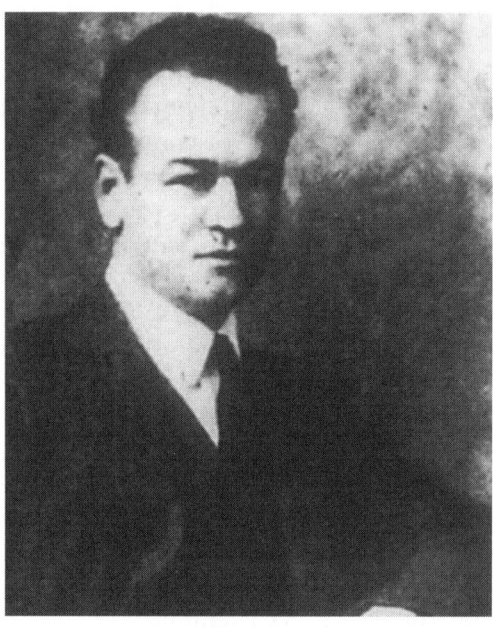

Cecil Murray

interest in psychosomatic illness and increased his awareness of emotional contributions to the onset and course of IBD. Sullivan's second series of 15 patients was featured by prolonged emotional conflict involving marital and fiscal difficulties. Five men were described as having a "mother complex." In 11 patients disease had begun within 48 hours of an emotional upset. In 1952, C. Wells[469] (Liverpool) rejected the psychosomatic hypothesis for ulcerative colitis ("nothing could be further from the truth"). Nevertheless, evolving from the psychoanalytical concepts of S. Freud in the 1920s, the rising interest in psychiatry worldwide, the leadership of Franz Alexander[631] at the Chicago Institute for Psychoanalysis and many other psychiatrists in the United States and in Europe during the 1930s, 1940s and 1950s,[632] psychogenic considerations dominated etiologic discussions of ulcerative colitis. Psychiatrists formulated an "ulcerative colitis personality," described as "immaturity of the patient, sensitivity, indecisiveness, dependence and inhibited interpersonal relationships" and upon emotional problems, such as the loss of a loved one, social rejection and maternal dominance. As late as 1962, psychiatrists, while recognizing the frequency of "other psychosomatic and psychiatric disorders," focused upon "a consistent pattern of weak, ineffective fathers and controlling, hostile, overprotective or domineering mothers." Prominent supporters of this concept included E. Wittkower[633] (1938), G.E. Daniels[634] (1942), Erich Lindemann[635] (1950) and J.W. Paulley[555] 1950, among many others.[636–638] H.I. Weinstock[639] of New York in 1962 reported the successful treatment of ulcerative colitis by psychoanalysis. D.G. Prugh[640] of the Children's Hospital, Boston, studying 12 children with ulcerative colitis, emphasized the role of emotional factors originating within the family constellation in the precipitous onset of the disease.

The early 20th century clinical reports implicating a psychogenic causation in ulcerative colitis were based upon the uncontrolled observations of psychiatrists and upon retrospective reviews of often incompletely documented hospital observations. Later opinions were based upon controlled clinical scrutiny and upon physiologic studies.[641,642] As noted earlier, R. Lium[183] of Boston produced hemorrhages and ulcerations in canine colonic explants in 15 dogs by the topical application of Shiga dysentery toxin and attributed the lesions to intense intestinal spasm initiated by the toxin ("increased parasympathetic activity") associated with depletion of protective colonic mucus. Utilizing a device to measure the frequency and intensity of rectal muscular contraction, the rectometrogram, Lium[643] noted intense and prolonged rectal muscular contractions in one patient with ulcerative colitis. The experiments of T.P. Almy and M. Tulin[644] of Cornell University, New York documented the significant physiological effects of emotional stress upon the normal colonic mucosa (hyperemia, vascular engorgement, increased secretion of mucus and augmented colonic motor activity). Such responses were intensified and more prolonged in the ulcerative colitis colon. Almy et al.[645] in 1949 described a systemic reaction comprising hypertension, sweating, sighing, pallor of the skin and increased motor activity of the lower sigmoid, vascular congestion of the colonic mucosa and increased secretion of mucus in seven healthy men under stress from mechanically produced headache or exposure to cold, "emotional conflict" or cholinergic stimulation and compared the colonic changes to those observed in patients with ulcerative colitis. The "hyper-dynamic" response and the diarrhea of disturbed colonic function included "increased rhythmic contractile activity of circular muscles in the cecum, ascending and transverse loops, while the descending and sigmoid colon ... assumed a rigid tubular shape due to longitudinal muscle activity ... This emptying reaction of the colon was evoked by words or events with special meaning to the individual, eliciting reactions of anger, resentment, guilt, humiliation and anxiety. A similar colonic response could be initiated or augmented by parasympathomimetic agents." A 1949 study of twenty patients with chronic ulcerative colitis, 12 males and 8 females (ages 14 to 45), by Mahoney, Bockus et al.[646] (Philadelphia) produced the following conclusions: "Patients suffering with ulcerative colitis are complex neurotics in whose early life there were major parent-child relationship disturbances and other traumatic experiences." "These patients present an abundance of neurotic traits commonly observed in the neuroses and other psychosomatic conditions ... None of the personality traits found in ulcerative colitis, when taken alone, are specific for this disease."

Wener, Hoff and Simon[647] of Montreal (Canada) in 1949 produced an "ulcerative colitis" in dogs by the prolonged administration of mecholyl. In 1950 Wener and Polonsky described engorgement and edema of a transverse colostomy in a patient with ulcerative colitis during periods of emotional tension,[648] and postulated "profound vascular disturbances caused by emotionally-triggered activation of the autonomic nervous system." Moeller and Kirsner[649] in 1954, seeking to confirm these observations, injected dogs repeatedly with parasympathomimetic drugs (methacholine, neostigmine) for one year and noted transient small superficial ulcerations in the colon mucosa, not ulcerative colitis. Similar findings were reported by Sleisenger et al.[650] An experimental fatal "colitis" allegedly resembling the nonspecific ulcerative colitis of man,[651] "induced" by "self-stimulation" of the central nervous system in three monkeys with electrodes implanted intracerebrally, was in accord with the psychogenic hypothesis for ulcerative colitis. Augmented parasympathetic activity was presumed to "trigger" central nervous system-intestinal interactions, involving complex neurotransmitter, humoral, and immune physiologic mechanisms.[243,652]

Opinions as to the presence and the significance of emotional disturbances in ulcerative colitis notwithstanding,[653-656] psychotherapy, conventional and occasionally psychoanalytical, was an important part of medical treatment during the 1930s, 1940s and 1950s. Treatment was prolonged and some patients remained in the hospital for months. Sperling[657] successfully treated children with ulcerative colitis by psychoanalysis. Groen and Bastiaans[658] of Amsterdam, Holland in 1951 described 35 patients with ulcerative colitis, 29 of whom were treated with "superficial" psychotherapy with favorable results. Psychoanalysis was not used and indeed rejected. "These patients need care, support and protection and we have attempted to give it to them in every aspect. Care was taken to be as kind to them as possible." In 1954, Grace, Pinsky and

Wolff[659] (New York Hospital) reported more favorable outcomes in terms of lower operability rate, fewer serious complications and lower mortality rate in a series of 34 patients with ulcerative colitis treated by therapy diminishing stress compared to a matched group of 34 patients in whom treatment consisted mainly of diet and medication. In 1954 and 1955, G. Engel,[660,661] University of Rochester, New York, reviewing psychosomatic hypotheses in ulcerative colitis, stated, "It is clear that none of the psychosomatic hypotheses so far advanced has fulfilled the requirements both of correctly identifying the somatic processes and of indicating how psychic processes are related to the somatic ..." Engel dismissed concepts of "parasympathetic over-reactivity" and suggested as a likely mechanism the response of the bowel mucosa to a "noxious agent" of microscopic or molecular size, including bacterial or viral agents, allergic phenomena, collagen disorder, "blood-borne chemical substances," genetic or "constitutional abnormalities" and "metabolic" or enzymatic disturbances.

In my experience, lacking effective therapeutic resources during the 1930s and 1940s, the psychiatric concept in the management of patients with ulcerative colitis was over-emphasized.[662] Patients and families were definitely helped by the emotional support provided by psychiatrists and physicians in coping with the illness, but sustained healing of ulcerative colitis was not observed. The disappearance of "personality defects" of the ulcerative colitis patient after successful medical or surgical therapy and the restoration of physical health, as described by B.V. White (Hartford, Conn.),[663] as had been suspected by many observers, was a pivotal observation. In the study of 13 patients, "depression, negativism and petulance disappeared and immaturity, dependency and hostility diminished." Feldman et al.,[664] in a study including two control groups of individuals (general population and consecutive concurrent admissions to the gastroenterology service), found no evidence of a dominant psychogenic relationship in 34 patients with ulcerative colitis. "In general, the control patients showed as much or more psychopathology than the ulcerative colitis cases." A clinical study of patients with ulcerative colitis in 1962 by Fullerton et al. (UCLA, Los Angeles)[665] focused on the psychophysiologic stress process in relation to IBD.

Clinical emphasis upon psychiatric factors in IBD diminished during the 1950s after the introduction of ACTH and adrenal steroids and the impressive, at times dramatic, clinical responses of patients to these compounds. Nevertheless, psychotherapy for ulcerative colitis continued. A striking experience with anaclitic psychotherapy was reported by S. Cobb in 1953[666] and expanded by Sifneos in 1964.[667] In 1970, Kirsner[668] observed: "The continuing unsettled role of psychogenic influences in the pathogenesis of ulcerative colitis reflects the preoccupation with earlier anecdotal psychiatric approaches and with subjective attempts to establish an exclusive or primary psychogenic etiology. Emotional disturbances are common in patients with ulcerative colitis and contribute to the exacerbation, chronicity and the severity of ulcerative colitis. However, they are not specific for ulcerative colitis and they reflect 'secondary emotional responses of the chronically ill patient'."

A. Karush et al.[669] of New York in 1977 summarized the position of many psychiatrists (and physicians), "We do not claim that ulcerative colitis is 'caused' by unusual reactions of the mind alone. We claim only that these reactions almost always play a vital role in the interaction of the four etiological determinants: genetic endowment, constitutional vulnerability, intrapsychic processes and the emotional environment. The intrapsychological processes may, for example, predispose to the actual development of the disease. In many cases, however, they may be secondary reactions to the disability caused by the disease ... They may also reflect a combination of causal ingredients, which seems to be the usual situation in chronic ulcerative colitis ... As do other humanist physicians, the psychiatrist, who works with somatic illness tries to view the patient as a whole and to see his illness as an outcome of many operant pathogenic factors." This viewpoint was accepted by many physicians.

In 1982 Helzer et al.[670] of North Carolina studied the lifetime prevalence of definitive psychiatric diagnoses in a series of 50 patients with ulcerative colitis. The frequency of psychiatric disorders (approximately 25%) was no higher than in a matched control population. In 1990 North, Alpers et al.[671] of Washington University, St. Louis, in a critique of 138 studies in the medical literature, found "serious flaws in research design, such as lack of control subjects, unspecified manner of data collection and abuse of diagnostic criteria."

In the year 2002, emotions and stress have gained physiologic credibility as contributing factors in human illness following E. Sternberg's[672,673] (National Institutes of Health) documentation of the integrative-CNS-neurohumoral immune-genetic mechanisms mediating the impact of emotional stress upon the gastrointestinal tract. As stated by Sternberg: "We understand the relationship between emotions and disease in terms of a balance. But now the balance consists of molecules and nerve signals instead of humors and magic ..." E.A. Mayer[674] of UCLA (Los Angeles) has summarized evidence indirectly supporting a role for stress-mediated activation of sympathetic (and parasympathetic) nerves in increasing the permeability of the gut, modifying the quantity of mucus and altering immune function in the reactivation of chronic ulcerative colitis. Stress also has been shown to increase bacterial adherence and diminish luminal lactobacilli, contributing to intestinal inflammation.

Crohn's disease

Psychogenic disturbances were less emphasized in Crohn's disease but opinions varied. Paulley,[675] Stewart[676] and Grace[677] were impressed with the relationship between emotional stress and the onset or relapse of Crohn's disease. Cohn et al.,[678] in a study of 12 patients, emphasized the dependency, passivity, immaturity, and obsessive worrying in Crohn's patients, as had been described by Paulley (Ipswich Hospitals).[679] Sperling[680,681] successfully treated young patients with regional enteritis by psychoanalysis. Kraft and Ardali[682] and Whybrow et al.,[683] on the other hand, studying children with regional ileitis, regarded the psychological difficulties as consequences of chronic, recurrent and frustrating illness. Crockett,[684] in a 1952 study of 16 patients, concluded: "Routine psychiatric examination does not give substantial support for the suggestion that emotional stress is a major etiological factor in Crohn's disease." In 1984 Helzer and his colleagues,[685] though finding "a diagnosable psychiatric disorder" (mostly depression) in 50% of 50 patients with Crohn's disease, concluded that the Crohn's disease and psychiatric illness "appeared to be independent of each other." An evaluation by F.P. McKegney, R.O. Gordon and S.M. Levine[686] of Yale concluded: "A two-phase study of 123 patients with either ulcerative colitis or Crohn's disease indicates a similarly high incidence of emotional disturbances and life crises prior to the illness onset in both somatic diseases. There are no significant differences between patients with the two diseases in a large number of demographic, psychosocial, personality, behavioral, psychiatric and physical disease characteristics. In both syndromes more severe emotional disturbances are associated with more severe physical disease ..."

Psychogenic Comment

The varying physician assessments of psychogenic disturbances in IBD reflect the limitations of the psychogenic evidence and individual physician attitudes as to the importance of "everyday" emotional disturbances in human illness. Emotional stress is common in patients with ulcerative colitis and Crohn's disease, as in other chronic, recurrent diseases and, though not necessarily causative, significantly influence the clinical course and the response to therapy, necessitating consideration of psychosocial factors in the treatment of IBD.[687] The similar neurohumoral and neurotransmitter peptide-producing cells in the central nervous system (pituitary gland, sensory ganglia) and in the gastrointestinal tract (e.g. VIP, somatostatin, substance P), the extensive neural innervations of the entire bowel wall, including the intestinal mucosa, and the enteric nervous system[688] provide many pathways for psycho-neuro-humoral-immunologic interactions between the brain and the gut[689] and for the individually-determined expression of emotional stress in inflammatory bowel disease. Renewed interest in the "stress system" and its relationship to human illness is providing useful new information.[690] The psycho-neuro-endocrinological effects upon the immune response have been described by G.F. Solomon[627] and Neal Miller.[691] Stead, Bienenstock and Stanisz[692] of McMaster University, Hamilton, Ontario, Canada examined the role of neuropeptides (e.g. substance P, somatostatin, nerve growth factor and vasoactive intestinal peptide) in the regulation of the mucosal immune system and stated: "Clearly there is good evidence that epithelium, nerves and mast cells interact in a functional manner in the gastrointestinal and respiratory tracts to promote specific, antigen-dependent, physiological changes."

The observations of Bass[693] apply to IBD: "All disease is the result of a complex interplay of biological, psychological and sociological variables. Each of these three classes of variables may play either a necessary or a contributory causal role. Thus, we should not be asking whether life events are related to the onset of illness but to what extent are life events related to the onset of this particular illness in this particular person at this particular time. This means that we should, in addition to life events, be measuring other variables that may have a bearing on the onset of illness."

Lysozyme

A concept allied to psychogenic hypotheses in the late 1940s and early 1950s involved the bacteriolytic and mucolytic enzyme lysozyme present in nasal secretions, saliva, and tears, discovered accidentally by A.B. Fleming[694] in 1922. H.G. Sammons[192] in his 1951 study of mucinases in ulcerative colitis had found increased amounts of lysozyme in the feces in ulcerative colitis. He associated the lysozyme with purulent material, the quantity decreasing after treatment with penicillin and streptomycin. K. Meyer et al.[695] (1948), Grace et al.[696] (1949) and Prudden and Meyer[697] (1950), all of New York, reported increases in the level of lysozyme in the blood and in the feces of patients with active ulcerative colitis and regional enteritis during periods of emotional stress, diminishing when the stress subsided. Lysozyme allegedly destroyed the protective colonic mucus, rendering the colon more vulnerable to invading bacteria and cytolytic substances. However, anti-lysozyme therapy was unimpressive in 18 patients with ulcerative colitis given 600 mg of purified sodium hexadecyl sulfate every four hours together with retention enemas of 100 cc of a (0.16%) suspension of the detergent twice daily to reduce the gut content of lysozymes.[698] S.J. Gray et al.[699] of the Brigham Hospital, Boston, in a 1950 study of 14 patients with active ulcerative colitis, decreased the elevated levels of fecal lysozyme by the oral administration of the detergent Aerosol OT, without altering the course of the disease. The increased lysozyme in active ulcerative colitis feces originates in the numerous polymorphonuclear cells of the inflammatory reaction as Sammons had surmised in 1951, and therefore is an accompaniment rather than a cause of IBD.

Interest in the role of lysozyme as a pathophysiological expression of emotional stress subsided after Kirsner's observation of large nonspecific increases in fecal lysozyme in the dog following electro-cautery of the rectal mucosa, the failure of large quantities of crystalline lysozyme to locally damage ileo-colonic pouches in dogs,[700] and the demonstrated inability of lysozyme to digest or dissolve human colonic mucus.[701]

MICROBIAL ASPECTS – ULCERATIVE COLITIS

L. Fleck[702] of Lvov, Poland credits M.T. Varro (116–127 BC) with the statement: "Minute animals that cannot be seen by the eye enter the body from the air, through the mouth and also through the nose and cause severe diseases." R.E. McGrew[703] adds: "The idea that entities too small to be seen exist and play a role in human illness" developed long before the 20th century, noting as major early contributors: Girolamo Fracastori of Italy, "On Contagion" (1546), Antonj Van Leeuwenhoek of Holland (1676), G. Bonomo (1687) (Italy), J. Henle of Zurich (1840), and P. Bretonneau of France (1850s). "As a discipline in its own light, bacteriology came of age in the third quarter of the nineteenth century" under the leadership of L. Pasteur[704] (1822–1895) of France and especially R. Koch[705] (1843–1910) of Germany. The subsequent development of bacteriology and its contributions to the recognition and understanding of human illness represent one of the major triumphs in the history of medicine.[706]

Bacterial causes of ulcerative colitis attracted attention early in the 20th century, when numerous bacterial pathogens of human disease were being discovered. In 1906 S. Flexner and J.E. Sweet (Rockefeller Institute for Medical Research, New York),[707] studying bacillary dysentery (not ulcerative colitis), observed small hemorrhages, ulcerations of the colon and a fibrinous exudate in rabbits injected intravenously with Shiga and Flexner dysentery bacilli or their toxins, especially the Shiga toxin ... "these lesions are due to the action of a toxin elaborated by the dysentery bacilli present in the diseased intestine, which toxin is first absorbed, in the main probably from the small intestine, and eliminated chiefly through the large intestine, which suffers injury through the act of excretion. In offering this view of the pathogenesis of dysentery ... the injury upon the tissues once inflicted in the manner mentioned, other micro-organisms than the dysentery bacillus doubtless come into action and complicate and increase the pathological effects of the dysentery toxin." In 1907 H. de R. Morgan[708] produced diarrhea in rats and rabbits fed a gram negative bacillus isolated from the feces of infants suffering with "summer diarrhea." A.J. Jex-Blake[709] in 1909 suggested Bacillus coli, B. proteus, B. pyocyaneus, B. lactis aerogenes, and streptococci, F.C. Wallis[710] (1909) oral streptococci, P.L. Mummery[711] (1911) E. coli and streptococci, and H. Rolleston[712] (1922), coliforms, among a variety of organisms. A. Bassler[713] (1933) of New York, after bacterial studies in 50 patients, emphasized a "mixed" infection with multiple organisms (hemolytic and non-hemolytic streptococci), H.F. Hewes[714] (1923), identifying ulcerative colitis as a "sequel to infectious diseases (pneumonia, influenza)," implicated multiple unspecified organisms. Bargen[715] (1924) emphasized the intestinal diplostreptococcus and only the Bargen organism received serious consideration (see later). A.F. Hurst[48] administered a "polyvalent anti-dysenteric serum" and J. Leusden[716] advocated an autologous vaccine of mixed fecal bacteria. Typhoid vaccine and autogenous vaccines of dysentery and fecal diplostreptococci also were administered,[98,717] with questionable benefit.[46]

"Focal infection" with endogenous bacteria was a popular concept of disease in the United States during the 1920s, implicating dental infections, "chronic cholecystitis" and "chronic appendicitis," as causes of varied abdominal symptoms, encouraging needless dental extractions and abdominal operations. L. Weinstein[718] of Boston in 1958 and S.L. Gorbach[719] of Boston in 1975 pointed out: "Bacterial elements of the normal gastrointestinal microflora were implicated in the pathogenesis of ulcerative colitis ... a prime example is the fecal streptococci of J.A. Bargen." Other organisms included Aerobacter aerogenes, Alcaligenes fecalis and Staphylococci.

The apparent precipitation of ulcerative colitis in several patients following the extraction of abscessed teeth aroused Bargen's interest in the possibility of oral bacteria as the cause of ulcerative colitis. At the same time (1919), bacteriologist E.C. Rosenow,[720] also at the Mayo Clinic, champion of the "principle of the selective localization of bacteria," was investigating the pathogenicity of diplostreptococci isolated from the mouth and from the feces. In 1924, J.A. Bargen[715] reported the occurrence of bloody diarrhea in rabbits injected intravenously with bacterial cultures prepared from the feces of patients with ulcerative colitis (presumably containing diplostreptococcus). Autopsy demonstrated petechial to massive submucosal hemorrhages and superficial ulcers involving much of the colon, "resembling human ulcerative colitis," and diplostreptococci were cultured from the ulcers. Bargen and Logan[721] in 1925 reported positive cultures from the rectal ulcerations in 80% of 68 patients. Colonic lesions developed in 45 of 139 animals injected with patient-derived diplostreptococci.

Cook[722] in 1931, in association with Rosenow, injected 60 rabbits with the diplostreptococci cultured from the abscessed teeth of patients with active ulcerative colitis. Sixty percent developed a "diffuse hemorrhagic infiltration of the colon." Cook also inoculated artificial cavities he created in the apices of the teeth of 15 dogs with the same diplostreptococci isolated from the teeth of patients with ulcerative colitis. Diarrhea developed in seven animals and rectal ulcerations were observed proctoscopically for as long as 8 to 16 months after the dental bacterial inoculation. Bargen[723] and others[724] then treated patients with an autologous vaccine of ulcerative colitis fecal discharges, containing diplostreptococci, with variable clinical benefit. In 1930 Bargen and his colleagues[725] utilized as intravenous therapy a serum prepared by injecting increasing amounts of freshly isolated strains of the diplostreptococcus into horses. This material later was replaced by an "antibody euglobulin solution" injected intramuscularly, and given to 50 patients with ulcerative colitis together with a vaccine of the diplostreptococcus, "greatly reducing the need for surgical ileostomy."

In 1931 R. Buttiaux and A. Sevin[726] of the Pasteur Institute (Lille, France) comprehensively reviewed bacterial possibilities in ulcerative colitis (36 pages) and, in support of Bargen's diplococcus, added an "enterococcus" of theirs. "En resume, nous pensons quo l'etiologie infectieuse de la colitie ulcereuse doit actuellement's interpreter de la facon suivante: il existe des colites chroniques qui relevant de germes specifiques de cette affection. Ces germes sont fort rares, on n'en connait actuellement que deux: celui de Bargen et le notre."

In 1932, H.A. Rafsky and P.J. Manheim[727] of New York and A. Hurst[728] of England in 1935 dismissed the "Bargen diplostreptococcus" as "simply a form of the normal enterococci present in all stools, often found in normal people," as shown later by Rodaniche, Palmer and Kirsner.[729] H.G. Rudner[96] of the University of Tennessee, Memphis reviewed early conflicting opinions as to bacterial causes of ulcerative colitis, particularly the evidence on the Bargen diplostreptococcus and bacillary dysentery. Subsequent studies by M. Paulson[730] of Johns Hopkins University, Baltimore and Mones-Gallart and Sanjuan[88] of Spain failed to confirm the 1924 observations of Bargen and the pathogenicity of the "Bargen diplostreptococcus" concept gradually lost scientific credibility. Interestingly, enteric and periodontal bacterial pathogens utilize similar invasion pathways to gain entrance into epithelial cells, via the protein "invasin;" both adhesin and invasin are encoded in the same gene.

Many other bacteria were implicated during the 1930s and subsequently, including the anaerobe spherophorus necrophorus[731] (later recognized as part of the normal flora of the bowel and the oropharynx), Bacillus morgagni, Pseudomonas maltophilia, ps. Aeruginosa, Proteus vulgaris, hemolytic and non-hemolytic E. coli, Klebsiella pneumoniae, Clostridium difficile, cell wall-defective variant of a pseudomonas-like microorganism and viruses (e.g. lymphopathia venereum). None fulfilled Koch's postulates and were discarded. Felsen (Bronx, New York)[732] in 1936, after a study of 553 patients (acute bacillary dysentery, ileitis and ulcerative colitis), again suggested a "common pathogenesis," i.e. bacillary dysentery, for acute and chronic "distal ileitis" and chronic ulcerative colitis, as he and Lynch had advocated in 1925,[733] Penner[734] of New York, among others, in 1936 found the evidence inconclusive.

E. histolytica was implicated following the 1933–34 Chicago epidemic of amebic dysentery.[735] Several patients with a previously confirmed amebic dysentery contracted during the epidemic actually presented in the 1950s as "typical ulcerative colitis." The sequence of events in these individuals theoretically appeared consistent with a "sensitization" of the bowel induced by the initial amebic infection, "priming" the colon for the later development of ulcerative colitis, see also C. Nagler-Anderson.[736] Subsequent studies failed to confirm a etiologic role for E. histolytica. J. Rachet and A. Busson[206] of Paris in 1950 suggested "La predisposition locale an sensibilite intestinale," increasing the vulnerability of the intestinal epithelium to various bacteria. J.H. Swartz and I. Jankelson of Boston,[737] finding increased amounts of geotrichum and monilia albicans in the stools of patients with ulcerative colitis (possibly secondary to antibacterial therapy), suggested a role for fungi in the chronicity of the disease; supporting evidence never developed.

Microbiological studies of the fecal flora in ulcerative colitis and regional enteritis in the 1940s were limited (e.g. incomplete panel of organisms, few anaerobic studies) and had little or no impact on either the understanding or the treatment of IBD. Pathogenic organisms were not found and aerobic bacterial counts, while increased, were mostly coliform organisms. Aerobic bacteria decreased during the oral administration of sulfonamides, partially compensated by increased numbers of gram positive enterococci and anaerobic bacteria, as shown in the 1942, 1943 and 1950 studies by Kirsner and his colleagues.[738–740] Fecal cultures at the Caroline Hospital[741] (Stockholm) "most commonly demonstrated an abundant flora of enterococci but this is by no means constant." Presuming an imbalance or "dysbiosis" of the normal intestinal microflora as a factor in IBD, Gorbach et al. of Boston,[742] in quantitative and qualitative microbiological studies of the fecal flora in 25 patients with untreated ulcerative colitis or regional enteritis (1968), found a normal microflora in mild or moderately ill patients with ulcerative colitis. Similar results were reported in 1978 by Keighley et al.,[743] Birmingham, England, examining surgically-resected colon tissue. Seneca and Henderson,[744] Columbia University, New York, reported an 85-fold increase over normal in the total number of organisms and a fiftyfold increase in the numbers of coliforms in the stools of patients with severe ulcerative colitis or with regional enteritis and postulated damaging proteolytic enzymatic activity from the large numbers of bacteria, injuring the intestinal mucosa and followed by secondary bacterial infection.

To determine the possible pathogenicity of E. coli organisms in ulcerative colitis, E. Mary Cooke of Westminster Hospital, London[745,746] in 1968 and 1974 compared strains of E. coli isolated from the feces of 47 patients with ulcerative colitis with 49 strains isolated from the feces of normal persons and 44 isolated from the feces of patients with acute diarrhea. The ulcerative colitis strains included a larger proportion of coliforms producing hemolysin and necrotoxin; belonged to one of a small number of O-groups and produced a severe tissue reaction in ligated segments of rabbit ileum, compared with strains from normal individuals and from patients with "simple" diarrhea. In 1980 Cooke and her colleagues[747] reported an increased incidence of fecal coliforms with in vitro adhesive and invasive properties in patients with ulcerative colitis. (Detailed studies of the normal human intestinal microflora have been published by R.M. Donaldson Jr.[748] and M.H. Floch, S.L. Gorbach and T.D. Luckey.[749])

The study of viral possibilities in ulcerative colitis has been handicapped by the technology and the complexity of "the viral world." Serological evidence of excessive exposure to known viruses (influenza, mumps, herpes, Cocksackie A, B, Echo, E-B, adenovirus[750]) in ulcerative colitis patients was negative. Recent serological studies for 19 common viruses, including measles, in two French families with a very high frequency of Crohn's disease also were negative.[751] The occasional increased titers of cytomegalovirus have been in malnourished, secondarily immunodeficient patients with severe Crohn's disease. A pilot attempt at virus recovery in 1961 by virologist J.T. Syverton[752] of the University of Minnesota with ulcerative colitis tissue from 14 patients with active ulcerative colitis airmailed by J.B. Kirsner of Chicago, utilizing six cell types (Hela, normal esophageal epithelium, normal liver, human amnion, monkey kidney and rabbit fibroblasts) failed to provide evidence for a pathogenic virus. Transfer studies to newborn mice and embryonated eggs also were negative. The clinical and proctoscopic similarity of ulcerative colitis to the colitis caused by lymphopathia venereum virus (chlamydia trachomatis) in the 1930s led in the 1940s to studies of a possible etiologic relationship by M. Paulson[753] in Baltimore and by E. Rodaniche, J.B. Kirsner and W.L. Palmer,[754] with negative results. Frei skin tests with mouse and human antigens were negative and the serum was negative for neutralizing antibodies against the virus. In 1950, R. Victor, J.B. Kirsner and W.L. Palmer[189] at proctoscopy injected extracts of actively diseased ulcerative colitis mucosa into the rectum of monkeys, with negative results.

The development of an ulcerative colitis type tissue reaction in the artificial vagina formed from the rectum in a 37-year-old woman with ulcerative proctosigmoiditis[755] and the simultaneous onset of ulcerative colitis in a 25-year-old woman's rectum and in a segment of colon previously used to construct an artificial vagina, removed from intestinal continuity,[756] suggested an inherent intestinal/colonic vulnerability to bacteria, as indicated also by the pouchitis following total colectomy and ileoanal anastomosis with J pouch in ulcerative colitis.

MICROBIAL ASPECTS – CROHN'S DISEASE

Infections of the terminal ileum and colon in animals have been associated with tissue changes "resembling" Crohn's disease,[757,758] including a fatal ileitis in the golden Syrian hamster, a spontaneous ileitis in rats, a regional enterocolitis in cocker spaniels[358] (1954), chlamydia trachomatis and mycobacterial infections of the terminal ileum in cattle, including mycobacterial paratuberculosis (Johne's disease,[759,760] a granulomatous enterocolitis in horses[364] (1974), a terminal ileitis in swine,[354] and a granulomatous colitis of Boxer dogs.[362] The febrile course of active Crohn's disease, the suppurative complications, the increased aerobic and anaerobic intestinal microflora and the occasional clinical response to antibiotics maintained clinical interest in a microbial etiology for Crohn's disease despite the failure to isolate an intestinal pathogen. In the 1932 Mt. Sinai series, intestinal tuberculosis was excluded by negative cultures and skin tests and the absence of tubercle bacilli in the tissue. In 1938 Pumphrey[761] of the Mayo Clinic investigated bacterial possibilities in 13 cases. Many gram-positive and gram-negative organisms were recovered but none predominated; dysentery organisms, tubercle bacilli or spirochetes were not found. The injection of cultures of streptococcus viridans isolated from the throats of two patients into rabbits did not produce colitis.

Other microorganisms implicated in Crohn's disease included: mycobacteria (M. Kansasii,[762] Mycobacterium avium paratuberculosis[763] isolated from the diseased intestine of two patients with Crohn's disease), a variety of anaerobic organisms (Eubacteria strains Me46, Me47, B. vulgatus, Peptostreptococcus, Aerobacter aerogenes, Coprococcus, Bifidobacteria), Campylobacter fetus ssp. jejuni, Yersinia enterocolitica and viruses; none achieved etiologic status. Because of a perceived histologic resemblance of the Crohn's disease granulomatous lesion to Boeck's sarcoidosis,[764] this possibility received transient consideration.[765] Nickerson-Kveim skin tests[766] were conflicting,[767] but a 1967 study by Fletcher and Hinton[768] of London found no diminution of the Mantoux reaction in Crohn's disease and normal tuberculin sensitivity; differentiating Crohn's disease from sarcoidosis and tuberculosis.

Detailed studies of the fecal flora in Crohn's disease by Wensinck[769] of Erasmus University, Rotterdam, Holland in 1975 demonstrated increased numbers of gram-positive coccoid rods (Eubacteria, Peptostreptococcus and Coprococcus) and gram-negative rods (Bacteroides and Fusobacterium) in comparison with the flora of healthy individuals. 1978 studies of the intestinal microflora by Keighley et al.[743] on resected samples of jejunum, ileum and colon from 30 patients with Crohn's disease revealed increases in E. coli and B. fragilis in the ileum and E. coli and lactobacilli in the colon. The abnormal ileal flora in Crohn's disease was unrelated to disease activity, diameter of the ileum or to excision of the ileocecal valve. Aerobic and anaerobic studies of the mucosa-associated bacterial flora by Peach et al.[770] of England in 1978 indicated no statistical difference in the numbers of bacteria associated with Crohn's disease tissue compared with histologically normal tissue from the same patients and from a control group of patients. Among the bacterial isolates, however, enterobacteria were more commonly associated with Crohn's tissue. In 1978 M.F. Kagnoff[771] of San Diego, California, referring to the implication of a cell wall defective bacterial variant of a pseudomonas microorganism as the etiologic agent, began his editorial: "The etiology of Crohn's disease has and continues to defy the sophisticated science of the 1970s." He concluded: ... "Perhaps the basic defect involves an abnormal host response to a single agent or a variety of agents."

Pathogens identified subsequently (E. coli 0157.H7, Aeromonas hydrophila, Plesiomonas shigelloides, Blastocystis hominis) renewed interest in microbial possibilities in IBD, including the slowly growing pleomorphic mycobacterial variant (Mycobacterium Linda),[772] widely distributed in the food chain (dairy products, beef), adherent E. coli strains,[773] bacterial components (lipopolysaccharides, peptidoglycans, oligopeptides), metabolic products (endotoxins), and "normal" intestinal bacteria (coliforms), without positive results. The injection of sterile non-viable bacterial (Group A streptococci) cell wall fragments into the cecal wall and ileal mesentery induced a "classic granulomatous inflammation" attributed to the peptidoglycan-polysaccharide complex.[368] Another bacterial cell wall constituent, A,E diaminopimelic acid, was identified in rectal biopsy tissue from patients with ulcerative colitis in 1965[774] but was not studied further. A long-term follow-up (five to eight years) of patients with yersinia terminal ileitis indicated no development of Crohn's disease.[775]

On the possible involvement of a prior infection with measles or vaccination against the measles virus in the development of Crohn's disease emphasized by Wakefield[776] (London), R. Logan[777] of England noted ... "the recent levelling off in Crohn's disease incidence ... in the face of increasing measles vaccination rates and the notable decline in measles incidence, provides no support for either as causes of Crohn's disease." An authoritative Canadian report in 1997 concluded that "current scientific data do not permit a causal link to be drawn between the measles virus and the chronic inflammatory bowel diseases."[778] A literature review by D.J. Robertson and R.S. Sandler, University of North Carolina (United States), does not support an association between measles virus and IBD.[779] Serological studies of exposure to rotavirus and Norwalk virus also were negative.[780]

The remote possibility of a transmissible agent was suggested clinically by the story of a 22-year-old woman with Crohn's disease for six years. The presence of Crohn's disease also in the patient's grandmother living in the same household implied a genetic susceptibility, except that the patient was adopted and not a natural offspring of the family. At least two additional similar experiences (Crohn's disease in grandmother and adopted granddaughter and mother and adopted daughter) have been observed. At least two dozen documented instances of inflammatory bowel disease[781-785] developing after many years of marriage (as long as 30 years) in the initially healthy spouse of an IBD mate (more often Crohn's disease) seemed consistent with the concept of "cross-infection with a virus" over prolonged time. However, no additional information has appeared on this potentially significant issue.

Search for a "transmissible agent" in Crohn's disease was undertaken in the early 1970s by Mitchell, Rees and Cave in London, utilizing the development of focal epithelioid and giant cell granulomata in animal footpads as an indication of "transmission." Cave[786] summarized this work as follows: "Homogenates of bowel and of lymph node affected by Crohn's disease were inoculated into the footpads of normal and immunologically deficient CBA mice.[787] Control mice from the same stock received homogenates prepared identically from normal lymph nodes removed during arterial grafting at operation for ligation of varicose veins. A significant proportion of the mice inoculated with Crohn's tissue slowly developed focal epithelioid and giant cell granulomata in their footpads. These histological changes were observed both early (26–46 days) and late (169–500 days). Similar results were obtained in mice rendered immunologically deficient by thymectomy at 6 weeks and whole body irradiation. Control mice did not develop these changes, with the exception of one immunodeficient animal in which the early granulomatous changes seen in the footpad were transient. Kveim tests were performed on the ears of all the mice using Hurley Type I suspension. Positive Kveim tests were observed in 6 of the 17 inoculated mice and were associated with granulomatous changes in the footpads ..." Subsequently, Taub and Siltzbach[788] (1971) of New York, using mice of the same strain (CBA), identified slowly-evolving epithelioid and giant cell granulomata in the footpads of 5 of 16 mice inoculated with homogenates of Crohn's tissue after periods of 1 to 8 months. In contrast, Bolton et al.[789] (1973), using TO mice and not CBA mice, failed to confirm these findings. Similar experiments in rats and guinea pigs also were negative.

In 1971 Mitchell and Rees[790] reportedly "achieved" a successful first passage in mice of homogenates prepared in an identical manner from mouse footpad tissues showing granulomatous changes 553–603 days following the injection of human Crohn's tissue. Slowly developing granulomatous changes were evident 151–365 days after inoculation. The apparent demonstration of a "transmissible agent" from Crohn's disease tissue prompted Cave to produce a more satisfactory animal model.[791,792] At laparotomy, two groups of three New Zealand White rabbits (NZW) were inoculated in the ileal wall with homogenates of frozen tissue from two separate donors with histologically confirmed Crohn's disease. A control homogenate was prepared identically from the terminal ileum of a right hemicolectomy specimen removed for carcinoma of the colon and was inoculated similarly into a group of three rabbits from the same stock. The evolution of macroscopic and microscopic changes was assessed at laparotomy with biopsy of the terminal ileum at 12, 24 and 36 weeks. The animals in all groups were killed and their tissues examined macroscopically and histologically after a mean interval of 42 weeks following inoculation. Macroscopic changes were limited to an ileal abscess, lymph node hyperplasia and ileal thickening in rabbits from one of the Crohn's-inoculated groups. Microscopically, two of the rabbits in this group showed granulomatous changes by 12 weeks; at 24 weeks all three rabbits showed granulomatous changes in the ileum, and granulomata also were present in the mesenteric lymph nodes in two of these animals and in the liver of one.

"... The transmissible agent ... is found in the ileum, the colon and the regional mesenteric lymph nodes and it persists for long periods as shown by successful late passage from mouse footpads. The agent can be passed through a 220 nm filter, which suggests that it may be a virus, a bacterium with a defective cell wall or a mycoplasma."

These intriguing observations stimulated extensive multicenter efforts in the United States to similarly identify a "transmissible agent" for Crohn's disease. However, the USA experiments did not confirm the British observations. The dependence upon animal footpads in microbial/viral transfer experiments was criticized and the experimental granulomas eventually were attributed to the unintended introduction of foreign material (hair, keratin, filter fiber) in many of the granulomas.[793] Experiments by J. Ahlberg et al.[794] (Karolinska Institute, Stockholm) also failed to demonstrate a "transmissible agent." In the Swedish studies, affected lymph nodes from 3 patients with Crohn's disease were homogenized and inoculated intramurally into the distal ileum of two piglets. Homogenates also were injected intramurally into the distal ileum of 15 rats and the results were compared with control animals injected with normal lymph node homogenates. There were no abnormalities macroscopically or microscopically.

Microbial Comment

No evidence was obtained in the early studies to suggest that either ulcerative colitis or Crohn's disease was a classic infectious disease (i.e. a specific pathogen acquired by direct contact with a patient), nor was there any evidence of an animal species serving as a reservoir for putative infectious agents. Nevertheless, the not infrequent onset of IBD following an acute enterocolonic infection (e.g. traveler's diarrhea) and such occurrences as the acute onset of Crohn's disease in two French families after drinking unpasteurized milk[795] and the clustering of Crohn's disease in Mankato, Minnesota,[796] and other localities (e.g. North Tees area) implicate a microbial agent (via contaminated water, milk or food) in precipitating IBD in individuals presumably vulnerable genetically and immunologically. In the Minnesota study in 1980, 285 of the 320 graduates of Mankato West High School were contacted. Seven instances of Crohn's disease were identified, presumably related to the prolonged and excessive contamination of the Mankato lakes, utilized for recreational swimming, by fecal coliform organisms. Van Kruiningen cites other instances of the clustering of Crohn's disease among unrelated individuals. Such experiences focus upon an altered intestinal microflora (microbial agents, antibiotics) and perhaps upon an altered intestinal epithelium. Multiple bacterial species apparently are involved, but as precipitants of the IBD tissue reaction, modified by immune and genetic influences, rather than as direct causes of the inflammation.

Sartor et al. (University of North Carolina)[797] (1998) summarized evidence for an abnormal immune response to a luminal microbial pathogen: "The hypothesis that aberrant immune responses to nonpathogenic luminal bacteria can cause colitis is supported by clinical observations that decreasing intestinal bacterial concentrations by various techniques can lead to clinical improvement and decreased intestinal inflammation. The role of normal resident bacterial flora in the development of chronic intestinal inflammation has been further demonstrated in several rodent models of experimental colitis, both induced and spontaneous. For example, HLA-B27 transgenic rats raised under specific-pathogen-free (SPF) conditions spontaneously develop colitis, gastritis, and arthritis, whereas transgenic rats do not develop these lesions when maintained under germfree conditions. Similarly, T-cell receptor-a knockout mice fail to develop colitis in the absence of normal bacteria. Colitis spontaneously develops in interleukin-2 (IL-2)-deficient mice under conventional housing conditions but is greatly attenuated in germfree conditions." In addition, the mitigation of experimentally-induced inflammatory bowel disease in guinea pigs by selective elimination of the aerobic gram-negative intestinal bacteria supported the view implicating the commensal intestinal microflora in the pathogenesis of IBD.[798]

The recent identification of a potentially pathogenic, adherent-invasive E. coli in the ileal mucosa of a patient with Crohn's disease, the emergence of "new" bacteria and viruses and "superbugs"[799] justify continued microbial consideration in IBD. Despite the negative evidence thus far, microbial agents (commensal bacteria coliforms, viral, bacterial constituent) are involved in the development of inflammatory bowel disease (directly in Crohn's disease) and as a "risk factor" in ulcerative colitis. The mechanism in Crohn's disease may be via a genetically altered response of the gut mucosal immune system to antigens in commensal or mucosal-adherent bacteria,[800] in the presence of an impaired mucosal barrier.[801,802] In ulcerative colitis, this may occur via epithelial antigens cross-reacting with antigens in commensal bacteria. M. Chiba et al.[803] of Akita, Japan suggested microbiological studies of the intestinal lymph follicle as a potential site of the microbial agent since "the macroscopically earliest lesion takes place in the lymph follicle."

The newer techniques of bacterial identification: DNA hybridization, genomic fingerprinting, search for extrachromosomal genetic elements (plasmid profiles, phages) and the polymerase chain reaction, should aid the search for new pathogens. The remarkable integrity of the normal gastrointestinal epithelium, exposed continuously to large numbers of "normal" aerobic and anaerobic bacteria and viruses, their constituents and metabolic products and to the many other elements of the complex gut content (in symbiosis with their human host's oral tolerance) remains a continuing challenge to the understanding of inflammatory bowel disease.

The microbiological aspects of IBD also have renewed interest in the potential therapeutic benefits of "restoring" the "normal" intestinal microflora by probiotics (B. acidophilus, Bifidobacteria, Lactobacillus, Nissle strain of E. coli) as adjuncts to conventional treatment,[804,805] described by Rettger and Chaplin of Yale (New Haven, Conn.) in 1921[806] and 1922[807] and Kopeloff in 1926.[808] According to Schrezenmeir and deVrese,[809] this concept originated much earlier. In a Persian version of the Old Testament (Genesis 18:8), it states that "Abraham owed his longevity to the consumption of sour milk." In 76 BC the Roman historian Plinius recommended the administration of fermented milk products for treating gastroenteritis.[810] Mechanisms of beneficial effect of probiotics include re-establishment of normal enteric microecology, restoration of normal intestinal permeability, enhancement of macrophage activity and gut-specific IgA responses, stimulation of the humoral immune response and perhaps as yet unidentified anti-bacterial pathogen action. These effects of probiotics are not exclusive to IBD and apparently are applicable also in children with atopic disease.[811]

IMMUNE MECHANISMS

Arnold R. Rich[812] of Johns Hopkins University (1893–1968), in his 1946 Harvey Lecture on Hypersensitivity in Disease, dates the earliest views on hypersensitivity and immunological reactions to Edward Jenner's[813] 1801 observation that "infection can alter the body in a manner that will cause its tissues to react with increased intensity to subsequent contact with the infective agent." Subsequently, E. Metchnikoff (1845–1916),[814,815] P. Ehrlich (1854–1915)[816] and C.E. Von Pirquet,[817] R. Koch (1843–1910), L. Pasteur (1822–1895), E. von Behring, among many other investigators, made early fundamental contributions to the understanding of immunity. Metchnikoff "was the first to understand the pivotal role of phagocytic cells in host defense ... and the first to formulate an immunologic theory."[818] The first known antibody, tetanus antitoxin, was described by Behring and Kitasato in 1890. "In the 1930s and 1940s, immunologists and biochemists, Landsteiner, Heidelberger, Marrack, Morgan and Kohler, established immunology on chemically secure foundations" (P. Medawer. Modern Immunology in Perspective). For further historical details see A.M. Silverstein – The History of Immunology in Fundamental Immunology, W.E. Paul, Editor, Raven Press, New York, 1984 and P. Graber – The Historical Background of Immunology in Basic and Clinical Immunology, D.P. Stites, J.D. Stobo, H.H. Fudenberg, J.V. Wells, Editors, Lange Medical Publications, Los Altos, California, 1984.

More than 100 years elapsed before the important role of the gastrointestinal tract in the immune homeostasis of the body was recognized.[819] Besredka[820] in 1919 demonstrated that oral "immunization of rabbits protected against otherwise fatal Shiga bacillus infection." Subsequent studies revealed "the efficacy of oral immunization in the prevention of dysentery." In 1922 Davies[821] documented the presence of fecal antibody in the stools of patients with bacillary dysentery before serum antibody appeared. From the 1920s to the early 1950s, numerous experiments demonstrated antibodies in the stools ("coproantibodies") indicating that locally produced (intestinal) rather than serum antibodies (systemic) determined intestinal mucosal resistance to infection.[822–825]

Heremanns[826] (Belgium) (1960), Tomasi et al.[827] (New York) (1965), and Tomasi and Bienenstock[828] (1968), (McMaster University, Hamilton, Ontario, Canada) later identified the secretory IgA class of immunoglobulins and their important role in the emerging field of mucosal immunity of the gastrointestinal tract. Gelzayd, Kraft and Kirsner[829] in 1968 demonstrated IgA within the apical portion of the cytoplasm of epithelial cells of normal rectal mucosal glands. Tomasi and Bienenstock[828] in 1968 described the components of the gastrointestinal mucosal immune "system" and their interactions with the neuroendocrine network of the gastrointestinal tract (the lymphoid tissue in Peyers patches and mesenteric lymph nodes, the lymphoid follicles beneath the epithelium in the mucosa, the many lymphocytes within the bowel epithelium, interepithelial lymphocytes, the eosinophils, macrophages and mast cells and the secretory IgA system of the gut). In principle, the mucosal immune system normally down-regulates the antigenic stimulus of the endogenous microflora and the intestinal content in the normal intestine to the level of "physiological" inflammation (the process of oral tolerance).[830] Later reviews further defined the immunological status of the gastrointestinal tract.[831,832]

Immunology of the gut, in relation to the pathogenesis of inflammatory bowel disease, developed, in part, in the context of early (1920s) considerations of "hypersensitivity" (allergy) of mucous membranes of the gastrointestinal tract to foods, pollens and other allergens.[833,834] During the 1920s and 1930s gastrointestinal allergy was implicated in various digestive disorders, including ulcerative colitis. Diagnosis then depended clinically upon the development of symptoms after multiple exposures to the suspected food, following symptom free periods when the food had been eliminated. Early in the 20th century, the recently developed Roentgen ray was utilized temporarily in the "diagnosis" of gastrointestinal allergy. Crispin[835] in 1915 described the roentgen appearance of angioneurotic edema of the pylorus. Duke[836] in 1921 noted by X-ray spasm and irritability of the stomach in response to a specific "food sensitivity." Similar reports[837,838] followed but, with the advance of science, this technique was abandoned. Diagnostic approaches to gastrointestinal allergy subsequently included skin tests, the direct observation of local allergic reactions at gastroscopy or proctoscopy, and the development of peripheral blood eosinophilia or leukopenia following the ingestion of an offending food.[839] A.F.R. Andresen[840,841] (Brooklyn, New York) and A.H. Rowe[842,843] (Oakland-San Francisco, California) independently comparing the ulcerative colitis tissue reaction to an eczematous-type allergic response, postulated an allergic basis for chronic ulcerative colitis (1920s) and for regional enteritis (1930s), implicating pollens and foods (milk, eggs, wheat, potato, orange, tomato, coffee, tea and chocolate). Elimination diets arbitrarily based upon "positive" skin tests to extracts of individual foods led to extreme dietary restrictions, with questionable clinical benefit. Rowe's "elimination" diet consisted of lamb, chicken, tapioca, white potato, rice, potato bread, carrots, squash, butter, salt, sugar and synthetic vitamins, eaten three times daily for weeks.

Since the gastrointestinal tract was the primary reacting tissue, Rider and Moeller[844] of San Francisco, California in 1962 injected extracts of wheat, eggs and milk directly into the rectal mucosa of patients with ulcerative colitis but the "nonspecific," inflammation-induced hyper-reactivity of the ulcerative colitis mucosa invalidated the mucosal responses. Taylor and Truelove[845] (Oxford) in 1961 noted circulating antibodies to milk proteins in ulcerative colitis and described five patients with ulcerative colitis in whom removal of milk and milk products from the diet was associated with clinical improvement.[846,847] The relapse of ulcerative colitis soon after the re-introduction of milk was interpreted as an immunological response to milk proteins although milk can be "irritating" to the bowel without invoking allergy or immunology[848] (e.g. lactase deficiency). Falchuk and Isselbacher[849] of Boston correctly related the circulating antibodies to dietary proteins in patients with inflammatory bowel disease to an increased intestinal epithelial permeability.

While allergy to foods occurs in unusually atopic adult individuals (for example, allergy to fish in an individual whose serum contains specific reagins transferrable to the skin of a normal person,[850]) convincing evidence of food allergy as the cause of "nonspecific" ulcerative colitis or Crohn's disease has not been reported. Pearson[851] and Anderson,[852] considering non-immunologically-related food sensitivity ("pseudo allergy"), later emphasized the weakness of food allergy-IBD concepts in adult illness. Katz, Spiro and Herskovic[853] (Yale University) in 1968 had found "precipitating substances" ("coproantibodies") in the stools of three of four children with "gastrointestinal milk sensitivity" (rectal bleeding), a recognized hypersensitivity disorder in children. Dupont and Heyman[854] of Paris have elaborated the scientific basis of "food protein-induced enterocolitis" (see also L. Mayer[855] and the American Gastroenterological Association[856]).

In 1938, I. Gray and M. Walzer[857,858] of New York produced an allergic reaction in the passively sensitized rectal mucosa of the rhesus monkey. After sensitization of the rectal mucous membrane with human serum containing atopic reagins, a local inflammatory reaction was induced within 10 to 15 minutes by feeding the specific protein (peanuts), characterized by pronounced erythema, edema and hyper-secretion of mucus. This observation was repeated in the mucosa of the ileum and the colon in man[859] (1940), documenting the immunological responsiveness of the gastrointestinal mucosa.

Immune and "autoimmune" mechanisms in the late 1940s were proposed in various diseases of unknown etiology. Alerted by the Gray-Walzer experiments and F.M. Burnett's 1949 Nobel prize-winning clonal selection theory of autoimmunity, a series of personal clinical experiences between 1936 and 1940 suggested the involvement of immune mechanisms also in ulcerative colitis. These events included (a) the abrupt onset of severe ulcerative colitis in a young woman who, with many others, had experienced acute food poisoning at a family picnic; everyone recovered within 24 to 48 hours except for the patient, who developed severe ulcerative colitis (1948) and later died; (b) the association of ulcerative colitis with other immune diseases (e.g. systemic lupus erythematosus,[860,861] Hashimoto's thyroiditis[862] and the association of ulcerative colitis with anti-erythrocyte antibodies[863,864]); (c) the ulcerative colitis developing years later in patients who had experienced an acute amebic dysentery during the 1933–34 Chicago epidemic (?priming "sensitization" of the bowel); (d) the familial occurrences of inflammatory bowel disease;[865] (e) the beneficial effects of ACTH and the adrenal corticosteroids;[866] and (f) the resemblance of the ulcerative colitis tissue reaction (edema, vascular congestion and infiltration of lymphocytes, plasma cells, eosinophils, neutrophils, mast cells and macrophages) to the histologic features of the immune-mediated reactions.

Despite the important observations of Besredka, Davies, Gray and Walzer, Bienenstock and Tomasi, among others, the immunologic resources of the gastrointestinal tract were not fully recognized in the 1950s and this area became a major research project of Kirsner et al. at the University of Chicago. Kirsner and Goldgraber demonstrated the responsiveness of the rabbit colon to the classic Arthus[867] and Shwartzman[868] reactions (see also Z. Maratka[869]). In 1957, Kirsner and Elchlepp,[870] utilizing the novel 1920 J. Auer[871] principle of local autosensitization to foreign protein, produced crystalline egg albumin immune complexes in rabbits. The immune complexes were localized to the distal bowel via the rectal instillation of a very dilute, non-inflammatory solution of formalin.[872] An ulcerative colitis promptly developed in precisely and only in those areas of the rectum demonstrated immunolo-

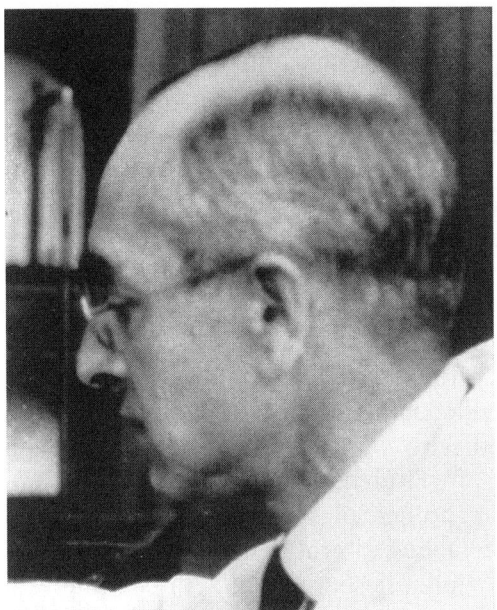

John Auer

gically to contain the immune complexes. Repeated "Auer–Kirsner" reactions in the colon produced "chronic ulcerative inflammation" of the bowel.[873] The Auer–Kirsner phenomenon was reproduced in 1963 by Callahan, Goldman and Burgess Vial[874] (Ann Arbor, Michigan) in colon-sensitized inbred mice and, with modifications, has been utilized as an experimental model of human ulcerative colitis.[875–878] Accinni et al.[879] (Rome, Italy, Buffalo, N.Y.) provided evidence for the intestinal localization of circulating immune complexes, inducing injury to the gastrointestinal tract. S.E. Kirkham et al.[880] of the Massachusetts General Hospital, Boston in 1986 produced an acute enteropathy in rats by the intravenous injection of pre-formed immune complexes (rat anti-bovine serum albumin – bovine serum albumin). The changes ranged from annular bands of serosal hyperemia to hemorrhage, epithelial necrosis and ulceration.

Gebbers and Otto[881] and Nielsen et al.[882] in 1978 demonstrated immune complexes in ulcerative colitis, but their role in the pathogenesis of the disease was unclear. The Gebbers (Hamburg) and Otto (Lucerne) study included immunohistochemistry, electron microscopy and ultracytochemistry and colonoscopically obtained mucosal biopsies in 63 young patients with ulcerative colitis. In active disease IgG was bound to the basement membrane of the surface epithelium together with ClQ and Cs and together with a massive infiltration of polymorphonuclear cells at the surface epithelium, findings interpreted as a local humoral and B cell immune phenomenon, perpetuating the disease. Circulating immune complexes also were demonstrated in Crohn's disease[883,884] and in bacillary and amebic dysentery.[885] R.D. Soltis et al.[886] of Madison, Wisconsin re-evaluated this question in 1979, utilizing four assays minimizing the technical problem of in vitro immunoglobulin aggregation. Their data suggested that circulating immune complexes either were not present in IBD patients or that they occurred infrequently and in low concentration. Other gastroenterologic immunologic experiments included the production of intestinal runt disease in newborn inbred mice and rats injected with adult spleen cells; the lesions did not resemble ulcerative colitis.[887] Elsewhere, delayed hypersensitivity to 2,4-dinitrochlorobenzene in guinea pigs and miniature swine produced lesions histologically resembling ulcerative colitis.[888]

James Gear[889] (Johannesburg, South Africa), interested in the concept of "autoallergic" disease, had stated in 1955: "Many important (autoallergic hyper-reactive) diseases of man may result from the action of autoantibodies developed against tissues made autoantigenic by some alteration in the tissue cells. Such an alteration may be caused by infections, drugs and other chemicals and by physical agents, including X-rays, heat and cold." Gear's interest in the problem developed when investigating homologous serum jaundice produced by certain batches of yellow fever vaccine. He noted a positive precipitin reaction when serum separated from blood collected during the acute phase of the illness was added to serum separated from blood during the convalescent phase of the illness, suggesting the reaction of an antigen (acute phase serum) with corresponding antibody (convalescent phase). When the convalescent serum was added to an extract of normal human liver, a similar precipitin reaction occurred, indicating that the antigen was a component of the liver. The rising interest in immunology and autoimmunity during the 1950s and 1960s now motivated a search for potentially damaging "colon autoantibodies" in ulcerative colitis and for a "specific" UC-colon antigen.

Kirsner and Bregman[890] (Chicago) (1960) preliminarily and O. Broberger and P. Perlmann[891] (Stockholm) (1959), in detail, utilizing the best methodology of the time, demonstrated heterogeneous hemagglutinating and precipitating anticolon "antibodies" in the sera of patients with ulcerative colitis. For the next two decades, the Swedish investigators at the Karolinska Institute and the Wenner-Gren Institute for Experimental

Biology, Stockholm, led the search for colon autoantibodies in ulcerative colitis and for evidence of pathogenetically-significant colonic autoimmunity. In the 1959 Broberger-Perlmann study, the sera of 30 children with ulcerative colitis contained a precipitating and hemagglutinating factor "reacting with one or several constituents of colon, liver and kidney." "The specificity of the antigenic extracts for ulcerative colitis is not absolute," and the sera of a few children with nephrosis, acute nephritis and rheumatoid arthritis also contained precipitating and hemagglutinating antibodies against substances in the phenol water extracts from colon, liver and kidney. "Preliminary experiments did not demonstrate cytotoxic effects for the ulcerative colitis sera." In a 1962 study,[892] sera from thirteen children with ulcerative colitis were examined by immunofluorescent methods for antibodies reacting with constituents of human colonic tissue. Three of 10 sera reacted positively when tested by the direct staining method; 6 of 13 sera reacted positively when tested indirectly with conjugates of rabbit antihuman gammaglobulin. Adsorption on epithelial basement membranes could not be demonstrated. These experiments were interpreted to demonstrate that the serum of children with ulcerative colitis contained gammaglobulin which also reacted with normal colonic antigen in situ. "Although there was no evidence that the circulating antibodies were of any pathogenic significance," the findings were evaluated as compatible with an immunologic pathogenesis.

In 1963, Broberger and Perlmann reported: "no damage of human fetal colonic cells in vitro from exposure to sera from children with ulcerative colitis[893] and specific cytotoxic activity could not be conferred upon normal white cells by pretreating them with patients' serum containing antibodies against colon antigens.[894] However, such an effect appeared upon exposure of the colon cells to an excess of whole blood cells from the peripheral blood of UC patients ... the effect of the lymphocytes seemed to be dependent on the presence, in the medium, of complement." In 1964, Broberger,[895] in the Annual Memorial Lecture of the American Gastroenterological Association, summarized to that time the contributions of the Swedish investigators. He indicated that since the antigen did not come from the same subject as the serum, the term "auto-antibodies" might not be fully justified; also that sensitization to colon-specific antigens "may be of importance for the tissue destruction in ulcerative colitis" but whether this phenomenon was primary or secondary was not known. He concluded: "At present, there is no evidence that immune reactions of this type are exclusively or even primarily responsible for the pathogenesis." It seemed more likely that "a variety of immune and nonimmune reactions contribute to the tissue damage." In 1965 S. Hammarstrom et al.[896] reported that "sera from patients with ulcerative colitis contained antibodies which hemagglutinate sheep red cells sensitized with phenol-water extracts from colon, cecum or feces of germ-free rats." These studies also indicated that "rat extracts (germfree inbred Swedish rats, multiple organs) contained a 'colon' antigen detected with antibodies, present in elevated titers in the sera of ulcerative colitis patients but not in the sera of controls."

Next, to avoid the problem of the inherent contamination of colon tissue with bacterial antigens from the intestinal microflora, in 1965, studies were made with extracts of the large intestine from germfree rats and sera from ulcerative colitis patients.[897] These extracts, in fact, contained antigen reacting with patients' sera, and antibodies which hemagglutinated sheep erythrocytes sensitized with phenol-water extracts from the large intestine of germfree rats. This antigen was similar to that of human colon and experiments with a crude lipopolysaccharide of E. coli 014 suggested a closer relationship between rat intestine and the human intestinal antigen. This lipopolysaccharide also contained, in addition to the type O specific antigen, large amounts of an heterogenetic antigen present in enterobacteriaceae. In 1966 Lagercrantz et al.[898] reported elevated titers of antibodies to an antigen from germfree rats, independent of the patient's age, but higher in females than males of the same age. There was no significant correlation between antibody titers and the duration or severity of the disease, the extent of colonic involvement and the presence of extra-colonic complications. Positive titers also were noted in 5 of 9 female patients with regional enteritis, in 7 of 9 male patients with regional enteritis and occasionally in other groups including two of eight sera from South African controls. The authors concluded that "these antibodies are secondary sequelae of the tissue lesions encountered in ulcerative colitis."

Other laboratories briefly joined in the search for evidence of autoimmunity in IBD.[899-902] Maratka and Wagner,[903] in reporting the presence of "anticolon autoantibodies," concluded: "The reaction was neither constant nor specific." In 1962, R.C. Nairn et al.[904] of Aberdeen, Scotland reported "an antigenic component specific for gastrointestinal mucosa, demonstrated by immunofluorescence and serological methods, using antisera from rabbits immunized with a microsomal fraction of normal human colon mucosa" found in the secretory region of the mucosal cell, apparently an acid mucopolysaccharide. "Similar antigenic material is present in the intestines of sheep, cattle, dogs and rats but not in rodents and not in any other organ studied in man or animals." This "antigen" was absent in patients with gastrointestinal carcinoma;[905] there was no further study of this material. Utilizing fluorescein-conjugated antibodies, Klavins[906] of the University of North Carolina, Durham, N.C. in 1963 demonstrated gammaglobulin combined with the colonic mucosal cells in biopsies from three of seven adults with ulcerative colitis and in one of four children with the disease, identifying the colonic epithelium as the site of an (undefined) antigen-antibody reaction. McGiven, Datta and Nairn[907] (Monash University, Melbourne, Australia) in 1967, reported: "Antibodies reactive with constituents of colon mucosa ... with possible significance in the pathogenesis of ulcerative colitis ... were induced by bowel organisms which share antigens with intestinal mucosa."

In 1967 Perlmann, Hammarstrom, Lagercrantz and Campbell[908] produced autoantibodies to germfree rat colon in rats and found that the antibodies were "specific" for three different colon determinants, including one common for both rat and human colon and a polysaccharide from E. coli 014 and concluded that a cross-reacting bacterial antigen may be an important contributing factor for autoantibody formation in ulcerative colitis. Lagercrantz et al.[909] (1968), investigating the origin of the "autoantibodies" in ulcerative colitis, found that the incidence and level of antibody titers to colon, assayed by indirect hemagglutination with a heat stable colon extract from germfree rats, was significantly higher in sera from patients with ulcerative colitis than in sera from healthy controls, patients with amebic liver abscess or those with bacillary dysentery. While sera from ulcerative colitis patients and controls were indistinguishable from normal in regard to the incidence and level of antibody titers to such antigens as Forsman antigen, Staphylococcus aureus S 209, Clostridium difficile, and several common strains of E. coli, UC sera additionally contained elevated titers of antibodies to a heat stable antigen of E. coli 014. Patients with amebic dysentery had normal titers of E. coli 014 antibodies. Hemagglutination inhibition experiments indicated that germfree rat colon and E. coli 014 shared common structures, including an heterogenetic antigen present in enterobacteriaceae. According to the Swedish investigators, this pattern of reactivity closely resembled that observed in rats made "autoimmune" to colon by the injection of newborn rabbit colon. Lagercrantz et al. had suggested that this antigen might give rise to anticolon antibody formation in ulcerative colitis through "loss of tolerance." Since this antigen also was present in healthy individuals, additional (unspecified) factors were required to explain the development of anti-colon autoimmunity in ulcerative colitis.

Summarizing, Lagercrantz, Hammarstrom, Perlmann, Broberger and Gustafsson stated: "While the occurrence of autoimmunity (in ulcerative colitis) is now well established, its cause is not yet understood. In most patients the serum contains anti-colon antibodies which react with a heat-stable gastrointestinal antigen of human or animal origin, chemically related to but immunologically distinct from the blood group (ABH) substances. The elevated anti-colon antibodies in ulcerative colitis are auto-antibodies and not merely the result of chronic colon damage. Antibody titers are not related to the clinical status of the patients, duration of the disease and other clinical variables ..."

In 1971, Lagercrantz, Perlmann and Hammarstrom[910] examined first-degree relatives of 93 patients with ulcerative colitis for the presence of anticolon antibodies, antibodies to colon-related E. coli 014 antigen and to an unrelated E. coli 075 antigen. Elevated titers to E. coli 014 antigen were found more often in female relatives of ulcerative colitis patients than control subjects. Male relatives did not differ significantly from controls. They concluded: "Taken with previously published evidence, these data are compatible with the hypothesis that a genetic disposition, together with environmental factors, such as cross-reactive bacterial antigens, may lead to autoimmunity in ulcerative colitis. The possible pathogenic significance of autoimmunity to colon in ulcerative colitis remains to be established." In 1977 Carlsson, Lagercrantz and Perlmann[911] reported that, in addition to anticolon autobodies in ulcerative colitis, elevated anticolon titers also were found in patients with liver cirrhosis, urinary tract infections, in gastroenteritis, and in patients with irritable colon, reflecting the heterogeneity of the material, ascribed to cross-reactivity with common antigen (enterobacteriaceae). Females with ulcerative colitis had higher titers than men with the disease.

At the University of Chicago, pursuing the question of autoantibodies to colon, anti-dog colon antibodies were produced by the injection of lyophilized dog colon mucosa into rabbits and iso-antibodies to rabbit colon were produced in rabbits injected with inflamed rabbit colon and Freund's complete adjuvant,[912] but auto-antibody cytotoxicity was not established. Elsewhere, colon "auto antibodies" were produced by the injection of colon tissue and bacteria. In accord with the findings of Lagercrantz et al. and Asherson and Holborow,[913] acting upon the demonstration of colonic "autoantibodies" and upon the possibility that the production of colonic autoantibodies in patients with ulcerative colitis might be stimulated by bacteria present in the bowel, Cooke et al.[914] injected E. coli (014) from the feces of patients with active disease into rabbits and induced antibodies in more than 50% of rabbits. However, there were no morphological changes in the mucosa of the rabbit intestine. The findings were interpreted as minimizing the significance of these autoantibodies in the pathogenesis of ulcerative colitis. One year later, Thayer et al.[915] found higher levels of antibodies to germfree rat feces, germfree rat colon and to E. coli 014 antibodies in patients with inflammatory bowel disease than in other diseases or in healthy controls, but without differentiating between ulcerative colitis and Crohn's disease of the colon, or between proctitis and universal ulcerative colitis.

Differing results were reported from other laboratories. Stefani and Fink (Veterans Administration Hospital, Hines, Illinois)[916] (1967) found that while both ulcerative colitis and normal lymphocytes were "sensitized" to E. coli 014, they were not sensitized to colonic mucosa, contradicting the earlier observation that ulcerative colitis lymphocytes sensitized to E. coli were simultaneously sensitized to autologous colon. S. Tabaqchali et al.[917] of St. Bartholomew Hospital, London in 1978 assayed for the presence of serum antibodies against 159 E. coli 0-antigens, in 30 patients with IBD (14 ulcerative colitis, 16 Crohn's disease) compared with 16 matched control subjects. Most IBD patients had agglutinating antibodies to multiple E. coli 0-antigens (e.g. E. coli 0136, 0144 0124) and in higher titers than controls simply as a reflection of the increased antigenic load. No specific 0-serotypes were associated with IBD. E. coli 014 antibodies were detected in only five patients and 0119 in none. There was no correlation between the numbers of E. coli agglutinins and the site, extent or severity of the disease. A 1973 study of 145 patients with ulcerative colitis by Marcussen and Nerup[918] of Copenhagen, Denmark had demonstrated circulating antibodies against "parts of colon epithelium" in 20% of patients but reproducibility of results was poor. A study from Australia[919] indicated that: "Patients with ulcerative colitis did not show a significant or selective increase in serum hemagglutinating antibodies to E. coli 014 lipopolysaccharide or to enterobacterial common antigen. In addition, patients with chronic liver disease, in whom there was no clinical evidence of colitis, had increased serum antibodies to these antigens ... These observations do not support the hypothesis that ulcerative colitis develops because members of the intestinal flora containing ECA stimulate or perpetuate autoimmune reactions to colonic epithelium in predisposed individuals."

In the search for potential "colon-damaging" antibodies during the 1950s and 1960s,[920] LeVeen et al. (1961)[921] Brooklyn, N.Y., in a limited experiment, utilized an antigen prepared from dog colon to produce dog colon antibodies in rabbits and ducks (actually anti-dog tissue serum). Injection of these colon "antibodies" in six dogs (two with rabbit antigen and four with duck antigens) induced bloody diarrhea from acute ulcerations in the colon. F.C. Shean et al. (UCLA, Los Angeles)[922] (1964) produced an "hemorrhagic colitis" in three of five dogs by the intravenous injection of rabbit anti-dog colon serum using colon removed from mongrel dogs at necropsy (without prior antibacterial treatment). The "anticolon serum" gave substantially identical precipitin patterns to rectum, colon, ileum, jejunum, duodenum and stomach. None of the three dogs reacted to the first dose; each reacted to the second injection. Attempts to induce chronic colitis by multiple injections of extracts of autologous colon mixed with Freund's adjuvant failed. In neither series of experiments was there conclusive immunological evidence of a colon-specific autoimmune reaction. J.J. Bernier, A. Lambling, G. Terris, and W. Cornelis[923,924] of Paris in 1962 and 1963 had induced bloody diarrhea in guinea pigs injected with large quantities of an anti-guinea pig colon serum. Again, these studies, while interpreted as autoimmune events, lacked conclusive immunologic evidence for a colon-specific antigen-antibody reaction.

K. Nordstoga (National Veterinary Institute, Oslo, Norway),[925] commenting on Sanarelli's[926] 1924 finding that necrotic lesions could be produced in the intestinal mucosa of rabbits by intravenous administration of cholera vibrio followed by injection of the culture filtrate of 'colon bacilli' (initial recognition of the Sanarelli-Shwartzman reaction) indicated that a fibrinous colitis may be easily induced in swine by a corresponding method, using viable Salmonella cholerae-suis and disintegrated cells of the same microbe. Capillary thrombosis was one of the main features in porcine fibrinous colitis. Chamovitz et al.[927] Philadelphia (1962) induced hemorrhagic necrosis of the rabbit colon by a single intravenous injection of E. coli 011.B4 endotoxin. Similar results were reported by Patterson et al.,[928] Galveston, Texas, utilizing a different dosage schedule of E. coli endotoxin. Question arises as to whether a Sanarelli-Shwartzman-type phenomenon might explain the earlier described experimental "autoimmune colitis."

Richardson and Leskowitz[929] (Boston, Mass.) in 1961 failed to produce autoimmunity to gastrointestinal tissue following the injection of rabbits, guinea pigs, rats, and mice with gastrointestinal antigens in Freund's adjuvant prepared from homologous stomach, small intestine and colon. McGiven, Ghose and Nairn[930] in 1967 found no evidence in support of a pathogenetic role for the intestinal autoantibodies, though they "may reflect underlying cellular activity by autoimmune lymphoid cells." In their studies of ulcerative colitis patients, utilizing hemagglutination, immuno-fluorescence, and tissue culture techniques, approximately one fifth manifested "intestinal specific" autoantibodies but these were not directed exclusively against colon mucosa. Rabin and Rogers[931] of Pittsburgh in 1976 concluded that "anti-intestinal antibody ... is not a factor in mediating inflammatory changes in the intestine of rabbits immunized with intestine." In 1978,[932] extending earlier studies of a model of ulcerative colitis produced by sensitization of the colon of guinea pigs with dinitrochlorobenzene (DNCB), rabbits were skin sensitized to DNCB and were challenged 10 days later with an intrarectal instillation of DNCB. After three days, mucosal ulceration, crypt abscesses and inflammatory infiltrate appeared in the lamina propria. Healing occurred after five weeks. Rabbits receiving repeated instillations of DNCB converted from a negative delayed hypersensitivity skin response to rabbit colon extract to a positive response. "Thus, a nonspecific cellular reaction in the colon produced histological changes 'compatible with ulcerative colitis' and leads to the production of lymphocytes which are sensitized to colon antigen." This paper prompted an editorial by J.W. Streilein[933] of Dallas, Texas on "Inflammatory Bowel Disease: T Lymphocytes may be the Culprits." Since the histologic appearance of ulcerative colitis is nonspecific, the reproduction of "nonspecific" histologic findings does not necessarily constitute an immune reaction.

R. Shorter et al.[934] (1972), recognizing the infant's immature intestinal defense system and more permeable intestinal epithelium permitting the entry of bacteria (enterobacteriaceae) and other antigens, and characterizing ulcerative colitis and Crohn's disease (IBD) as polar extremes of a single disease, suggested very early "priming" of the gut mucosal immune system, possibly via a gastroenteritis, "preparing" the bowel for later reaction to a constituent of the normal intestinal flora and precipitating "inflammatory bowel disease." In the Shorter hypothesis, bacterial antigens gained access to the intestinal epithelium during infancy, before the normal mucosal block to their uptake was established, creating a potential hypersensitivity state. The subsequent interaction of enterobacterial antigens and "sensitized" (intestinal) T. lymphocytes released proinflammatory biological mediators, initiating the IBD tissue reaction. While "most people probably were immunologically primed to react to enterobacterial antigens given the proper challenge," the occurrence of IBD in some individuals similarly exposed was theoretically attributed to an "innate, individual, possibly genetic, susceptibility."

The 1979 observation of Whorwell et al.,[935] Southhampton, U.K., that approximately 30% of 51 patients with ulcerative colitis had never been breast fed in comparison with 12% of controls, confirmed similar observations by Acheson and Truelove[936] (1961) and by Wright and Truelove[937,938] (1965, 1966) on early weaning in patients with ulcerative colitis, implied a latent early "sensitization" of intestinal immune defenses among children, consistent with the Shorter hypothesis. Since human breast milk, containing secretory IgA, protects against bacterial invasion of the gastrointestinal tract in infants and promotes normal development of the infant intestinal mucosa, the lack of breast milk early in life could be a factor in modifying the immune status of the gut mucosal immune system. The occurrence of an earlier gastroenteritis in 10.5% of patients with Crohn's disease, independent of breast-feeding or bottle-feeding, contrasting with 0.9% for controls, in Whorwell's study also was consistent with Shorter's "priming" concept of the gut mucosal immune system as an antecedent to IBD.

In other aspects of the complex immune process, complement has had an uncertain role in the immunologic response of the intestine. In 1963, Thayer and Spiro[939] of Yale, in a study of 15 patients with ulcerative colitis found normal values for serum complement in the 10 patients whose disease was in remission, elevated in one quiescent case and in the four acutely ill patients. J. Fletcher[940] of Central Middlesex Hospital, London (1965) also reported normal or elevated serum complement in 14 of 15 patients with active ulcerative colitis. In 1975 Ward and Eastwood[941] of Edinburgh reported elevated serum C_4 levels in patients with active ulcerative colitis. In 1975 Hodgson et al.[942] found increased concentrations of C_3 in sera from patients with active ulcerative colitis; Teisberg and Gjone[943] in 1975 reported increased levels of C_c, C_4 and C_3PA in 25 patients with ulcerative colitis; Ross et al.[944] Birmingham, England in 1979 also noted increased levels of C_3 and C_4 in patients with active IBD. The high or normal serum complement levels in ulcerative colitis were in contrast to the low levels of serum complement in classic autoimmune conditions.

The immunology of the gastrointestinal tract and of ulcerative colitis and Crohn's disease had become a major IBD research activity.[945] K.E. Fichtelius and his colleagues[946,947] (Uppsala and Karolinska Institute, Sweden) had described the immune-related properties of lymphocytes of the intestinal mucosa and the circulating blood lymphocytes. Such concepts evolved as "specific lymphocyte-mediated (NK cells) cytotoxicity for autologous and allogeneic colonic epithelial cells,"[948–950] in ulcerative colitis attributed to a lymphotoxin released by the interaction of IBD lymphocytes with colonic target cells,[951–952] a reaction eliminated by total colectomy. In a 1980 study, Kemler and Alpert[953] of Boston reported significantly greater in vitro toxicity of circulating mononuclear cells from patients with IBD for colon epithelial cells compared with cells from healthy controls, irrespective of the clinical activity of IBD.

S.P. James and W. Strober[954] of the National Institutes of Health (Institute of Allergy and Infectious Diseases) (1986), reviewing cytotoxic lymphocytes and intestinal disease, noted "that NK cells are infrequent in the intestine and that NK activity of intestinal lymphocytes is low ..." In studies of human disease, there has been no major difference in cytolytic activity of intestinal lymphocytes from patients with active or inactive IBD, patients with colon cancer and various control patients. They concluded: "The weight of data suggests that NK cells acting as direct cytolytic cells are not important in intestinal disease." In 1995 Elson,[955] University of Alabama, Birmingham, also found this cytotoxicity "unexplained or puzzling ... The finding of substantial lamina propria ADCC (or NK cell) cytotoxicity toward autologous epithelial cells is at odds with the relative lack of K or NK effector cells in the mucosa ... The role that cells cytotoxic for colon cells play in inflammatory bowel disease remains unknown ..."

Serum concentrations of the major immunoglobulins, except for the nutritionally related decreases in serum albumin and the numbers and proportions of circulating T and B lymphocytes generally were normal and did not correlate with the activity or severity of IBD. Bicks, Kirsner and Palmer,[956] in a paper electrophoresis 1959 study of 63 patients with ulcerative colitis, had found decreased serum albumin and nonspecific elevations in A_2 and γ-globulins. Soergel and Ingelfinger[957] in a similar 1961 study of 39 patients with ulcerative colitis reported an absolute decrease in serum albumin and an absolute increase in A_2 globulin. There were no alterations in the γ-globulins and no supporting evidence for an immune mechanism in ulcerative colitis.

Early studies of tissue immunoglobulins in inflammatory bowel disease also yielded variable results of uncertain significance. Probably representing local immune-related manifestations of the inflammatory process, gut-associated immunocytes producing IgA, IgM or IgG were greatly increased in the intestinal lamina propria in both ulcerative colitis and Crohn's disease but in numbers comparable to those found in bacterial colitis. In 1966 Crabbe and Heremans,[958] Louvain, Belgium, had reported large numbers of plasma cells containing IgD in the rectal mucosa of a patient with ulcerative colitis. Gelzayd et al.[959] (1968) found in ulcerative colitis, "that although IgA cells predominated over IgM, IgG and IgD-containing cells, the population density of IgA cells in the lamina propria of the rectal mucosa was lower than in normal rectal tissue" and IgA often was present in extracellular sites. Brandtzaeg et al.[960] (Oslo, Norway) (1974) reported increased numbers of IgA, IgM and IgG-containing plasma cells in colonic tissue specimens from patients with ulcerative colitis. Brandtzaeg also compared 8 patients with active ulcerative colitis with 6 control patients without overt inflammation. "The average total numbers of mucosal IgA and IgM immunocytes in areas with persisting glands were raised 2.2 and 5.2 times, respectively." "The average total numbers of mucosal IgG immunocytes in such cases was raised about 30 times, and the submucosa, in addition, contained a dense immunocyte population with 84% IgG cells," indicative of an intensified local immune response.

In 1979 Brandtzaeg and Baklien,[961] discussing the immunopathology of the intestinal lesion in Crohn's disease, concluded that "a pronounced local activation of the B-cell system takes place associated with an intense secretory Ig response." In 1980 Rosenkrans, Meijer, van der Wal, et al.[962] of Holland, in an excellent morphometric immunoperoxidase study, confirmed the increased number of IgG cells in the colitis mucosa with IgA cells, the major immunoglobulin cell type. A 1987 study by Kett, Rognum and Brandtzaeg[963] of mucosal subclass distribution of immunoglobulin G-producing cells found a significantly higher number of IgG_1 immunocytes in ulcerative colitis than in Crohn's disease. Conversely, the number of IgG_2 immunocytes was significantly higher in Crohn's disease than in ulcerative colitis; differences thought to be important in the pathogenesis of UC and CD. R.P. MacDermott,[964] then at Washington University, St. Louis, related the elevated IgG_1 in serum and in ulcerative colitis colon tissue to an autoimmune mechanism and the increased serum and intestinal IgG_2 in Crohn's disease a response to carbohydrate and bacterial antigens. While serum concentrations of IgE were normal in most patients with ulcerative colitis,[965] Heatley, Calcraft, Fifield et al.,[966] Cardiff, Wales, reported large numbers of IgE-producing cells in rectal biopsies of patients with proctitis and suggested "an immediate hypersensitivity reaction" as one of the mechanisms involved in the pathogenesis of proctitis. However, the anti-IgE compound, disodium chromoglycate, was ineffective therapeutically.

In another immune-related aspect, with variable results, Bendixen[967] (Copenhagen, Denmark) in 1967, proposing a cell-mediated immune mechanism in IBD, reported "specific" inhibition of the in vitro migration of leukocytes in ulcerative colitis by (ulcerative colitis) colonic and jejunoileal mucosal homogenates (nature, specificity?), interpreted as reflecting hypersensitivity to an (unidentified) constituent of normal colonic or jejuno-ileal mucosa. Leukocytes from patients with Crohn's disease did not show this reactivity. Sachar et al.[968] in 1973 described impaired lymphocyte responsiveness in IBD. In 1975, Fixa et al.[969] (Jradia Kralove, Czechoslovakia) reported inhibition of leukocyte migration by "antigens" from human colon and by E. coli 014 in patients with ulcerative colitis; the characteristics of the antigens were not described. S.G. Meuwissen[970,971] of Amsterdam, Holland, pursuing this observation in Crohn's disease in 1975 and 1977, observed decreased in vitro lymphocyte activity, after exposure to a "cocktail" of five antigens in 54 patients, contrasting with the responses of 20 healthy controls and less activity than the responses of 18 patients with malabsorption and malnutrition without IBD. Skin reactivity to the intradermal injection of the same five antigens also was diminished, prompting the conclusion "that depression of the anamnestic cellular immune response is a basic feature in Crohn's disease."

Contradictory results were reported by others. In 1973 Asquith, Kraft and Rothberg[972] had found lymphocyte responses to nonspecific mitogens highly variable. Diminished lymphocyte responses also were demonstrable in normal individuals. In 1974 A.G. Bird and S. Britton[973] at the Karolinska Institute found no evidence for decreased lymphocyte reactivity in patients with Crohn's disease. The in vitro lymphocyte proliferative response of Crohn's disease patients in response to PHA and to tuberculin did not differ from normal. There was no evidence for impaired T-cell responsiveness in mesenteric lymph nodes compared with circulating lymphocyte activity in the same patient or in control groups and the proportion of lymphocytes forming rosettes with sheep erythrocytes (a marker for human T cells) was similar to controls. On the other hand, substantial evidence supported the link between malnutrition and reduced cell-mediated immunity.[974] The observations of J. Schwab,[975] University of North Carolina, on suppression of the immune response by microorganisms and of Rhodes, Bartholomew and Jewell[976] on the inhibition of leukocyte motility by drugs used in the treatment of ulcerative colitis indicated the many factors involved in secondary, immune-related reactions. Investigators continued to extend knowledge of immune phenomena associated with IBD but, as reviews[977-981] indicated, there were no immunologic "breakthroughs."

More recently, the possible "autoimmune" significance of the 40K Das antigens present on the plasma membrane of colonic epithelial cells, found only in patients with ulcerative colitis, associated with Ig immunoglobulins bound to colonic tissue[982–984] renewed interest in colonic autoimmunity. The presence of "autoantibodies" reactive to the Mr-40,000 protein-epitope noted also in the captive cottontop tamarin (S. oedipus) with colitis and the expression of the Mr-40,000 protein only in the colonic epithelium, as observed in human ulcerative colitis, appeared more consistent with an environmentally acquired abnormality of microbial origin. The Das antigen subsequently was identified as a two peptide protein with a molecular weight of 40 KD. The amino acid sequence of each peptide matched with the cytoskeletal tropomysins, "microfilamental proteins present in all eukaryocytic cells with organ specific isoforms." Overall, these studies demonstrated the presence of colon tissue-bound disease-specific IgG (CCA-IgG) in the colonic tissue of patients with ulcerative colitis. Similar IgG was found circulating in the serum of UC patients. The question yet remains as to whether these peptides act as autoantigens in ulcerative colitis.[985]

Numerous studies during the 1960s, 1970s and 1980s had demonstrated in patients with IBD a wide variety of circulating "antibodies" and "reactants:" antinuclear factors, IgM antibodies, cross-reactive with E. coli, antibodies against surface antigens in mucus-secreting colonic epithelial cells, fetal colonic tissue and against colonic epithelium from germfree rats, and antibodies to intestinal epithelial antigens in patients with IBD and their relatives.[986,987] These heterogeneous antibodies were not present in all patients with IBD, did not correlate with the age or sex of the patient, a family history of IBD, the extent, duration or severity of IBD and were not pathogenic for colon epithelial cells in vitro or in vivo.[988] IBD serum also contained "antibodies" to cow's milk protein, gastric parietal cells, bile ductule epithelium, pancreatic homogenates, rheumatoid factor, anti-erythrocyte antibodies, antibodies to thyroglobulin, adrenal antibodies, small intestinal mucous cells, and various proteins, including orosomucoid, haptoglobin, ceruloplasmin, transferrin and bovine albumin, reflecting the increased intestinal permeability ("leakiness") of the chronically inflamed bowel.[989,990] The agglutinins to bacteria and the elevated serum antibodies to antigens of seven enteric bacterial pathogens in patients with active Crohn's disease further reflected the increased intestinal permeability in CD and the nonspecific heterogeneity of the antibody responses.[991,992]

Calabresi et al.[993] of New Haven, Conn. (Yale), utilizing the fluorescent antiglobulin technique, had demonstrated circulating antinuclear globulins in ulcerative colitis in 1961. In 1990 antineutrophil cytoplasmic IgG antibodies were demonstrated in patients with ulcerative colitis[994] and their healthy relatives, less often in Crohn's disease or in the infectious colitides, and initially were proposed as a marker of genetic susceptibility to ulcerative colitis. However, serum antineutrophil cytoplasmic antibodies also were demonstrated in the captive cottontop tamarin colitis, consistent with an acquired abnormality rather than a genetic marker.[995] Their presence and titers were not correlated with disease activity or with the site of the inflammation.[996] Targan,[995] Cedars Sinai Hospital, Los Angeles, added: "Colombian cottontop tamarins neutrophils contain antigens recognized by immune globulins from the ANCA-positive serum of patients with ulcerative colitis. However, cottontop tamarins do not generate serum IgG reactive to cottontop or human neutrophils ..." Serum antineutrophil cytoplasmic antibodies also were demonstrated in patients with primary sclerosing cholangitis and in a few instances of biliary cirrhosis but not in patients with hepatitis B or C.

Overall, the early immunologic studies had revealed significant gastrointestinal-immunologic relationships:[997] the importance of the gastrointestinal lymphoid tissue in the immunologic homeostasis of the body; the close association of the secretory IgA system with gastrointestinal tract defenses, and the common mucosal immunologic system involving the bronchus, breast and bowel.[998] However, with advancing immunologic knowledge and technology, the limitations of the early immunologic experiments became evident: the lack of damaging effects of colon autoantibodies upon colonic epithelial cells, the inability to identify a specific ulcerative colitis colon antigen and the variable reproducibility of early immune studies. Sachar, Auslander and Walfish[999] (Mt. Sinai, New York) in their 1980 comprehensive review of past IBD immunologic studies concluded: "With respect to the evidence implicating immune mechanisms in the tissue damage of ileitis and colitis, we can conclude that the disease process probably induces immune aberrations in the host and that the inflammatory reaction may even be mediated in part via immune effector pathways. To date, however, the case for any primary pathogenetic role of immunological factors in IBD remains unproven." In 1991, Targan, Karp and Shanahan,[1000] in an overview of the immunopathogenesis of inflammatory bowel disease, re-emphasized the inconclusive and often conflicting early immunologic data on colon autoantibodies and colonic autoimmunity.

Immunologic investigation now turned to the nature of oral tolerance and the intriguing concept of defective immune regulation of the endogenous microbial flora by the intestinal mucosal immune system, a "dysfunction" attributed by Mayer and Eisenhardt[1001] of Mt. Sinai (NY) Hospital to the possibility "that there may be an intrinsic defect in intestinal epithelial cells of patients with IBD, resulting in their inability to normally stimulate suppressor T cells in an antigen overloaded environment." "In contrast to normal enterocytes, 42/42 Crohn's and 35/38 ulcerative colitis-derived epithelial cells stimulated CD^{4+} T cells, whereas 65/66 and 9/9 normal and inflammatory control enterocytes respectively stimulated CD^{8+} T cells ... Furthermore, IBD enterocytes from both histologically involved and uninvolved tissue were similar in their ability to selectively activate CD^{4+} T cells."

In 1991, MacDermott and Elson[1002] listed important IBD-related immunologic advances as: the gut mucosal immune system, the protective role of secretory IgA, the biology of the intraepithelial lymphocytes (the first immune cells to encounter pathogens invading epithelial surfaces), the role of the M-cell in antigen sampling, the function of Peyer's patches as inductive immunologic sites, the immunoregulatory cytokines, and the regulatory role of neuropeptides in intestinal immune responses.

Comment

Although early immunological studies had demonstrated a central role for the gastrointestinal tract in the immunological defenses of the body,[1003] fifty years (1950–2000) of research have not fully clarified the immunologic status of inflammatory bowel disease and have not produced conclusive evidence for an intrinsic defect in the immunologic defenses of the IBD patient, antedating the onset of IBD. Most, if not all, of the immunologic phenomena described thus far appear to represent secondary events, associated with a chronically activated gut mucosal immune system.[1004] With the advance of immunologic knowledge and technology,[1005] the limitations of the initial "immune" studies became increasingly apparent and their importance as primary immune events (e.g. lymphocyte cytotoxicity, inhibition of leukocyte migration) declined. The pathogenetic significance of the circulating "autoantibodies" in ulcerative colitis and Crohn's colitis also diminished.[1006–1008] Seibold and Scheurlen[1009] concluded in 1999: "None of the antibodies is of pathogenetic relevance but may be the consequence of a disturbed regulation of the immune system."

The antinuclear cytoplasmic antibodies in ulcerative colitis and the antibodies to saccharomyces cerevisiae mannan in Crohn's disease also appeared to represent responses to disease rather than primary disease "markers." Rutgeerts and Vermeire[1010] stated: "Ulcerative colitis-asso-

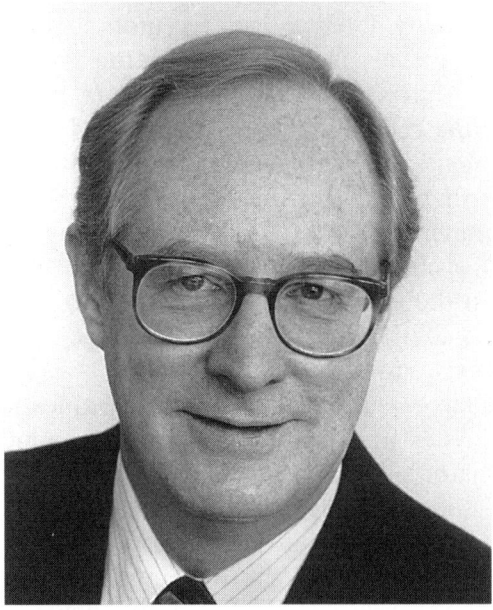

C.O. Elson

ciated ANCA (probably representing cross-reactivity with enteric bacterial antigens) ... is produced by B cells on the colonic mucosa and react with a 50 KDa nucleus envelope protein of neutrophils. ASCA associated with Crohn's disease react to yeast cell-wall phosphopeptido-mannans (present also in the cell wall of mycobacteria and Candida albicans) ..."

While evidence documenting the incorporation of viral antigen from an experimental porcine adenovirus into the epithelium of the small intestine[1011] and the presence of bacterial constituents within the bowel wall (e.g. diaminopimelic acid) provided biological opportunities for "an acquired colonic auto-immunogenicity" in ulcerative colitis, conclusive evidence of colonic autoimmunity in IBD is yet to be documented. Shanahan and Targan[1012] concluded in 1992 that "although autoimmunity might contribute to the perpetuation of disease, the primary mechanism of tissue injury probably does not involve a direct autoimmune assault on a specific target cell." Interestingly, "natural autoimmunity can also be a factor of health."[1013]

Immunological issues of current IBD interest include further characterization of the Th_1 (Crohn's disease) and Th_2 (ulcerative colitis) immune-cytokine responses, the nature of oral tolerance[1014] and its potential therapeutic applicability, T cell antigen receptors,[1015] antigen processing by the intestinal epithelial cells,[1016] including the interaction of intestinal epithelial cells and intraepithelial lymphocytes in host defense,[1017] the role of non-immune cells (fibroblasts, muscle and vascular endothelial cells), the interactions of the gut mucosal system with the neuroendocrine system,[1018] with the enteric nervous system,[1019] cytokine regulation of gut mucosal immune function,[1020] and the role of the IL-6S IL-6R system in the persistence of chronic intestinal inflammation.[1021] Recent observations indicate that the epithelial cell plays an active role in the immune response and is capable of producing upregulating cytokines (e.g. IL-2, IL-4, IL-6) and downregulating PG_2, NO and TGF-β cytokines. New technological resources, such as the microarray expression technology to determine "the genes and pathways underlying regulation of autoimmune/inflammatory disease ... especially immune pathways which may play a role in susceptibility and resistance to such illness,"[1022,1023] reflect the progress to be anticipated in the future.[1024–1027]

Citing C.O. Elson (1999), "... the working pathogenetic hypothesis, especially for Crohn's disease, suggests a dysregulated immune response of the mucosal immune system to normal (commensal) enteric bacterial antigens." "... Regardless of the specific immune cells driving the process in IBD, a final common pathway of inflammation, involves cells and cytokines of the innate immune system, with many manifestations of active disease mediated through their production of cytokines and other inflammatory mediators." As the gastrointestinal immunologic frontiers advance, the microbial-neurogenic-immune and genetically-influenced interactions with the intestinal epithelium represent significant approaches to the etiopathogenesis of ulcerative colitis and Crohn's disease.

M CELL

Two additionally important aspects of the immune-mediated inflammatory response in IBD involve the intestinal M cell and epithelial permeability. The M (membranous, microfold) cell is a specialized epithelial cell characterized by luminal surface microfolds rather than microvilli overlying the gut-associated (also bronchial-associated) lymphoid tissues, which transport bacterial, viral or food antigens from the intestinal lumen to the extracellular space, allowing access to lymphocytes, macrophages and plasma cells and to the mucosal immune system.[1028–1030] The M cell was identified in 1923 when K. Kumagai,[1031] Nagoya, Japan, demonstrated the uptake of ink, carmine dye, powdered erythrocytes and living or dead mycobacteria from the intestinal lumen into the rabbit appendix and/or Peyer's patches via specialized cells in the intestinal epithelium. In 1965 J.F. Schmedtje,[1032] Tufts University, Boston, Mass., studying the epithelium of the rabbit appendix, designated such cells overlying lymphoid follicles as "lympho-epithelial cells." R.L. Owen and A.L. Jones[1033] of San Francisco (1974) coined the term M cells. Their important status in inflammatory bowel disease, especially as to the recognition and transepithelial transport of bacterial and viral antigens to the mucosal immune system, continues under investigation.[1034–1036] The immunologically-presenting antigen-presenting dendritic cells also are under investigation.[1037]

EPITHELIAL PERMEABILITY

The permeability of the normal gastrointestinal wall to unaltered protein has been known for many years.[1038] Human intestinal permeability in relation to disease was first evaluated by J. Fordtran et al.[1039] (Houston, Texas) in 1965, I.S. Menzies of England in 1974[1040] and by W.A. Walker (Boston) in 1975[1041] but their studies did not include inflammatory bowel disease. In 1982 Pearson et al.[1042] used mannitol and lactulose as screening probe molecules to measure intestinal permeability in children and documented a sixfold increase in permeability (lactulose) in active small bowel Crohn's disease. J. Madara and his colleagues[1043] (Emory University, Atlanta, Georgia) have extensively studied the intestinal epithelial structure as it relates to barrier function and the state of this barrier in active inflammation (IBD).

The barrier function of the intestine (permeability) as a factor in the pathogenesis of gastrointestinal disease did not attract interest until the 1970s and since then has increased in importance. In 1986 and 1992 D. Hollander and his colleagues, (University of California, Irvine, California)[1044,1045] using polyethylene glycol-400 as a permeability probe, demonstrated increased intestinal permeability in many patients with Crohn's disease and postulated the increased entry of bacteria and bacterial products into the intestinal wall, initiating or participating in the inflammatory reaction. Of particular interest was the increased intestinal permeability in 25% of healthy relatives of Crohn's disease patients, presumably of genetic origin. Although numerous studies confirmed these observations, the mechanism of the increased intestinal permeability in Crohn's disease related in part to microbial action and to the use of NSAIDS remains under investigation. A. Darfeuille-Michaud et al.[773] suggested that entero-adherent E. coli strains in ileal mucosa may disrupt the intestinal barrier by synthesizing a hemolysin. Environmental stress increases gastrointestinal permeability transiently in rats, mediated by glucocorticoids.[1046] Stress also may increase intestinal permeability via neuronal activation of mucosal mast cells.[1047]

Irvine and Marshall[1048] of McMaster University, Hamilton, Ontario, Canada recently described the course of a 24-year-old woman with a family history of Crohn's disease, who had an increased gut permeability at age 13 recognized "as part of a cross-sectional cohort study in patients and their first degree relatives." Repeated study at age 21 because of diarrhea and weight loss revealed ileocolonic Crohn's disease requiring steroids; an unequivocal instance of an intestinal permeability defect preceding the onset of Crohn's disease. Further progress in clarifying the important role of epithelial permeability in IBD depends in part on the development of more selective probes with regard to the anatomic regions of involvement with Crohn's disease[1049] and increased understanding of the physiological regulation of intercellular tight junctions in the small intestine.[1050] Burns et al.,[1051] Seattle, Washington, recently have demonstrated that certain microbial pathogens may breach the epithelial barrier by direct transit through the absorptive villus enterocyte. Garcia-Lafuente et al.[1052] have shown that bacteria colonizing the rat colon mucosa may increase intestinal permeability to hydrophilic compounds and render the mucosa susceptible to injury.

INFLAMMATION (CYTOKINES, LYMPHOKINES)

Interest in the biology of inflammation and its interaction with immune mechanisms dates back more than 100 years to studies of phagocytosis by Elie Metchnikoff[1053] in 1883 and to the observations on humoral immunity by Paul Ehrlich[816] (1908).

During the 1950s and 1960s, the tissue reaction of ulcerative colitis was variously attributed to enzymes (e.g. pancreatic trypsin), fibrinolytic agents, mast cell products, especially histamine, 5-hydroxytryptamine and bradykinin (see also Stenson[1054]). Valy Menkin of the Fearing Research Laboratories, Boston, and later Temple University, Philadelphia[1055,1056] in 1931 and 1944 had described a biologic agent, necrosin, capable of causing cellular inflammation and had identified a variety of other inflammation-related molecules, including leukotoxin, pyrexin and leukopexin[1057] but these findings were never applied to the problem of IBD. Interest subsequently extended to phospholipase A and the cell-membrane-based arachidonic acid cascade and to studies with animal models of IBD demonstrating an increased eicosanoid production by the inflamed intestinal tissue, including increases in products of both the cyclooxygenase and lipooxygenase limbs of the arachidonic acid cascade.

As noted by M.B. Grisham: "McCord and Fridovich,[1058] Durham, North Carolina, in 1969 were the first to discover the enzyme superoxide dismutase (SOD) and to recognize the superoxide anion free radical is produced in mammalian systems. Up to that time, no one actually had believed that reactive free radicals could be generated in living systems. Bernard Babior[1059] of Boston was the first to demonstrate that activated polymorphonuclear cells (PMNs) produce large quantities of the superoxide anion radical. The importance of PMN-derived free radicals later was confirmed using PMNs from patients with chronic granulomatous disease. Following the publication of this paper, many investigators[1060,1061] related inflammatory tissue injury to reactive oxygen molecules. "The first demonstration that reactive oxygen metabolites could play a major role in intestinal pathophysiology was reported by D.N. Granger and colleagues,[1062] Mobile, Alabama, who demonstrated that post-ischemic microvascular injury in the small bowel could be attenuated by the intravenous administration of superoxide dismutase." Today, reactive nitrogen metabolites, in addition to reactive oxygen metabolites, also are implicated in the IBD inflammation.[1063]

Grisham and Granger[1064] also were among the first to consider the possibility that immunologically-activated phagocytic leukocytes (e.g. PMNs, eosinophils, macrophages) could be important contributors to the mucosal injury characterizing intestinal and colonic inflammation. They also demonstrated the inhibitory effect of 5 aminosalicylic acid upon free oxygen radicals with healing of intestinal lesions. In 1975, Gould[1065] of England found increased levels of the cyclooxygenase prostaglandins (PGE_2) in the stools of patients with ulcerative colitis. Sharon et al.,[1066] Jerusalem, Israel, extended these observations in 1978 and also noted elevated levels of prostaglandins of the cyclooxygenase pathway in the colonic mucosa, the serum and the stools of patients with ulcerative colitis. In 1984 Sharon and Stenson,[1067] Washington University, St. Louis, demonstrated a 50-fold increase in the leukotriene LTB_4 and mono HETEs in the colonic mucosa of ulcerative colitis and postulated a proinflammatory role for LTB_4 in both ulcerative colitis and Crohn's disease. Subsequent studies with a specific inhibitor of LTB_4 demonstrated significant healing of experimental colonic inflammation[1068] but therapeutic studies in patients were unimpressive.

The interrelationship of the immune response in IBD with the inflammatory process and the regulatory role of the cytokines-lymphokines produced by immunologic effector cells and lamina propria cells now was recognized as extremely important in understanding the nature of intestinal inflammation. Cytokines are low molecular weight soluble peptides produced by various "producer" cells responding to inducing stimuli (e.g. cancer, autoimmunity), influencing the behavior of particular target cells in specific surface receptors. Lymphokines is the arbitrary term applied to cytokines produced by immune cells. Cytokines act in an autocrine or paracrine manner, participate in the regulation of the immune response and help orchestrate the complex process of inflammation. Lymphokines/cytokines are major determinants of immune responsiveness to antigens crossing the epithelium ... capable of stimulating cell growth and differentiation, inducing acute phase reactants and modulating the effects of inflammatory cells.[1069] Cytokines are identified as proinflammatory (IL-1β, IL-8, IL-6 and TNF-α) and anti-inflammatory (IL-4, IL-10, IL-11, TGF-β) and immunologically as Th_1 (IL-2, IFN-γ, TNF-β) and as Th_2 (IL-4, IL-6, IL-10). Interest in lymphokines/cytokines dates to the 1972 discovery of a factor produced by macrophages stimulating T cell responses to antigens,[1070] later designated as interleukin-a (IL-1) (perhaps known earlier in the 1940s as endogenous pyrogen[1071] and to the discovery of interleukin-2 (IL-2) by Paetkau et al.,[1072] Alberta, Canada, and by Chen and di Sabato[1073] (Nashville, Tennessee) in 1976. In 1985, according to G. Majno,[1074] (Worcester, Massachusetts) approximately 50 cytokines/lymphokines were identified, including interleukins 1 through 10, tumor necrosing factor, transforming growth factors, platelet activating factor (PAF) and colony stimulating factor (CSF). In addition, experimental therapeutic approaches with protective anti-inflammatory molecules (e.g. IL-10)[1075] are in progress. Today, many more biological molecules (pro-, anti-inflammatory, aggressive/protective) have been identified (e.g. defensins,[1076,1077] integrins, statins, selectins, claudins, annexins, laminins, intimins, aquaporins, microcins) and more are yet to be identified.

As noted earlier, initial studies identified proinflammatory LTB_4 and interleukin-1 and the possible cytoprotective prostaglandin E_2 in inflammatory bowel disease. "The numerous biologic activities of interleukin-1,[1078] in particular, implicated interleukin-1 as a key participant in both the distinctive and restorative processes that follow infection or injury." Of interest in relation to the increased tendency of the Crohn's disease process to involve the distal ileum and the neoterminal ileum is the observation by

Lilja et al.,[1079] Malmo, Sweden, that "mast cells may be an important source of TNF-α production in all layers of the ileal wall." Research on lymphokine/cytokine profiles, their interactions with the products of activated macrophages, and mast cells (histamine, prostaglandins, leukotrienes) and with the neurohumoral and neurotransmitter peptides of the enteric nervous system, the role of molecules, such as nitric oxide, the IκB, NF-κB system,[1080] and other biologically active molecules (TNF-α, INF, IL-7, IL-10, IL-12, IL-15, IL-16, IL-18) in the tissue reaction of ulcerative colitis and of Crohn's disease today is the most active area of investigation in IBD.

A further advance in understanding the complex network of immune-cytokine responses in IBD has been recognition of Th_1-type and Th_2-type inflammatory-immune responses.[1081] As summarized by Chen et al. (Hong Kong):[1082] "On antigen challenge, Th-helper cells differentiate into two functionally distinct subsets, Th_1 and Th_2, characterized by the different effector cytokines that they secrete." See also T.R. Mossman and R.I. Coffman.[1083] Th_1 cells produce interleukin-(IL)-2, interferon-γ (IFN-γ and lymphotoxin B which mediate proinflammatory functions critical for the development of cell-mediated immune response, whereas Th_2 cells secrete cytokines such as IL-4, IL-5 and IL-10 that enhance humoral immunity. Th_1 characterizes the Crohn's disease type of tissue reaction; Th_2 defines the ulcerative colitis response. W. Strober et al. (NIH)[1084] in 1998 outlined the pathogenesis of mucosal inflammation in murine models of inflammatory bowel disease and its relationship to Crohn's disease. In a recent workshop on advances in the molecular cell biology of inflammation, W. Doe,[1085] Australian National University, Canbarra City, Australia, emphasized four elements of the mucosal inflammatory response: the expression of adhesion molecules, the activation of mucosal inflammatory cells, the anti-inflammatory and immuno-suppression roles of IL-10 and the regulation and expression of IL-1 and IL-1 receptor antagonist.

The important transcription factor NFκB discovered in 1986[1086] is of particular interest today because of its regulation of multiple genes and biological responses, including TNF-α and its involvement in various human diseases, including IBD.[1087] Nuclear factor kappa B, representing a family of pleiotropic transcription factors, is present in the cytoplasm of most cells. NFκB controls a variety of cellular genes regulating transcriptional activity of various promoters of proinflammatory cytokines, cell surface receptors and adhesion molecules involved in intestinal inflammation. Although many regulatory peptides and other bioactive molecules

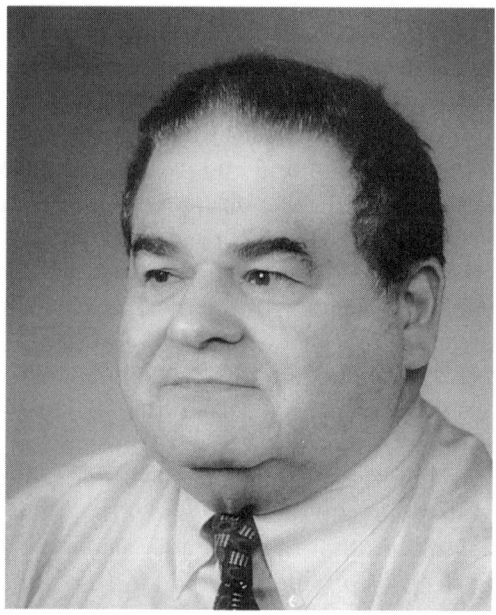

Warren Strober

that contribute to the amplification in IBD and its downregulation have been identified, many more are expected;[1088] multiple targets for future therapeutic intervention. Further investigation of the Th_1 and Th_2 cytokine patterns and the nature of the intracellular signalling pathways, as illustrated by the results of blockade of NFκB activation in animal models of IBD, will provide additional opportunities to target pivotal mediators of inflammation in IBD. Reinshagen et al.,[1089] University of Ulm, Germany, in 1999 concluded: "The sensory enteric nervous system is involved in the regulation of inflammation by releasing proinflammatory and anti-inflammatory sensory neuropeptides in response to the inflammatory stimulus ... this system is under the control of neurotrophic mediators such as nerve growth factor which might serve as the prototypic mediator of neuro-immune interactions in the gut."

As noted by Fiocchi (Case Western Reserve University, Cleveland, Ohio), "There is no evidence for congenital abnormalities of cytokine synthesis in UC or CD ... hence, a non-primary defect of soluble mediators production is not the cause of IBD ... However, ... cytokines are almost certainly involved in IBD pathogenesis." "Their actual production in vitro and abnormal levels in vivo translate evidence for some abnormality of immunoregulation in inflammatory control, implicating them in the mechanism of disease ... as indicated by the favorable clinical response to their blockade or to the administration of anti-inflammatory cytokines ..." Fiocchi adds, "the seemingly endless complexity of these substances contains critical clues to the basic mechanisms of disease and potential new approaches to more specific therapeutic interventions," a viewpoint emphasized further by Standiford,[1090] Bregenholt,[1091] Papadakis and Targan,[1092] and by Kubes and McCafferty.[1093] Comprehensive information on cytokines, chemokines, growth factors, eicosanoids and other bioactive molecules has been published by D.K. Podolsky and C. Fiocchi[1094] and by H.J.F. Hodgson.[1095]

GENETIC ASPECTS OF INFLAMMATORY BOWEL DISEASE – EARLY OBSERVATIONS

The first published instances of familial IBD from the 1909 London symposium on ulcerative colitis: (a) brother and sister, (b) father and sibling, and (c) father and sister of a third patient were dismissed as "coincidences."[34] A French instance of "familial" ulcerative colitis was reported at the 1935 Brussels Congress of Gastroenterology. Individual case reports by Kirsner[425] (1948), P. Sherlock and T. Almy[1096] in 1963, Barker[1097] (1962), the 1963, 1971 and 1973 studies by Kirsner et al.,[865,1098,1099] and by R. McConnell[1100] (1966) increased clinical interest in "familial IBD." Reports[1101–1103] of "familial" inflammatory bowel disease in twins[1104–1106] further indicated a genetic influence in IBD.

Ulcerative Colitis

In 1936 Moltke[1107] had described 5 families with ulcerative colitis (mother and daughter, 2; brother and sister, 2; and father and daughter, 1). Many similar reports followed.[1108–1110] Sloan, Bargen and Gage[89] (1950) noted 26 positive family histories among 2000 patients. Paulson[1111] and Kirsner and Palmer[135] (1954) each reported 6 family occurrences. Banks, Korelitz and Zetzel,[1112] Beth Israel Hospital, Boston (1957), identified 9 families among 244 patients. The seven families studied by Houghton and Naish[552] (1958) included father (ileocolitis) and daughter (ulcerative colitis); father and daughter, 2: and 2 brothers, 1 with ileocolitis and Bacon[1113] (1958), 3 familial instances: (a) twin brothers and sister, (b) mother and son and (c) two cousins.

Additional clinical studies of "familial" IBD followed. Schlesinger and Platt[1114] (1958) obtained a family history of ulcerative colitis in 17% of 60 children with ulcerative colitis; almost one-fourth of the series were of Jewish origin, fourfold higher than the usual ethnic distribution of the hospital population. The 1963 Chicago study included multiple family occurrences in 66 of 1084 patients with ulcerative colitis. An unusual sequence of events involved two brothers, who developed ulcerative colitis each succumbing to carcinoma of the colon within 15 years after onset of the disease (Gassaniga and Gassaniga[1115] 1962).

Crohn's Disease

Crohn and Yarnis[380] in 1958 wrote: "Ulcerative colitis ... rarely occurs in more than one member of a family ... on the other hand, regional ileitis or enteritis occurs in multiple instances of blood-related family members sufficiently often to warrant attention," and they recorded 12 instances of familial involvement including three family groups (a) young woman, brother and half-brother with ileitis and father with ulcerative colitis; (b) ileitis, segmental colitis and ulcerative colitis in three adult siblings; and (c) a child and her two blood-related aunts with ileitis, confirmed at operation.

Early familial instances of regional enteritis were reported by many observers. One of the Houghton-Naish families included a brother with regional enteritis and a sister with ileocolitis. Aronson and Ruoff[1116] in 1969 reported the occurrence of Crohn's disease in a father and both siblings. In the family reported by Kuspira et al.,[1117] six members were affected, spanning three generations.

Familial Patterns – UC and CD

Familial distributions of IBD involved first-degree relatives (parent, child or siblings) more often than second-degree or third-degree relatives[1099] (aunts, uncles, nieces and nephews). In the 1963 Chicago study for ulcerative colitis, 50 of the 89 family members were brothers and sisters and cousins, approximately the same generation as that of the probands and 11 were grandparents. For regional enteritis, 15 of the 22 family members involved brothers, sisters and first cousins.

de Matteis[1118] (1963) summarized 5 reports on ulcerative colitis comprising 20 parent-child combinations; mother and child were involved in 16 and father and child in 4. Among 32 reports on Crohn's disease involving 72 familial instances, mother and child were affected in 7 instances and father and child in 3, suggesting a maternal predominance.

The involvement of father and son, though less common, nevertheless excluded a role for sex-linked genes.

The occurrence of IBD in three or more members of the same family, a possibility estimated as one in 12 billion, strongly supported a genetic influence. Early three family member reports cited by McConnell[1100] and Kirsner[1099,1119] included Moltke (1936): brother, sister and maternal aunt; Brown and Schieffley (1939): 2 sisters and 1 brother; Houghton and Naish (1958): (a) ulcerative colitis in 3 members of 1 family, (b) mother and 3 daughters with ulcerative colitis and a nephew with regional enteritis; Jackman and Bargen[1110] (1942): (a) mother, son and mother's brother; (b) mother and 2 daughters with ulcerative colitis and nephew with regional enteritis; and Bacon[1113] (1958): twin brothers and a sister and in the 1963 Chicago study: (a) mother, brother and sister with ulcerative colitis; (b) 2 sisters and a grandfather with ulcerative colitis; (c) 3 sisters with ulcerative colitis; and (d) 3 sisters and 1 brother with ulcerative colitis. The later occurrences of Crohn's disease (or ulcerative colitis) in the initially healthy mate of a patient with Crohn's disease (or ulcerative colitis) raised the intriguing question of a communicable infectious agent (?viral) acquired after prolonged intimate contact.[1120]

Thayer's personal communication (1972) on an unusual family included a 21-year-old male with ulcerative colitis since the age of 8 who developed a carcinoma of the descending colon. A maternal aunt developed ulcerative colitis at the same time. One year after the death of the index patient, his brother, 2 years younger developed ulcerative colitis and required colectomy and ileostomy. The 8 members of the Morris family[1121] (1965) represented 3 generations, all with ulcerative colitis, 4 males and 4 females, a distribution compatible with the influence of an autosomal dominant gene.

The 7 affected members of the Ashkenazi Jewish family studied by Sherlock et al., Cornell Medical School, New York[1096] (1963), included 5 with regional enteritis and 2 with ulcerative colitis. The index patient was a woman of 48 with regional enteritis of 25 years' duration. Regional enteritis was present in a sister aged 47, brothers, 53 and 55 and in a male first cousin, aged 72. Ulcerative colitis was present in a married sister aged 46 and a nephew aged 16. Seven uninvolved relatives of the family had varying degrees of deafness.

Intermingling of Diseases (UC, CD) – Twins

Ulcerative colitis was more likely to occur than Crohn's disease among the families of probands with ulcerative colitis and the same relationship held for probands with Crohn's disease. However, the disease distribution was mixed in approximately 25% of families. In the 1971 Chicago study, 31 of the 103 positive families included mixed inflammatory bowel disease. The intermingling of IBD, noted by many observers,[1099] suggested a pathogenetic relationship between the two diseases.

The survey of monozygotic twins demonstrated moderate concordance for ulcerative colitis and strong concordance for Crohn's disease, powerful evidence for a genetic influence in inflammatory bowel disease. Discordance was more common for ulcerative colitis than for Crohn's disease.[1122] J. Purrmann et al.[1123] in 1986 reported monozygotic triplets with Crohn's disease of the colon developing within a period of 11 months. Both parents were free of digestive disease. The predominance of concordance in monozygotic twins and discordance in dizygotic twins strengthened the likelihood of a genetic influence in the development of Crohn's disease. The association of ulcerative colitis and Crohn's disease with genetically-mediated conditions, such as for ulcerative colitis: ankylosing spondylitis,[1124,1125] Turner's syndrome[1126] and for Crohn's disease:[1127] Chediak–Higashi syndrome,[1128] psoriasis,[1129] erythrocyte glucose-6-phosphate dehydrogenase deficiency (especially among Jewish patients)[1130,1131] and the Hermansky–Pudlak syndrome[1132] added to the evidence (see Kirsner[1099] for details).

V. Binder et al.[1133] (1966), by questionnaire, compared 152 patients with ulcerative colitis and a control group matched by sex, age, and social class. The colitis series included 8 families with additional affected members (5.3%); whereas the control group had 1 family (0.73%). In the 1971 Chicago study,[1098] a positive family history for IBD was documented in 113 of 646 personally examined patients, 17.5%. As further validation, 150 of the 646 patients were selected at random and were matched by age, sex, race, religion and social status with 50 apparently healthy individuals from the community. A positive family history was noted in 11% of the patients and in 4% of the controls. In 1969 Burch, deDombal and Watkinson[1134] (Leeds, England), in a detailed mathematical analysis of the age patterns for ulcerative colitis in seven series of patients from England (three), New Zealand, Norway and the United States, concluded that ulcerative colitis was an "autoaggressive" (autoimmune) disease initiated by "random events" occurring in genetically predisposed individuals.

Part III – Etiology and Pathogenesis of IBD   165

Genetic Possibilities

In the 1960s, the major histocompatibility antigens held responsible for the strongest antigenic barrier to graft acceptance were controlled by the HLA (Human Leukocyte Ceptum A) gene complex located on the short arm of chromosome 6; so named since the histocompatibility antigens were first detected serologically on the leukocytes and later found to be present on all nucleated cells. It includes four closely linked but distinct and highly polymorphic loci (A, B, C, D). Since the major histocompatibility complex controls a spectrum of genes involved in immune regulation, associations between HLA genes (particularly Class II gene products) and disease susceptibility have been actively investigated in IBD.[1135] IBD genetic considerations included a polygenic mode of inheritance,[1099] "a specific form of somatic gene mutation in mesenchymal stem cells ... (and) the emergence of a 'forbidden clone' of cells whose 'mutant' humoral products attack the colonic mucosa,"[1136] a recessive gene with incomplete penetrance,[1137] a "rare additive major gene,"[1138] and a T-cell antigen receptor gene.[1139] Gene clusters ordinarily involved in the expression of immune responses with possible relevance to IBD included HLA genes on chromosome 6, immunoglobulin heavy chain markers on chromosome 14, immunoglobulin light chain marker on chromosome 2, complement-controlling genes on chromosomes 6 and 19 and T cell antigen receptor genes on chromosomes 14 (alpha chain). The spontaneous development of inflammatory bowel disease in transgenic rats expressing HLA B_{27} and human B2m provided an interesting model to explore genetic possibilities in IBD.[1140]

Genetic Comment

The early clinical observations indicated that ulcerative colitis and Crohn's disease were not classic genetically transmissible disorders. Inheritable protein, enzymatic, metabolic defects or chromosomal abnormalities were not yet demonstrated, ABO blood groups secretor status was normal; there was no consanguinity and there were no Mendelian ratios. Nonetheless, increasing clinical evidence supported a genetic influence in at least 15 to 20% of patients with inflammatory bowel disease, much more so in Crohn's disease than ulcerative colitis,[1141,1142] and the newer experimental models have provided strong evidence in support of this concept. Initial surveys of histocompatibility haplotypes HLA A, B, C, and DR, other than revealing ethnic-related differences, did not demonstrate a dominant or specific HLA distribution in IBD, with the exception of HLA B_{27} in patients with ulcerative colitis and ankylosing spondylitis, a possible association between HLA-DR2 phenotype in Japanese patients with ulcerative colitis between DR or B44C$_w$5 phenotype with Crohn's disease and HLA DQB-1 genotype in children with Crohn's disease. Rotter and Yang[1143] summarized the increasing evidence to 1993.

Evidence recently (1998) was obtained for loci on chromosomes 3, 7 and 12 linked to IBD overall, loci on chromosomes 2 and 6 in ulcerative colitis and linkage with chromosome 16 in Crohn's disease only,[1144] with considerable variability in relation to ethnicity (e.g. chromosome 12). Genetic linkage studies identified susceptibility gene loci on chromosome 6 (possibly for ulcerative colitis), chromosome 16 (definitely for Crohn's disease) and a locus on chromosome 1 (1p,3q) in the immigrant Iraqi Chaldean population living near Detroit, Michigan).[1145] To date, seven genome-wide searches for disease susceptibility genes have been performed, including two reported in abstract form, demonstrating multiple genetic loci in IBD. With the single exception on chromosome 1, precise localization sufficient to undertake positional cloning efforts has been difficult. As noted by Brant,[1146] Johns Hopkins University, "potential loci with evidence of replication have been identified in at least six regions (chromosomes 1, 4q, 6p-MHC region, 12, 14q and 16 and perhaps the natural resistance associated macrophage protein 2 [NRAMP2]." Of added interest is the recent Belgian study by Colombel and his colleagues at the Hematology, Immunology and Cytogenic Center, Valencienne, France, composed almost completely of "pure CD families." In this group of 54 families, linkage was not demonstrated on chromosomes 3, 7, 12 and 16 and currently evaluated as indicative of genetic heterogeneity.[1147] Genetic research programs also are investigating profiles related to intestinal epithelial integrity, the role of tobacco, molecules mediating the inflammatory reaction, and severe Crohn's disease (IBD1 locus on chromosome 16[1148,1149]), recently identified as a mutation in Nod2, a susceptibility locus on chromosome 3p, and susceptibility to severe ulcerative colitis associated with polymorphism in the MHC gene IKBL.[1150]

The development of new methods of genetic investigation, including tunneling electron microscopy to physically identify individual DNA bases, restriction fragment length polymorphism analysis of genomic DNA, methods to define the functions of the T cell antigen receptor,[1151] recombinant DNA and monoclonal antibody methodology, the polymerase chain reaction[1152] (PCR) capable of rapidly amplifying a single molecule of template DNA several millionfold, mitochondrial DNA[1153] and PCR-based microsatellite mapping technology, now provide powerful resources to clarify the molecular events involved in gene regulation of antigen processing by the IBD intestinal epithelium. The complex genetic aspects of IBD, involving multiple genes (multilocus/oligogenic inheritance) and in different etiologic combinations (genetic heterogeneity), constitute an increasingly active area of cooperative investigation and together with studies on the aggregation of familial interactive environmental risk factors,[1154] eventually should identify individual profiles of genetic vulnerability and genetic resistance to IBD. Sartor[1155] suggested that "genetically determined overly aggressive immune responses to ubiquitous resident luminal bacterial constituents cause chronic intestinal inflammation. This dysfunctional response can be mediated by either defective immunoregulation or abnormal epithelial barrier function/healing."

Encouraging progress has been made towards delineating the role of genetic factors in the etiopathogenesis of inflammatory bowel disease (e.g. the IBD1 locus on chromosome 16 for Crohn's disease) but much is yet to be learned. To cite A.G. Motulsky,[1156] "there are few or no clues as to how a mutant gene causes disease – much more needs to be learned about the mechanisms of pathogenesis, gene-gene interactions, epistatic factors and the specific environmental factors in gene-environmental interactions ... many scientific approaches are required to understand the pathway from genotype to phenotype." Genetic studies now include statistical and epidemiologic genetics, molecular genetics, biochemical genetics, pharmacogenetics, and functional genomics.[1157]

CONCLUDING COMMENTARY

The chronological events described for ulcerative colitis and for Crohn's disease reveal "old" rather than "new" diseases, at least several centuries old. Though their etiology and pathogenesis remain unknown, much has been learned of their clinical and biologic nature. The onset of IBD has been associated with varying circumstances: childhood hygiene, enteric infections, the use of antibiotics,[1158,1159] emotional crises, fast foods,[1160] non-steroidal anti-inflammatory drugs, oral contraceptives, cessation of smoking (UC), and excessive smoking (CD), "precipitating" rather than causative events, often associated with significant changes in the intestinal microflora. A feature of the "nonspecific" inflammatory bowel diseases, in addition to their chronicity and recurrent nature, is the frequency and diversity of the complications.[1161] In the colon, hemorrhage, toxic dilatation, perforation and cancer of the colon and rectum clearly are direct consequences of the IBD tissue reaction. The systemic complications, ranging from autoimmune hemolytic anemia, thrombocytosis, ankylosing spondylitis, "metastatic" Crohn's disease, pyoderma gangrenosum, and iritis to retardation of growth in children, nephrolithiasis, cholelithiasis, sclerosing cholangitis, and hepatic disease, in addition to genetic influences, represent disease mechanisms, yet to be fully defined.

Malnutrition, a prominent feature of ulcerative colitis and Crohn's disease early in the 20th century[1162] and the colonic ulcerations developing in animals made deficient in pantothenic acid, pyridoxine, folic acid or vitamin A, initially implicated nutritional deficits in the development of IBD. Later hypotheses included allergy (milk, wheat), cornflakes,[1163] cytotoxicity of processed fats, the overuse of sugars, (increased intestinal bacteria[1164]) and insufficient intake of dietary fiber[1165] but convincing evidence for foods as the cause of either ulcerative colitis or Crohn's disease previously had not been published.[1166] J.M. Rhodes of Liverpool, U.K., at a recent international IBD meeting, indicated that food antigens and food nanoparticles are under active consideration as contributory factors in inflammatory bowel disease.

The changing epidemiological patterns, the increases of IBD during the latter part of the 19th century, especially in northern Europe and England, extending to the United States in the early 20th century, the prominence of ulcerative colitis during the first half and of Crohn's disease during the second half of the century continuing into the 21st century, their frequency in industrialized "northern" countries, their subsequent emergence in previously lagging areas worldwide,[1167,1168] their occurrence in individuals immigrating from low IBD incidence (rural) to higher incidence (urban) areas, and the occasional geographic sites of greatly increased IBD incidence, such as the central Canadian province of Manitoba (14.6/100,000 incidence and 198.5/100,000 prevalence[1169]) implicate environmental factors (?microbial agents, industrial pollutants) not confined to any ethnic group or to any geographic region.

The apparent rarity of IBD in third world countries with a high incidence of specific intestinal infections and parasitic infestations is of particular interest. A modest 1994 attempt to correlate inflammatory bowel disease and domestic hygiene in infancy in England[1170] included 364 IBD patients with matched controls (133 Crohn's disease and 231 ulcerative colitis), utilizing the availability of a hot water tap and bathroom in the childhood home as "evidence" of a "sanitized" environment. While the results supported the hypothesis of delayed early exposure to enteric infections as a contributing factor in the development of Crohn's disease (not ulcerative colitis), the limitations of this study are apparent. Interestingly, mice previously exposed to helminthic infestations apparently are protected against experimentally-induced intestinal inflammation[1171,1172] via the induction of a functional T cell anergy or a parasite-induced interleukin-10 response.[1173] (See the related observations of Shi et al.[1174] on a helminth-induced mucosal Th_2 response.) The 1981 epidemiologic observations of Gutensohn and Cole (Harvard School of Public Health, Boston)[1175] on "childhood social environment and Hodgkin's disease" may be pertinent to IBD risk. They state: "Risk is therefore associated with a set of factors that tend to decrease or delay early exposure to infections and this association might be explained by a viral origin of the disease, with age at infection as a major modifier of risk." On the other hand, the clustering of Crohn's disease, as in the French and Minnesota experiences, clearly implicates a microbial mechanism.

Another unexplained observation is the suggested protective effect of appendectomy against ulcerative colitis;[1176] more pronounced if appendectomy had been performed before the age of 20 years,[1177–1180] and for appendicitis or lymphadenitis (not for nonspecific abdominal pain[1181]), prompting immunological speculation, involving the possible role of the lymphoid follicles of the appendix. Mizoguchi et al.[1182] of the Massachusetts General Hospital, Boston, Mass. found that appendectomy at 1 month of age suppressed the development of experimental IBD in TCR-α mutant mice, possibly related to decreased numbers of mesenteric lymph node cells. The concept of a "neuroimmune appendicitis"[1183] also is intriguing in this context. Mast cell/nerve cell interactions also influence epithelial cell function. The recurrences of Crohn's disease in the neo-terminal ileum after intestinal resection and re-anastomosis[1184–1186] may be related to the increased density of mast cells in the ileum (submucosa, muscularis propria) expressing TNF-α and to the increased number of microbial adhesion sites.

A frequent question for ulcerative colitis and Crohn's disease is whether they are independent conditions[1187,1188] or related entities and whether proctitis is an independent disorder. Ward[1189] of Edinburgh in 1977, echoing earlier beliefs as to IBD heterogeneity, understandably ventured: "It is unlikely that the cause of Crohn's disease will ever be discovered, because the disease does not have the characteristics of a single cause either extrinsic or intrinsic." Epistemologically, human illness results from the complex interaction of many antecedent events, widely separated from each other in time.[1190] Because these events, though similar, vary quantitatively and temporally and because the capacity of individual patients to adapt to the stress of illness varies[1191] "... every disease, in a general sense, comprises many illnesses of varying pathogenesis ... important in understanding why a disease follows a different path and responds to a treatment in one patient and not in another."

The two prototype diseases (UC and CD) share comparable epidemiologic and demographic features except for the infrequency of active lifetime smokers (UC) and the frequency of former smokers among patients with ulcerative colitis, contrasting with the excess of active cigarette smokers among patients with Crohn's disease. Clinically, the focal lesions, involvement of the upper gastrointestinal tract, perianal abscess and fistula formation and histologically prominent lymphoid tissue are typical of Crohn's disease. However, as noted by Carpenter and Talley,[1192] the earlier "differential" features of IBD are no longer absolutely differentiating. Colonic Crohn's disease may be confluent, resembling ulcerative colitis. The healing of ulcerative colitis produces a patchy tissue reaction, suggestive of focal Crohn's disease, and mucosal inflammation, once regarded as an exclusive feature of ulcerative colitis, has been observed in "early" Crohn's colitis. Ulcerative colitis and Crohn's disease probably are separate though related, multifactorial and multistage entities with overlapping morphologic and demographic features. Indeterminate colitis is observed in 10 to 15% of patients usually presenting as ulcerative colitis with Crohn's disease features, clarification of indeterminate colitis may provide important clues to the relationship between the two diseases.

Despite the many immunological studies of the 1960s, 1970s, and 1980s, the immunologic status of ulcerative colitis and of Crohn's disease remains incompletely understood. The earlier described immunologic phenomena, including "colonic autoimmunity," lymphocyte cytotoxicity and cellular hyporesponsiveness, represent secondary manifestations of a complex intestinal tissue reaction rather than primary events. The increased titers of serum anti-neutrophil cytoplasmic antibodies[994,1193,1194] considered unique to ulcerative colitis, representing cross-reactivity with endogenous enteric bacterial antigens[1195] have been noted in other conditions. The antibodies against goblet cells in patients with ulcerative colitis and their first degree relatives are more common in ulcerative colitis than in Crohn's disease but there are numerous exceptions. Such markers of Crohn's disease: increased colon tissue levels of angiotensin I and II,[1196] anti-endothelial cell antibodies in Crohn's disease[1197] and not in ulcerative colitis, antibodies to a trypsin-sensitive antigen in pancreatic juice,[1198] the increased IgA mannan antibodies to a soluble antigen of the yeast Saccharomyces cerevisiae,[1199,1200] also are present in autoimmune liver disease[1201] and probably reflect concurrent rather than antecedent events in Crohn's disease.

The etiologic hypotheses of the early 20th century:[1202] nutritional deficiencies, (conventional) bacterial infection, psychosomatic illness, intestinal "protective" deficits and "colonic autoimmunity" (ulcerative colitis), have been replaced by concepts based upon significant new knowledge of the intestinal epithelium:[1203] the mucosal immune system, the neurophysiologic impact of emotional disturbances upon the bowel, increased understanding of commensal-host-intestinal microbial relationships,[1204] Paneth cell biology,[1205] the molecular basis of intestinal inflammation (proinflammatory/anti-inflammatory imbalance) and the complex genetic mechanisms in human disease. Despite earlier negative evidence, the possibility of an unconventional pathogen[1206] or a microbial mechanism definitely remains in the etiologic spectrum, especially for Crohn's disease. Important predisposing circumstances include: prior antigenic (microbial) experience of the intestinal mucosal immune system (?early age enteric infection), an intrinsic or acquired defect in the intestinal epithelium,[275,1207] increased intestinal permeability to bacteria, viruses, and to other antigens, and a genetically-influenced immunologically (gut mucosal immune system) vulnerable individual.[1208]

The IBD tissue reaction comprises a series of coordinated proinflammatory events mediated by cytokines and lymphokines of the lipooxygenase pathway, insufficiently balanced by protective anti-inflammatory molecules, with important contributions by activated macrophages and inflammatory cells (polymorphonuclear cells, lymphocytes, eosinophils, mast cells, Paneth cells, and cells of the innate immune system, the vascular endothelium and matrix metalloproteinases). The individuality of the clinical course: earlier onset among IBD families, increased clinical severity, particular complications (e.g. perianal fistulas in Crohn's disease), and responses to treatment (including biologic therapy)[1209] probably reflect genetically-influenced variations in the inflammatory reaction and in host response rather than multiple independent diseases.

The etiopathogenesis of ulcerative colitis and Crohn's disease involves two stages:[1210] first, the primary IBD tissue reaction, probably initiated by a microbial mechanism generating local autoimmune reactions (key factors: genetic endowment, immune dysregulation and environmental "triggers"), and secondly, enteric bacterial infection of the vulnerable intestinal mucosa, initiating a cascade of inflammatory reactions comprising activation of nonspecific inflammatory cells, proinflammatory cytokines and lymphokines and activation of the intestinal vascular endothelium and local immunologic reactions. Microbiological mechanisms are involved in both ulcerative colitis and Crohn's disease. As observed by Gorbach[1211] of Boston: "The lumen of the distal ileum and colon contains the highest concentrations of microorganisms (10^8–10^{10}) in the normal flora and these are the (usual) sites of active inflammation in IBD ... The luminal bacteria produce chemotactic formylated oligopeptides, such as F-met-leu-phc (FMLP) and cell-wall polymers such as lipopolysaccharide (LPS, endotoxin) and peptidoglycan-polysaccharide (PG-PS) complexes. These bacterial products are important activators of inflammatory cells and stimulate secretion of soluble inflammatory mediators. Various bacteria and their products cross the more permeable ulcerated intestinal mucosa in IBD, gaining access to the gut mucosal immune system, initiating tissue inflammation amplified by Th_1 molecules in Crohn's disease and Th_2 in ulcerative colitis. Secondary invasion and translocation of bacteria occur in tissues of such patients."

As noted by Duchmann et al.,[1212] Mainz, Germany, "increasing evidence suggests that an abnormal immune response to constituents of the normal intestinal flora may be crucial for the development and/or maintenance of chronic intestinal inflammation." Also human "flora-specific T cells in the intestine are activated by discrete glycoprotein antigens and at least some of these T cells cross-react with different bacterial species." Elson and his colleagues[1213] have shown that "T cells reactive with conventional antigens of the enteric bacterial flora can mediate chronic inflammatory bowel disease." Ringel and Drossman,[1214] University of North Carolina, re-emphasizing the contribution of psychosocial factors in IBD, had postulated a "dysregulation of homeostatic systems (i.e. neural, endocrine, immune and inflammatory) in a biologically predisposed host rather than as conditions caused by specific etiologic factors."

As Elson[1215] has summarized, "(recent) animal models (especially transgenic, "knockout") have been particularly valuable in dissecting the interactions among the early immune, environmental and genetic factors that appear crucial to induction of the disease"...: the newer mouse models already have confirmed the central role of CD^{4+} T cells in disease pathogenesis. They have shown that enteric bacterial antigens can drive the disease and that CD^{4+} T cells reactive with these antigens are the major effector cells. The experimental models also indicate that multiple genes contribute to susceptibility to IBD. Because such genes can be manipulated more readily in the animal models than they can in humans, it is likely that colitis susceptibility genes will first be isolated and cloned in mice. Lastly, the models already have suggested two novel forms of therapy for patients and more are almost certain to follow.

Much progress has been made in the understanding of human disease, including the inflammatory bowel diseases, during the past fifty years, but much more is yet to be learned. The study of ulcerative colitis and Crohn's disease today involves more advanced clinical and scientific knowledge, more fundamental scientific disciplines, sophisticated technology and more accomplished clinicians and investigators than in the past. The challenge for the 21st century will be to fully utilize these resources in the enlightened investigation of ulcerative colitis and Crohn's disease towards their ultimate conquest.

REFERENCES

Epidemiology IBD – Smoking and IBD

542. Winkelstein Jr. W. Interface of epidemiology and history: A commentary on past, present and future. Epidemiol Rev 2000;22:2–6.
543. Snow J. On the mode of communication of cholera. London Medical Gazette 1849;44:230–42, 745–52.
544. Budd W. Typhoid fever – its nature, mode of spreading and prevention. London: Longmans Green, 1873 (Reprint, New York: Grady Press, 1931).
545. McKeown T. The origins of human disease. New York: B Blackwell, 1988:83.
546. Kantor JL. Common affections of colon, their origin and their management. Bull NY Acad Med 1929;5:757–88.
547. Spriggs EI. Chronic ulceration of the colon. Q J Med 1934;27:3:549–78.
548. Sedlack RE, Nobrega FT, Kurland LT, Sauer WG. Inflammatory colon disease in Rochester, Minnesota, 1935–1964. Gastroenterology 1972;62:935–41.
549. Sedlack RE, Whisnant J, Elveback LR, Kurland LT. Incidence of Crohn's disease in Olmsted County, Minnesota, 1935–1975. Am J Epidemiol 1980;112:759-63.
550. Rose JD, Roberts GM, Williams G, Mayberry JF, Rhodes J. Cardiff Crohn's disease jubilee – the incidence over 50 years. Gut 1988;29:346–51.
551. Melrose AG. The geographic incidence of chronic ulcerative colitis in Britain. Gastroenterology 1955;29:1055–60.
552. Houghton EAW, Naish JM. Familial ulcerative colitis and ileitis. Gastroenterologia 1958;89:65–74.
553. Ustvedt HJ. Ulcerative colitis: a study of all cases discharged from Norwegian hospitals in the ten year period 1945–55. In: Pemberton J, Willard H, eds. Recent studies in epidemiology. London: Oxford Press, 1958:23–34.
554. Acheson ED. The distribution of ulcerative colitis and regional enteritis in United States veterans with particular reference to the Jewish religion. Gut 1960;1:291–3.
555. Paulley JW. Ulcerative colitis. A study of 173 cases. Gastroenterology 1950;16: 566–76.

556. Acheson ED, Nefzger MD. Ulcerative colitis in the United States army in 1944 – epidemiology: Comparisons between patients and controls. Gastroenterology 1963;44:7–19.
557. Weiner HA, Lewis CM. Some notes on the epidemiology of nonspecific ulcerative colitis. An apparent increase in incidence in Jews. Am J Dig Dis 1960;5:406–18.
558. Birnbaum D, Groen JJ, Kollner G. Ulcerative colitis among the ethnic groups in Israel. Arch Int Med 1960;105:843–8.
559. Acheson ED. Ulcerative colitis and regional enteritis in Jews. Hebrew Med J 1963;1:308–10.
560. Gilat T, Ribak J, Benaroya Y, Zemishlang Z, Weissman I. Ulcerative colitis in the Jewish population of Tel-Aviv Jafo. I. Epidemiology. Gastroenterology 1974;66: 335–42.
561. Odes HS, Fraser D. Ulcerative colitis in Israel: Epidemiology, morbidity and genetics. Public Health Rev 1989-90;17:297–319.
562. Odes HS, Fraser D, Hollander L. Epidemiological data of Crohn's disease in Israel: Etiological implications. Public Health Rev. 1989-90;17:321–35.
563. Roth MP, Petersen GM, McElree C, Feldman E, Rotter JI. Geographic origins of the Jewish patients with inflammatory bowel disease. Gastroenterology 1989; 97:900–4.
564. Fahrlander H, Baerlocher C. Clinical features and epidemiologic data on Crohn's disease in Basle area. Scand J Gastroenterol 1971;6:657–62.
565. Keighley A, Miller DS, Hughes AO, Langman MJ. The demographic and social characteristics of patients with Crohn's disease in the Nottingham area. Scand J Gastroenterol 1976;11:293–6.
566. Salem SN, Shubair KS. Nonspecific ulcerative colitis in Bedouin Arabs. Lancet 1967;1:473–5.
567. Mir-Madjlessi SH, Forouzandeh B, Ghadimi R. Ulcerative colitis in Iran: a review of 112 cases. Am J Gastroenterol 1985;80:862–6.
568. Billinghurst JR, Welchman JM. Idiopathic ulcerative colitis in the African – a report of four cases. Br Med J 1966;1:211–13.
569. Al-Nakib B, Radhakrishnan S, Jacob GS, Al-Liddawai H, Al-Ruwaih A. Inflammatory bowel disease in Kuwait. Am J Gastroenterol 1984;79:191–4.
570. Segal I, Tim LO, Hamilton DG, Walker AR. The rarity of ulcerative colitis in South African blacks. Am J Gastroenterol 1980;74:332–6.
571. Jena GP. Idiopathic ulcerative colitis in a Zimbabwean African patient. S Afr J Surg 1980;18:157–9.
572. Giraud RM, Luke I, Schmaman A. Crohn's disease in the Transvaal Bantu: A report of 5 cases. S Afr Med J 1969;43:610–13.
573. Bartholomew C, Butler A. Inflammatory bowel disease in the West Indies. Br Med J 1979;2:824–5.
574. Ratzlaff N, Jacobs WH. Regional enteritis in the American negro. Am J Gastroenterol 1970;53:252–8.
575. Samuels AD, Weese JL, Berman PM, Kirsner JB. An epidemiologic and demographic study of inflammatory bowel disease in black patients. Am J Dig Dis 1974;19:156–60.
576. Fahrländer H. Ulcerative colitis – a review of 172 cases. German Med Monthly 1967;12:140–55.
577. Evans JG, Acheson ED. An epidemiological study of ulcerative colitis and regional enteritis in the Oxford area. Gut 1965;6:311–24.
578. Iversen E, Bonnevie O, Anthonisen P, Riis P. An epidemiological model of ulcerative colitis. Scand J Gastroenterol 1968;3:593–610.

579. Binder V, Both H, Hansen PK, Hendriksen C, Kreiner S, Torp-Pedersen K. Incidence and prevalence of ulcerative colitis and Crohn's disease in the county of Copenhagen 1962–1978. Gastroenterology 1982;83:563–8.
580. Norlen BJ, Krause U, Bergman L. An epidemiological study of Crohn's disease. Scand J Gastroenterol 1970;5:385–90.
581. Monk M, Mendeloff AI, Siegel CI, Lilienfeld A. An epidemiologic study of ulcerative colitis and regional enteritis among adults in Baltimore. I. Hospital incidence and prevalence 1960–1963. Gastroenterology 1968;54(Suppl):822–4. II. Social and demographic factors. Gastroenterology 1969;56:847–57.
582. Mendeloff AI. The epidemiology of idiopathic inflammatory bowel disease. In: Kirsner JB, Shorter RG, eds. Inflammatory bowel disease. Philadelphia: Lea and Febiger, 1975:3–19.
583. Garland CF, Lilienfeld AM, Mendeloff AI, Markowitz JA, Terrell KB, Garland FC. Incidence rates of ulcerative colitis and Crohn's disease in fifteen areas of the United States. Gastroenterology 1981;81:1115–24.
584. Rogers BH, Clark LM, Kirsner JB. The epidemiologic and demographic characteristics of inflammatory bowel disease: An analysis of a computerized file of 1400 patients. J Chronic Dis 1971;24:743–73.
585. Kyle J. Crohn's disease. New York: Appleton-Century-Crofts, 1972.
586. Calkins BM, Lilienfeld AM, Garland CF, Mendeloff AI. Trends in incidence rates of ulcerative colitis and Crohn's disease. Dig Dis Sci 1984;29:913–20.
587. Calkins BM, Mendeloff AI. Epidemiology of inflammatory bowel disease. Epidemiol Rev 1986;8:60–91.
588. Brahme F, Lindstrom C, Wenckert A. Crohn's disease in a defined population: An epidemiological study of incidence, prevalence, mortality and secular trends in the city of Malmo, Sweden. Gastroenterology 1975;69:342–51.
589. Tragnone A, Corrao G, Miglio F, Caprilli R, Lanfranchi GA. Incidence of inflammatory bowel disease in Italy. Int J Epidemiol 1996;25:1044–52.
590. Langman MJS. Chronic nonspecific inflammatory bowel disease in the epidemiology of chronic digestive disease. Chicago: Yearbook Inc., 1979:80–102.
591. Lee ECG. Crohn's workshop. A global assessment of Crohn's disease. London: HM and M Publishers, 1981.
592. Segal I, Tim LO, Hamilton DG, Mannell A. The Baragwanath experience of Crohn's disease and intestinal tuberculosis in the black population. In: Lee ECG, ed. Crohn's workshop. A global assessment of Crohn's disease. London: HM and M Publishers, 1981:107–15. (Cited by Lee, reference 591).
593. Faustino G. Crohn's disease in Brazil (cited by Lee, reference 591).
594. Ghaffar AY, Wahba ME. Ulcerative colitis in Egypt. J Egypt Med Assoc 1959;42:509–16.
595. Chuttani HK, Nigam SP, Sama SK, Dhanda PC, Gupta PS. Ulcerative colitis in the tropics. Br Med J 1967;4:204–7.
596. Yamase K, Masuda K, Shimada S, Yamada Y. Regional enteritis in Japan – a review of 548 cases. Int Surg 1967;47:497–502.
597. Devlin HB, Datta D, Dellipiani AW. The incidence and prevalence of inflammatory bowel disease in North Tees Health District. World J Surg 1980;4:183–93.
598. Colombel JE, Salomez JL, Cortot A, Marti R, Lemaire B, Beuscart R, et al. Incidence of inflammatory bowel disease in northwestern France. Nord Pas-de-Calais. Scand J Gastroenterol Supplement 1980;170:22–4.
599. Probert CS, Jayanthi V, Pinder D, Wicks AC, Mayberry JF. Epidemiological study of ulcerative proctocolitis in Indian migrants and the indigenous population of Leicestershire. Gut 1992;33:687–93.
600. Whalen G. Epidemiology of inflammatory bowel disease. Med Clin North Am 1990;74:1–12.

601. Boller R. Erfahrungen an 89 colitis-ulcerosa-fallen ber abteilung boller im allgemeinen krankenhaus Wien. Gastroenterologia 1956;86:693–6. Cited by Ekbom A. Epidemiology of inflammatory bowel disease. In: Bistrian BR, Walker-Smith JA, eds. Inflammatory bowel diseases. Basel, Switzerland: S Karger, 1999.
602. Samuelsson SM. Ulcerosa colit och proktit. Department of Social Medicine, Thesis, University of Uppsala 182, 1976.
603. Harries AD, Baird A, Rhodes J. Nonsmoking: a feature of ulcerative colitis. Br Med J 1982;284:706.
604. Bures J, Fixa B, Komarkova O, Fingerland A. Nonsmoking: a feature of ulcerative colitis. Br Med J 1982;285:440.
605. de Castella H. Nonsmoking: A feature of ulcerative colitis. Br Med J 1982; 284:1706.
606. Roberts CJ, Diggle R. Nonsmoking: a feature of ulcerative colitis. Br Med J 1982; 285:440.
607. Jick H, Walker AM. Cigarette smoking and ulcerative colitis. N Engl J Med 1983; 308:261–3.
608. Boyko EJ, Koepsell TD, Perera DR, Inui TS. Risk of ulcerative colitis among former and current cigarette smokers. N Engl J Med 1987;316:707–10.
609. Benowitz NL. Drug therapy. Pharmacologic aspects of cigarette smoking and nicotine addiction. N Engl J Med 1988;319:1318–30.
610. Green JT, Richardson C, Marshall RW, Rhodes J, McKirdy HC, Thomas GA, et al. Nitric oxide mediates a therapeutic effect of nicotine in ulcerative colitis. Aliment Pharmacol Ther 2000;14:1429–34.
611. Kessler II, Diamond EL. Epidemiologic studies of Parkinson's disease. I. Smoking and Parkinson's disease. A survey and explanatory hypothesis. Am J Epidemiol 1971;94:16–25.
612. Mendeloff AI, Calkins BM. The epidemiology of idiopathic inflammatory bowel disease. In: Kirsner JB, Shorter RG, eds. Inflammatory bowel disease. Philadelphia: Lea and Febiger, 1988:3–34.
613. Thomas DC. Genetic epidemiology with a capital "E". Genet Epidemiol 2000; 19:289–300.
614. Pekkanen J, Pearce N. Environmental epidemiology: Challenges or opportunities. Environ Health Perspect 2001;109:1–5.
615. Willett W. Nutritional epidemiology, 2nd edn. New York: Oxford University Press, 1998.

Psychogenic Aspects (UC, CD) – Lysozyme

616. Moschowitz E. The psychogenic origin of organic disease. N Engl J Med 1935; 212:603–11.
617. Palmer WL. The patient, the physician, and the gut – a consideration of mind and matter. Dallas Medical J 1966;52:500–4.
618. Wolf S. The central nervous system regulation of the colon. Gastroenterology 1966;51:810–24.
619. Cabanis PJG. On the relations between the physical and moral aspects of man. In: Mora G, ed. Vol. 1, Saidi, MD. Trans. Baltimore: Johns Hopkins University Press, 1981.
620. Darwin C. Expression of emotion in men and animals. London: John Murry, 1872.
621. Pavlov I. Conditioned reflexes (Trans GV Anrep). New York: Oxford University Press, 1927.

622. Cannon WB. Bodily changes in pain, hunger, fear and rage, 2nd edn. New York: Appleton, 1929.
623. Dupont JR, Sprinz H. The effect of endotoxin on abdominal sympathetic ganglia. Acta Neuroveg 1965;27:121–30. Discussion of paper "The central nervous system regulation of the colon." Wolf S. Gastroenterology 1966; 51(part 2):810–24.
624. Cohnheim J. Vorlesungen ueber allgemeine pathologie, Vol. 2. Berlin: A. Hirschwald, 1882:125.
625. Moreau A. Ueber die folgen der durchschreidung der dasmnereun. Med Zentralbl. 1868;14:209–11. Cited by Sprinz (Reference 623) and Cohnheim (Reference 624).
626. Sullivan AJ. Emotions and diarrhea. N Engl J Med 1936;214:299–305.
627. Solomon GF. Psychoneuroendocrinological effects on the immune response. Ann Rev Microbiol 1981;35:155–84.
628. Mohr F. Die wechselwirkung korperlicher und seelischer faktoren im krankheits-geschehen. Klin Wochschr 1927;6:772–6.
629. Murray CD. Psychogenic factors in the etiology of ulcerative colitis. Am J Dig Dis 1930;180:239–48.
630. Sullivan AJ, Chandler CA. Ulcerative colitis of psychogenic origin: Report of six cases. Yale J Biol Med 1932;4:779–86.
631. Alexander F. The influence of psychologic factors upon gastrointestinal disturbances. I. General principles, objectives and preliminary results. Psychoanal Q 1934;3:501–39.
632. Weiss E, English OS. Psychosomatic medicine, 2nd edn. Philadelphia: WB Saunders Co., 1949.
633. Wittkower E. Ulcerative colitis, personality studies. Br Med J 1938;2:1356–60.
634. Daniels GE. Psychiatric aspects of ulcerative colitis. N Engl J Med 1942; 226:178–84.
635. Lindemann E. Modifications in the course of ulcerative colitis in relationship to changes in life situations and reaction patterns. In: Wolff HG, Wolf Jr. SG, Hare CC, eds. Life stress and bodily disease, Vol. 29. Baltimore: Williams and Wilkins Company, 1950:706–23.
636. Groen J, VanderValk JM. Psychosomatic aspects of ulcerative colitis. Gastroenterologia 1956;86:591–608.
637. Paull A, Hislop IG. Etiological factors in ulcerative colitis. Birth, death and symbolic equivalents. Int J Psychiatry Med 1974;5:57–64.
638. McDermott J, Finch S. Ulcerative colitis in children. Am Acad Child Psychiatry 1967;6:512–17.
639. Weinstock HI. Successful treatment of ulcerative colitis by psychoanalysis – a survey of 28 cases with follow up. J Psychosom Dis 1962;6:243–9.
640. Prugh DG. The influence of emotional factors on the clinical course of ulcerative colitis in children. Gastroenterology 1951;18:339–54.
641. Grace WJ, Wolf S, Wolff HG. Life situations, emotions and chronic ulcerative colitis. JAMA 1950;142:1044–8.
642. Grace WJ, Wolf S, Wolff HG. The human colon. New York: PB Hoeker, Inc., 1951:225–7.
643. Lium R. Observations on the etiology of ulcerative colitis. IV. The rectometrogram and the rectal reactions of eight normal subjects and one patient with ulcerative colitis before and after spinal anesthesia. Am J Med Sci 1939;197: 841–7.
644. Almy TP, Tulin M. Alterations in colonic function in man under stress. I. Experimental production of changes simulating the irritable colon. Gastroenterology 1947;8:616–26.

645. Almy TP, Hinkle LE, Berle B, Kern Jr. F. Alterations in colonic function in man under stress. III. Experimental production of sigmoid spasm in patients with spastic constipation. Gastroenterology 1949;12:437–49.
646. Mahoney VP, Bockus HL, Ingram M, Hundley JW, Yaskin JC. Studies in ulcerative colitis. I. A study of the personality in relation to ulcerative colitis. Gastroenterology 1949;13:547–63.
647. Wener J, Hoff HE, Simon MA. Production of ulcerative colitis in dogs by the prolonged administration of mecholyl. Gastroenterology 1949;12:637–47.
648. Wener J, Polonsky A. The reaction of the human colon to naturally occurring and experimentally induced emotional states: Observations through a transverse colostomy in a patient with ulcerative colitis. Gastroenterology 1950;15:84–94.
649. Moeller HC, Kirsner JB. The effect of drug induced hypermotility on the gastrointestinal tract of dogs. Gastroenterology 1954;26:303–11.
650. Sleisenger MH, Lewis CM, Pert JH, Roseman DR, Nickel Jr. WF, Almy TP. Use of parasympathetic stimulation in the production of bloody diarrhea in dogs with comment on relation of red cell and colon cholinesterase. Gastroenterology 1958;34:582–97.
651. Porter RW, Brady JV, Conrad DG, Mason JW. Occurrence of gastrointestinal lesions in behaviorally conditioned and intracerebral self-stimulated monkeys (abstract). Fed Proc 1957;16:101–2.
652. Probert L, Anagnostides AA. The neuroendocrine system of the gut. In: Anagnostides AA, Hodgson HJF, Kirsner JB, eds. Inflammatory bowel disease. London: Chapman and Hall, 1991:239–61.
653. Crohn BB. Psychic factors affecting the course of chronic ulcerative colitis (editorial). Gastroenterology 1949;12:325–7.
654. Feiereis H, Kamrowski H, Rohrmoser HG. Colitis ulcerosa und psyche. Arch Psychiatrie Nervenkrankheiten 1962;202:657–77.
655. Mendeloff AI, Monk M, Siegel CI, Lilienfeld A. Illness experience and life stresses in patients with irritable colon and with ulcerative colitis. N Engl J Med 1970;282:14–17.
656. Almy TP. Psychiatric aspects of chronic ulcerative colitis and Crohn's colitis. In Kirsner JB, Shorter RG, eds. Inflammatory bowel disease, 1st edn. Philadelphia: Lea and Febiger, 1975:37–46.
657. Sperling M. Psychoanalytic study of ulcerative colitis in children. Psychoanal Q 1946;15:302–29.
658. Groen J, Bastiaans J. Psychotherapy of ulcerative colitis. Gastroenterology 1951;17:344–52.
659. Grace WJ, Pinsky RH, Wolff HG. Treatment of ulcerative colitis. Gastroenterology 1954;26:462–8.
660. Engel GL. Studies of ulcerative colitis. II. The nature of the somatic processes and the adequacy of psychosomatic hypotheses. Am J Med 1954;16:416–33.
661. Engel GL. Studies of ulcerative colitis. III. The nature of the psychologic process. Am J Med 1955;19:231–56.
662. Kirsner JB, Palmer WL. Therapeutic problems in ulcerative colitis. Med Clin North Am 1953;37:249–59.
663. White BV. Effect of ileostomy and colectomy on personality adjustment of patients with ulcerative colitis. N Engl J Med 1951;244:537–40.
664. Feldman F, Cantor D, Soll S, Bachrach W. Psychiatric study of a consecutive series of 34 patients with ulcerative colitis. Br Med J 1967;3:14–17.
665. Fullerton DT, Kollar EJ, Caldwell AB. A clinical study of ulcerative colitis. JAMA 1962;181:463–71.

666. Cobb S. Anaclitic treatment in a patient with ulcerative colitis. Am J Med 1953; 14:731–5.
667. Sifneos PE. Ascent from chaos. Cambridge, Mass.: Harvard University Press, 1964.
668. Kirsner JB. Ulcerative colitis – 1970 – recent developments. Scand J Gastroenterol Suppl 1970;6:63–91.
669. Karush A, Daniels GE, Flood C, O'Connor J, Druss R, Sweeting J. Psychotherapy in chronic ulcerative colitis. Philadelphia: WB Saunders, 1977.
670. Helzer JE, Stillings WA, Chammas S, Norland CC, Alpers DH. A controlled study of the association between ulcerative colitis and psychiatric diagnoses. Dig Dis Sci 1982;27:513–18.
671. North CS, Clouse RE, Spitznagel EL, Alpers DH. The relation of ulcerative colitis to psychiatric factors: A review of findings and methods. Am J Psychiatry 1990; 147:974–81.
672. Sternberg EM. Emotions and disease – from balance of humors to balance of molecules. Nature Med 1997;3:264–7.
673. Sternberg EM. Neural-immune interactions in health and disease. J Clin Invest 1997;100:2641–7.
674. Mayer EA. The neurobiology of stress and gastrointestinal disease. Gut 2000; 47:6:861–9.
675. Paulley JW. Regional ileitis (letter). Lancet 1948;1:923.
676. Stewart WA. Psychosomatic aspects of regional enteritis. NY State J Med 1949; 49:2820–4.
677. Grace WJ. Life stress and regional enteritis. Gastroenterology 1953;23:542–53.
678. Cohn EM, Lederman II, Shore E. Regional enteritis and its relation to emotional disorders. Am J Gastroenterol 1970;54:378–87.
679. Paulley JW. Crohn's disease. Lancet 1958;ii:959–60.
680. Sperling M. The psycho-analytic treatment of a case of chronic regional ileitis. Int J Psychoanal 1960;41:612–18.
681. Sperling M. Psychosomatic disorders in childhood. New York: Jason Aronson, 1978:61–101.
682. Kraft IA, Ardali C. Psychiatric study of children with diagnosis of regional ileitis. Southern Med J 1964;57:799–802.
683. Whybrow PC, Kane FJ, Lipton MA. Regional ileitis and psychiatric disorder. Psychosom Med 1968;30:209–21.
684. Crockett RW. Psychiatric findings in Crohn's disease. Lancet 1952;1:946–9.
685. Helzer JE, Chammas S, Norland CC, Stillings WA, Alpers DH. A study of the association between Crohn's disease and psychiatric illness. Gastroenterology 1984;86:324–30.
686. McKegney FP, Gordon RO, Levine SM. A psychosomatic comparison of patients with ulcerative colitis and Crohn's disease. Psychosom Med 1970;32:153–66.
687. Cassileth BR, Lusk E, Strouse TB. Psychosocial status in chronic illness. N Engl J Med 1984;311:506–11.
688. Gerson MD, Erde SM. The nervous system of the gut. Gastroenterology 1981; 80:1571–94.
689. Wood JD. Communication between minibrain in gut and enteric immune system. News Physiol Sci 1991;6:64–9.
690. Chrousos GP, Gold PW. The concepts of stress and stress system disorders. JAMA 1992;267:1244–52.
691. Miller NE. Effects of emotional stress on the immune system. Pavlovian J Biol Sci 1985;20:47–52.
692. Stead RH, Bienenstock J, Stanisz AM. Neuropeptide regulation of mucosal immunity. Immunol Rev 1987;100:333–59.

693. Bass C. Life events and gastrointestinal symptoms. Gut 1986;27:123–6.
694. Fleming A. On a remarkable bacteriolytic element found in tissues and secretions. Proc Royal Soc London 1922;93:306–17.
695. Meyer K, Gellhorn A, Prudden JF, Lehman WL, Steinberg A. Lysozyme activity in ulcerative alimentary disease. Am J Med 1948;5:496–502.
696. Grace WJ, Seton PH, Wolf S, Golff HG. Studies of human colon, variations in concentration of lysozyme with life situation and emotional state. Am J Med Sci 1949;217:241–51.
697. Prudden JF, Meyer K. Lysozyme (mucolytic activity) in chronic ulcerative colitis with a preliminary report on antilysome therapy. In: Bockus HL, ed. Postgraduate gastroenterology. Philadelphia: WB Saunders Co., 1950.
698. Prudden JF, Lane N. Studies on the mechanism of alimentary lysozyme production. Gastroenterology 1950;15:104–9.
699. Gray SJ, Reifenstein RW, Connolly EP, Spiro HM, Gordon Young JC. Studies on lysozyme in chronic ulcerative colitis. Gastroenterology 1950;16:687–97.
700. Moeller HC, Marshall HC, Kirsner JB. Lysozyme production in response to injury of the gastrointestinal tract in dogs. Proc Soc Exp Biol Med 1951;76:159–61.
701. Jerzy Glass GB, Pugh BL, Grace WJ, Wolf S. Observations on the treatment of human gastric and colonic mucus with lysozyme. J Clin Invest 1950;29:12–19.

Microbial Aspects (UC)

702. Fleck L. Epistemological conclusions from the established history of a concept. In: Trenn TS, Merton RK, eds. Translated by Bradley F, Trenn TJ. Genesis and development of a scientific fact. Chicago, IL: University of Chicago Press, 1979:20–51. Originally published as Entstehung und Entwicklung einer wissenschaftlichten Tatsache: Einfuhrung in die Lehre vom Denkstil und Denkkollektiv. Basel, Switzerland: Benno Schwabe and Co., 1935.
703. McGrew RE (with Margaret P. McGrew). Encyclopedia of medical history. New York: McGraw-Hill Book Company, 1985.
704. Pasteur L. Memoire sur la fermentation appelee lactique. C R Acad Sci (Paris) 1857;45:915–16.
705. Koch R. Zur untersuchungen von pathogenen. Organismen Mittelheil Kais Gesundbeitsamte 1881;1:1–48.
706. Lederberg J. Infectious history. Science 2000;288:287–93.
707. Flexner S, Sweet JE. The pathogenesis of experimental colitis and the relation of colitis in animals and man. J Exp Med 1906;8:514–35.
708. de R. Morgan H. Upon the bacteriology of the severe diarrhea of infants. Br Med J 1907;2:16–19.
709. Jex-Blake AJ, Higgs FW. Statistics of ulcerative colitis. Proc Royal Soc Med 1908–1909;2:119–24. Cited by Bargen JA (Reference 715).
710. Wallis FC. The surgery of colitis. Br Med J 1909;1:10–13.
711. Mummery PL. The varieties of colitis and their diagnosis by sigmoidoscope examination. Br Med J 1911;2:1685–6.
712. Rolleston H. Discussion on ulcerative colitis. Proc Royal Soc Med 1922;16:91–6.
713. Bassler A. The bacteriology of ulcerative colitis. Med J Rec 1933;138:472–8.
714. Hewes HF. Infectious colitis. Boston Med Surg J 1923;188:994–9.
715. Bargen JA. Experimental studies on the etiology of chronic ulcerative colitis (preliminary report). JAMA 1924;83:332–6.

716. Leusden JT. Observations on colitis ulceration with a contribution to the knowledge of the pathogenetic effects of colon bacilli. Nederlandisch Tijdschr v Geeneesk 1921;2:2890–905.
717. Lups S. Vaccine therapy in ulcerative colitis. Am J Dig Dis Nutr 1935;2:65–90.
718. Weinstein L. Bacteriologic aspects of ulcerative colitis. Gastroenterology 1958; 40:323–30.
719. Gorbach SL. Intestinal microflora in idiopathic inflammatory bowel disease – implications for etiology and therapy. In: Kirsner JB, Shorter RG, eds. Inflammatory bowel disease, 1st edn. Philadelphia: Lea and Febiger, 1975:47–59.
720. Rosenow EC. Studies on elective localization, focal infection with special reference to oral sepsis. J Dent Res 1919;1:205–68.
721. Bargen JA, Logan AH. The etiology of chronic ulcerative colitis. Experimental studies with suggestions for a more rational form of treatment. Arch Int Med 1925;36:818–29.
722. Cook TJ. Focal infection of the teeth and elective localization in the experimental production of ulcerative colitis. J Am Dent Assoc 1931;18:2290–301.
723. Rankin FW, Bargen JA, Buie LA. The colon, rectum and anus. Philadelphia: WB Saunders Co., 1932:219–27.
724. Fradkin WZ, Gray I. Chronic ulcerative colitis. Report of vaccine therapy. JAMA 1930;94:849–52.
725. Bargen JA, Rosenow EC, Fasting GFC. Serum treatment for chronic ulcerative colitis. Arch Int Med 1930;46:1039–47.
726. Buttiaux R, Sevin A. Sur l'etiologie des colites ulcereuses (etude clinique et experimental). Ann Inst Pasteur 1931;47:173–219.
727. Rafsky HA, Manheim PJ. The significance of the Bargen organism as an established factor in ulcerative colitis. Am J Med Sci 1932;183:252–6.
728. Hurst AF. Ulcerative colitis. Guy's Hosp Rep 1935;85:317–55.
729. Rodaniche EC, Palmer WL, Kirsner JB. The streptococci present in the feces of patients with nonspecific ulcerative colitis and the effect of oral sulfanomide compounds upon them. J Infect Dis 1943;72:222–7.
730. Paulson M. Chronic ulcerative colitis with reference to a bacterial etiology. Exp Stud Arch Int Med 1928;41:75-96.
731. Dack GM, Heinz TE, Dragstedt LR. Ulcerative colitis. Study of bacteria in the isolated colons of three patients by culture and by inoculation of monkeys. Arch Surg 1935;31:225–40.
732. Felsen J. The relationship of bacillary dysentery to distal ileitis, chronic ulcerative colitis and nonspecific intestinal granuloma. Ann Int Med 1936;10: 645–69.
733. Lynch JM, Felsen J. Nonspecific ulcerative colitis. Arch Int Med 1925;35:433–56.
734. Penner A. On the possible relation of bacillary dysentery to nonspecific ulcerative colitis. Am J Dig Dis Nutr 1936;3:740–3.
735. Fradkin WZ. Ulcerative colitis – bacteriological aspects. NY J Med 1957;37:249–53.
736. Nagler-Anderson C. Tolerance and immunity in the intestinal immune system. Crit Rev Immunol 2000;20:103–20.
737. Swartz JH, Jankelson IR. Incidence of fungi in stools of nonspecific ulcerative colitis. Am J Dig Dis 1941;8:211–14.
738. Kirsner JB, Rodaniche EC, Palmer WL. The use of sulfaguanidine in non-specific ulcerative colitis and other infections of the bowel. Am J Dig Dis 1942;9:229–33.

739. Rodaniche EC, Kirsner JB, Palmer WL. Effect of the oral administration of sulfonamide compounds on the fecal flora of patients with non-specific ulcerative colitis. Gastroenterology 1943;1:133–9.
740. Marshall HD, Kirsner JB, Palmer WL. The variable effect of sulfonamides on fecal flora in patients with chronic ulcerative colitis. Gastroenterology 1950;14: 418–24.
741. Svartz N. The pathogenesis and treatment of ulcerative colitis. Acta Med Scand 1951;141:172–84.
742. Gorbach SL, Nahas L, Plaut AG, Weinstein L, Patterson JF, Levitan R. Studies of intestinal microflora. V. Fecal microbial ecology in ulcerative colitis and regional enteritis: Relationship to severity of disease and chemotherapy. Gastroenterology 1968;54:575–87.
743. Keighley MRB, Arabi Y, Dimock F, Burdon DW, Allan RN, Alexander-Williams J. Influence of inflammatory bowel disease on intestinal microflora. Gut 1978;19: 1099–104.
744. Seneca H, Henderson E. Normal intestinal bacteria on ulcerative colitis. Gastroenterology 1950;15:34–9.
745. Cooke EM. Properties of strains of Escherichia Coli isolated from the faeces of patients with ulcerative colitis, patients with acute diarrhoea and normal persons. J Pathol Bacteriol 1968;95:101–13.
746. Cooke EM, Ewins SP, Hywell-Jones J, Lennard-Jones JE. Properties of strains of Escherichia Coli carried in different phases of ulcerative colitis. Gut 1974;15: 143–6.
747. Dickinson RJ, Varian SA, Axon ATR, Cooke EM. Increased incidence of fecal coliforms with in vitro adhesive and invasive properties in patients with ulcerative colitis. Gut 1980;21:787–92.
748. Donaldson Jr. RM. Normal bacterial populations of the intestine and their relation to intestinal function. N Engl J Med 1964;270:938–46, 994–1000, 1050–6.
749. Floch MH, Gorbach SL, Luckey TD. Intestinal microflora. Am J Clin Nutr 1970; 23:1425–6.
750. Grotsky HW, Hirshaut Y, Sorokin C, Sachar D, Janowitz HD, Glade PR. Epstein-Barr virus and inflammatory bowel disease. Experientia 1971;27:1474–5.
751. Van Kruiningen HJ, Mayo DR, Vanopdenbosch E, Gower-Rousseau C, Cortot JF. Virus serology in familial Crohn's disease. Scand J Gastroenterol 2000;35:403–7.
752. Syverton JT. Enteroviruses. Gastroenterology 1961;40:2:331–7.
753. Paulson M. Intracutaneous responses, comparable to positive Frei reactions, with colonic exudate from chronic ulcerative colitis cases with positive Frei tests. Am J Dig Dis 1936;3:667–73.
754. Rodaniche EC, Kirsner JB, Palmer WL. Lymphogranuloma venereum in relation to ulcerative colitis. JAMA 1940;115:515–19.
755. Metz A. Ein fall von colitis ulcerosa in einer vagina artificialis. Gastroenterologia 1962;98:113–16.
756. Descos L, Gillon J, Andre C, Papazian A, Lesbros F, Rochet Y, et al. Simultaneous onset of ulcerative colitis in the rectum and in a segment of colon used for colpopoiesis. Dis Colon Rectum 1981;24:532–4.
757. Nielsen K. Regional enteritis in domestic animals. In: Engel A, Larson T, eds. Regional enteritis (Crohn's disease). Stockholm: Nordiska Bokhandelns Forlag, 1971:266–78.
758. Mayberry JF, Rhodes J, Heatley RV. Infections which cause ileocolic disease in animals – are they relevant to Crohn's disease? Gastroenterology 1980;78: 1080–4.

759. Johne HA, Frothingham L. Ein eigenthumlicher fall von tuberculose beim rind. Dtsch Z Thiermed Vergleichende Pathol 1895;21:438–54.
760. Patterson DS, Allen WM. Chronic mycobacterial enteritis in ruminants as a model of Crohn's disease. Proc Royal Soc Med 1972;65:998–1001.
761. Pumphrey RE. Studies on the etiology of regional ileitis. Proc Staff Meet Mayo Clin 1938;13:539–41.
762. Burnham WR, Lennard-Jones JE, Stanford JL, Bird RG. Mycobacteria as a possible cause of inflammatory bowel disease. Lancet 1978;2:693–6.
763. Chiodini RJ, Van Kruiningen H, Thayer WR, Merkay RS, Coutu JA. Possible role of mycobacteria in inflammatory bowel diseases. I. An unclassified mycobacteria species isolated from patients with Crohn's disease. Dig Dis Sci 1984;29: 1073–9.
764. Phear DV. The relation between regional ileitis and sarcoidosis. Lancet 1958;2: 1250–1.
765. Willoughby JMT, Mitchell DN, Wilson JD. Sarcoidosis and Crohn's disease in siblings. Lancet 1963;2:650–3.
766. Siltzbach LE, Ehrlich JC. The Nickerson-Kveim reaction in sarcoidosis. Am J Med 1954;16:790–803 citing Nickerson DA and Kveim A.
767. Karlish AJ, Cox EV, Hampson F, Hemsted EH. The Kveim test in Crohn's disease, ulcerative colitis and coeliac disease. Lancet 1972;1:438–9.
768. Fletcher J, Hinton JM. Tuberculin sensitivity in Crohn's disease. A controlled study. Lancet 1967;2:753–4.
769. Wensinck F. The fecal flora of patients with Crohn's disease. Van Leeuwenhoek Arch 1975;41:214-215. Cited by Van de Merwe JP. A possible role of eubacterium and peptostreptococcus species in the aetiology of Crohn's disease. In: Pena AS, Weterman IT, Booth CC, Strober W, eds. Recent advances in Crohn's disease. The Hague: Martinus Nijhoff, 1981:201–6.
770. Peach S, Lock MR, Katz D, Todd IP, Tabaqchali S. Mucosal-associated bacterial flora of the intestine in patients with Crohn's disease and in a control group. Gut 1978;19:1034–42.
771. Kagnoff MF. On the etiology of Crohn's disease. Gastroenterology 1978;75:526–7.
772. Chiodini RJ, Van Kruiningen HJ, Merkal RS, Thayer Jr. WR, Coutu JA. Characteristics of an unclassified mycobacterium species isolated from patients with Crohn's disease. J Clin Microbiol 1984;20:966–71.
773. Darfeuille-Michaud A, Neut C, Barnich N, Lederman E, DiMartino P, Gambiez L, et al. Presence of adherent Escherichia Coli strains in ileal mucosa of patients with Crohn's disease. Gastroenterology 1998;115:1405–13.
774. Bregman E, Kirsner JB. Amino acids of colon and rectum. Possible involvement of diaminopimelic acid of intestinal bacteria in antigenicity of ulcerative colitis colon. Proc Soc Exp Biol Med 1965;118:727–31.
775. Persson S, Danielson D, Kjellander J, Wallenstein S. Studies of Crohn's disease. I. The relationship between yersinia enterocolitica infection and terminal ileitis. Acta Chir Scand 1976;142:84–90.
776. Wakefield AJ, Pittilo RM, Sim R, Cosby SL, Stephenson JR, Dhillon AP, et al. Evidence of persistent measles virus infection in Crohn's disease. J Med Virol 1993;39:345–53.
777. Logan RF. Inflammatory bowel disease incidence: Up, down or unchanged? Gut 1998;42:309–11.
778. Health Canada – association between measles infection and the occurrence of chronic inflammatory bowel disease. Can Commun Dis Rep 1997;23:1.
779. Robertson DJ, Sandler RS. Measles virus and Crohn's disease: A critical appraisal of the current literature. Inflamm Bowel Dis 2001;7:51–7.

780. Greenberg HB, Gebhard RL, McClain CJ, Soltis RD, Kapikian AZ. Antibodies to viral gastroenteritis viruses in Crohn's disease. Gastroenterology 1979;76:349–50.
781. Whorwell PJ, Eade OE, Hossenbocus A, Bamforth J. Crohn's disease in a husband and wife. Lancet 1978;2:186–7.
782. Kirsner JB. Later development of inflammatory bowel disease in the healthy spouse of a patient. (Letter to Editor) N Engl J Med 1982;307:1148.
783. Purrmann J, Cleveland S, Miller B, Strohmeyer G. Crohn's disease in a married couple. Hepato-Gastroenterology 1987;34:132–3.
784. Murray CJW, Thomson ABR. Marital idiopathic inflammatory bowel disease. J Clin Gastroenterol 1988;10:95–7.
785. Bennett R, Rubin PH, Present DH. Inflammatory bowel disease (IBD) in husbands and wives. Gastroenterology 1988;94:A811.
786. Cave DR. The aetiology of Crohn's disease. In: Truelove S, Goodman MJ, eds. Topics in gastroenterology. London: Blackwell Scientific, 1975:357–72.
787. Mitchell DN, Rees RJ. Agent transmissible from Crohn's disease tissue. Lancet 1970;2:168–71.
788. Taub RN, Siltzbach LE. Induction of granulomas in mice by injection of a transmissible agent from Crohn's disease. In: Iwa K, Itosoda Y, eds. Proc. VI Internet Conference Sarcoidosis 1972. Tokyo, Japan: University of Tokyo Press, 1971:1122–4.
789. Bolton PM, Owen E, Heatley RV, Williams WJ, Hughes LE. Negative findings in laboratory animals for a transmissible agent in Crohn's disease. Lancet 1973;2:1122–4.
790. Mitchell DN, Rees RJ. Sarcoidosis and Crohn's disease. Proc Royal Soc Med 1971;64:944–6.
791. Cave DR, Mitchell DN, Kane SP, Brooke BN. Further animal evidence of a transmissible agent in Crohn's disease. Lancet 1973;2:1120–2.
792. Cave DR, Mitchell DN, Brooke BN. Experimental animal studies of the etiology and pathogenesis of Crohn's disease. Gastroenterology 1975;69:618–24.
793. Thayer WR. Executive summary of the AGA-NFIC sponsored workshop on infectious agents in inflammatory bowel disease. Dig Dis Sci 1979;24:781–4.
794. Ahlberg J, Bergstrand O, Gillstrom P, Holmstrom B, Kronevi T, Reiland S. Negative findings in search for a transmissible agent in Crohn's disease. Acta Chir Scand 1978;482:45–7.
795. Van Kruiningen HJ, Colombel JF, Cartun RW, Whitlock RH, Koopmans M, Kangro HO, et al. An indepth study on Crohn's disease in two French families. Gastroenterology 1993;104:351–60.
796. Van Kruiningen HJ, Freda BJ. A clustering of Crohn's disease in Mankato, Minnesota. Inflamm Bowel Dis 2001;7:27–33.
797. Sellon RK, Tonkonogy S, Schultz M, Dielsman LA, Grenther W, Balish E, et al. Resident enteric bacteria are necessary for development of spontaneous colitis and immune system activation in interleukin-10-deficient mice. Infect Immun 1998;66:5224–31.
798. Van der Waaij D, Cohen BJ, Anver MR. Mitigation of experimental inflammatory bowel disease in guinea pigs by selective elimination of the aerobic gram-negative intestinal microflora. Gastroenterology 1974;67:460–72.
799. Ferber D. Superbugs on the hoof? Science 2000;288:792–4.
800. Dubos R, Schaedler RW, Costello R, Hoet P. Indigenous, normal and autochthonous flora of the gastrointestinal tract. J Exp Med 1965;122:67–75.
801. Gewirtz AT, Simon Jr. PO, Schmitt CK, Taylor LJ, Hagedom CH, O'Brien AD, et al. Salmonella typhimurium translocates flagellin across intestinal epithelia, inducing a proinflammatory response. J Clin Invest 2001;107:99–109.

802. Fleckenstein JM, Kopecko DJ. Breaking the mucosal barrier by stealth: An emerging pathogenic mechanism for enteroadherent bacterial pathogens. J Clin Invest 2001;107:27–30.
803. Chiba M, Komatsu M, Izuka M, Masamune O, Hoshina S, Kono M. Microbiology of the intestinal lymph follicle: A clue to elucidate causative microbial agents in Crohn's disease. Med Hypotheses 1998;51:421–7.
804. Campieri M, Gionchetti P. Probiotics in inflammatory bowel disease: New insight to pathogenesis or a possible therapeutic alternative? Gastroenterology 1999;116:1246–60.
805. Shanahan F. Probiotics and inflammatory bowel disease: Is there a scientific rationale? Inflamm Bowel Dis 2000;6:107–15.
806. Rettger LF, Chaplin HA. Treatise on the transformation of intestinal flora, with special reference to the implantation of bacillus acidophilus. New Haven, Conn.: Yale University Press, 1921.
807. Rettger LF, Chaplin HA. Bacillus acidophilus and its therapeutic application. Arch Int Med 1922;29:357–67.
808. Kopeloff N. Lactobacillus acidophilus. Baltimore, MD: Williams and Wilkins, 1926.
809. Schrezenmeir J, deVrese M. Probiotics, prebiotics and synbiotics – approaching a definition. Am J Clin Nutr 2001;73:(Suppl):361S–4S.
810. Bottazzi V. Food and feed production with microorganisms. Biotechnology 1983;5:315–63.
811. Kalliomaki M, Salmonen S, Arvilommi H, Kero P, Koskinen P, Isolauri E. Probiotics in primary prevention of atopic disease: A randomized placebo-controlled trial. Lancet 2001;357:1076–9.

Immune Mechanisms – M Cell – Epithelial Permeability – Inflammation

812. Rich AR. Hypersensitivity in disease. The Harvey Lecture Series with special reference to periarteritis involving rheumatic fever, disseminated lupus erythematosus, and rheumatoid arthritis. 1946–47;42:106–47.
813. Jenner E. An inquiry into the causes and effects of the variolae vaccinae. A disease discovered in some of the counties of England, particularly Gloucestershire, and known by the name of the cow pox. London: Lancet, 3rd edn, DN Shury, 1801:13.
814. Metchnikoff E. Lectures on the comparative pathology of inflammation. New York: Dover, 1968 (originally published 1893).
815. Metchnikoff E. Immunity in infective diseases. London: Cambridge University Press, 1905.
816. Ehrlich P. Experimental researches on specific therapy: On immunity with special reference to the relationship between distribution and action of antigens, and experimental researches on specific therapy. In: Himmelweit F, ed. Collected papers, Vol. 3. London: Pergamon Press, 1956-60 (originally published 1908).
817. Von Pirquet CE. Allergy. Arch Intern Med 1911;7:259–88.
818. Chernyak L, Tauber AI. The birth of immunology: Metchnikoff, the embryologist. Cell Immunol 1938;117:218–33.
819. Bienenstock J. The physiology of the local immune response. In: Asquith P, ed. Immunology of the gastrointestinal tract. London: Churchill Livingstone, 1979: 3–13.

820. Besredka A. La vaccination contre les etats typhoides par la voie buccale. Ann Inst Pasteur 1919;33:882–903.
821. Davies A. An investigation into the serological properties of dysentery stools. Lancet 1922;2:1009–12.
822. Burrows W, Elliott ME, Havens I. Studies on immunity to Asiatic cholera. IV. The excretion of coproantibody in experimental enteric cholera in the guinea pig. J Infect Dis 1947;81:261–81.
823. Harrison PE, Banvard J. Coproantibody excretion during enteric infection. Science 1947;106:188–9.
824. Barksdale WL, Ghode A, Okabe K. Coproagglutinus in ulcerative colitis. J Infect Dis 1951;89:47–51.
825. Pierce AE. Specific antibodies at mucous surfaces. Vet Rev Annot 1959;5:17–36.
826. Heremanns JF. Les globulines seriques du systeme gamma, leur nature et leur pathologie. Brussels: Arcia, 1960.
827. Tomasi TB, Tan EM, Solomon A, Prendergast RA. Characteristics of an immune system common to certain external secretions. J Exp Med 1965;121:101–24.
828. Tomasi TB, Bienenstock J. Secretory immunoglobulin. In: Dixon FJ, Kunkel HJ, eds. Advances in immunology, Vol. 9. New York: Academic Press, 1968:1–96.
829. Gelzayd EA, Kraft SC, Kirsner JB. Distribution of immunoglobulins in human rectal mucosa. I. Normal control subjects. Gastroenterology 1968;54:334–40.
830. Spiekermann GM, Walker WA. Oral tolerance and its role in clinical disease. J Pediatr Gastroenterol Nutr 2001;32:237–55.
831. Kraft SC, Kirsner JB. Immunological apparatus of the gut and inflammatory bowel disease. Gastroenterology 1971;60:922–51.
832. Ferguson A. Immunological role of the gastrointestinal tract. Scott Med J 1972;17:111–18.
833. Kirsner JB, Goldgraber MB. Hypersensitivity, autoimmunity and the digestive tract. Gastroenterology 1960;38:536–62.
834. Kirsner JB. The immunologic response of the colon. JAMA 1965;191:809–14.
835. Crispin EL. Visceral crises in angioneurotic edema. Collected papers, Mayo Clin Mayo Found 1915;7:823–35.
836. Duke W. Food allergy as a cause of abdominal pain. Arch Int Med 1921;28:151–65.
837. Eyermann CH. X-ray demonstration of colonic reaction in food allergy. J Mo Med Assoc 1927;24:129–35.
838. Rowe AH. Roentgen studies of patients with gastrointestinal food allergy. JAMA 1933;100:394–400.
839. Schloss EM. Intubation studies in intestinal allergy. Am J Med 1949;7:156–67.
840. Andresen AFR. Gastrointestinal manifestations of food allergy. Med J Rec 1925;122(Suppl):271–5.
841. Andresen AFR. Ulcerative colitis – an allergic phenomenon. Am J Dig Dis 1942;9:91–8.
842. Rowe AH. Chronic ulcerative colitis: Allergy in its etiology. Ann Int Med 1942;17:83–100.
843. Rowe AH. Chronic ulcerative colitis – an allergic disease. Ann Allergy 1949;7:727–51.
844. Rider JA, Moeller HC. Food hypersensitivity in ulcerative colitis – further experience with an intramucosal test. Am J Gastroenterol 1962;37:497–507.
845. Taylor KB, Truelove SC. Circulating antibodies to milk proteins in ulcerative colitis. Br Med J 1961;2:924–9.
846. Truelove SC. Ulcerative colitis provoked by milk. Br Med J 1961;1:154–60.
847. Wright R, Truelove SC. Circulating antibodies to dietary proteins. Br Med J 1965;2:142–4.

Part III – Etiology and Pathogenesis of IBD

848. Sewell P, Cooke WT, Cox EV, Meynell MJ. Milk intolerance in gastrointestinal disorders. Lancet 1963;2:1132–5.
849. Falchuk KR, Isselbacher KJ. Circulating antibodies to bovine albumin in ulcerative colitis and Crohn's disease. Gastroenterology 1976;70:5–8.
850. Prausnitz P, Kustner H. Studien uber die uberemp findluchkeit. Z Bakt Orig 1921;86:160–8.
851. Pearson DJ. Pseudo food allergy. Br Med J 1986;292:221–2.
852. Anderson JA. Non-immunologically-mediated food sensitivity. Nutr Rev 1984; 42:109–16.
853. Katz J, Spiro HM, Herskovic T. Milk-precipitating substance in the stool in gastrointestinal milk sensitivity. N Engl J Med 1968;278:1191–4.
854. Dupont C, Heyman M. Food protein-induced enterocolitis syndrome: Laboratory perspectives. J Pediatr Gastroenterol Nutr 2000;30:Suppl:S50–7.
855. Mayer L. Putting up a different front for food hypersensitivity. Gastroenterology 1997;113:1034–8.
856. American Gastroenterological Association. Guidelines for the evaluation of food allergies. Gastroenterology 2001;120:1023–5.
857. Gray I, Walzer M. Studies in mucous membrane hypersensiteveness. III. The allergic reaction of the passively sensitized rectal mucous membrane. Am J Dig Dis Nutr 1938;4:707–12.
858. Walzer M, Gray I, Straus HW, Livingston S. Studies in experimental hypersensitiveness in the Rhesus monkey: Allergic reaction in passively locally sensitized abdominal orga. J Immunol 1938;34:91–5.
859. Gray I, Harten M, Walzer M. Studies in mucous membrane hypersensiveness: allergic reactions in passively sensitized mucous membrane of ileum and colon in humans. Ann Int Med 1940;13:2050–6.
860. Kurlander DJ, Kirsner JB. Association of chronic "nonspecific" inflammatory bowel disease with lupus erythematosus. Ann Int Med 1964;60:799–813.
861. Brown C, Haserick J, Shirey E. Chronic ulcerative colitis with systemic lupus erythematosus. Cleveland Clin Q 1956;23:43–6.
862. Brearley KS, Spiers SD. Autoimmune disease of the thyroid and colon: With a report of a case of chronic ulcerative colitis in association with Hashimoto's disease and penicillin allergy. Med J Aust 1962;1:789–95.
863. Lorber M, Schwartz LI, Wasserman LR. Association of antibody-coated red blood cells with ulcerative colitis: Report of four cases. Am J Med 1955;19:887–94.
864. Fong S, Fudenberg H, Perlmann P. Ulcerative colitis with anti-erythrocyte antibodies. Vox Sang 1963;8:668–79.
865. Kirsner JB, Spencer JA. Family occurrences of ulcerative colitis, regional enteritis and ileocolitis. Ann Int Med 1963;59:133–44.
866. Kirsner JB, Palmer WL. Effect of corticotropin (ACTH) in chronic ulcerative colitis. JAMA 1951;147:541–9.
867. Goldgraber MB, Kirsner JB. The Arthus phenomenon in the colon of rabbits. AMA Arch Pathol 1959;67:556–71.
868. Goldgraber MB, Kirsner JB. The Shwartzman phenomenon in the colon of rabbits. A serial histologic study. AMA Arch Pathol 1959;68:539–52.
869. Maratka Z. Experimentally produced changes in digestive tract in rabbits, guinea pigs and dogs by means of Shwartzman phenomenon. Casop lek Cesk 1951;90:11-14.
870. Kirsner JB, Elchlepp J. The production of an experimental colitis in rabbits. Trans Assoc Am Physicians 1957;70:102–19.
871. Auer J. Local autoinoculation of the sensitized organism with foreign protein as a cause of abnormal reactions. J Exp Med 1920;32:427–44.

872. Kraft SC, Kirsner JB, Fitch F. Histologic and immunohistochemical features of the Auer colitis in rabbits. Am J Pathol 1963;43:913–27.
873. Kirsner JB, Elchlepp JG, Goldgraber MB, Ablaza J, Ford H. Production of an experimental ulcerative colitis in rabbits. Arch Pathol 1950;68:392–408.
874. Callahan WS, Goldman RG, Burgess Vial A. The Auer phenomenon in colon-sensitized mice. J Surg Res 1963;3:395–403.
875. Hodgson HJF, Potter BJ, Skinner J, Jewell DP. Immune-complex mediated colitis in rabbits. Gut 1978;19:225–32.
876. Hodgson HF, Potter BJ, Jewell DP. Immune complexes in inflammatory bowel disease. Clin Exp Immunol 1977;29:187–96.
877. Mee AS, McLaughlin JE, Hodgson HJF, Jewell DP. Chronic immune colitis in rabbits. Gut 1979;20:1–5.
878. Jewell DP, MacLennan IC. Circulating immune complexes in inflammatory bowel disease. Clin Exp Immunol 1973;14:219–26.
879. Accinni L, Brentjens JR, Albini B, Ossi E, O'Connell DW, Pawlowski IB, et al. Rabbits with chronic serum sickness. Am J Dig Dis 1978;23:1098–106.
880. Kirkham SE, Bloch KJ, Bloch MB, Perry RP, Walker WA. Immune complex-induced enteropathy in the rat. I. Clinical and histologic features. Dig Dis Sci 1986;31:737–43.
881. Gebbers JO, Otto HF. Evidence for local immune complexes in ulcerative colitis. Acta Gastroenterol Belg 1978;41:329–50.
882. Nielsen H, Binder V, Daugharty H, Svehag SE. Circulating immune complexes in ulerative colitis. I. Correlation to disease activity. Clin Exp Immunol 1978;31:72–80.
883. Doe WF, Booth CC, Brown DL. Evidence for complement-binding immune complexes in adult coeliac disease, Crohn's disease and ulcerative colitis. Lancet 1973;1:402–3.
884. Fiasse R, Lurhuma AZ, Cambiaso CL, Masson PL, Dive C. Circulating immune complexes and disease activity in Crohn's disease. Gut 1978;19:611–17.
885. Koster FT, Tung KS, Gilman RH, Ahmed A, Rahaman MM, Williams Jr. RC. Circulating immune complexes in bacillary and amebic dysentery. J Clin Lab Immunol 1981;5:153–7.
886. Soltis RD, Hasz D, Morris MJ, Dodd Wilson I. Evidence against the presence of circulating immune complexes in chronic inflammatory bowel disease. Gastroenterology 1979;76:1380–5.
887. Reilly RW, Kirsner JB. Runt intestinal disease. Lab Invest 1965;14:102–7.
888. Rosenberg EW, Fischer RW. DNCB allergy in the guinea pig colon. Arch Dermatol 1964;89:99–103.
889. Gear J. Autoantibodies and the hyper-reactive state in the pathogenesis of disease. Acta Med Scand 1955;152(Suppl 306):39–55.
890. Bregman E, Kirsner JB. Colon "antibodies" in ulcerative colitis. (abstract) J Lab Clin Med 1960;56:785.
891. Broberger O, Perlmann P. Autoantibodies in human ulcerative colitis. J Exp Med 1959;110:657–74.
892. Broberger O, Perlmann P. Demonstration of an epithelial antigen in children by means of fluorescent antibodies from children with ulcerative colitis. J Exp Med 1962;115:13–26.
893. Broberger O, Perlmann P. In vitro studies of ulcerative colitis. I. Reactions of serum from patients with human fetal colon cells in tissue culture. J Exp Med 1963;117:705–15.
894. Perlmann P, Broberger O. In vitro studies of ulcerative colitis. II. Cytotoxic action of white blood cells from patients in human fetal colon cells. J Exp Med 1963;117:717–33.

895. Broberger O. Immunologic studies in ulcerative colitis. Gastroenterology 1964; 47:229–40.
896. Hammarstrom S, Lagercrantz R, Perlmann P, Gustafsson BE. Immunological studies in ulcerative colitis. II. Colon antigen and human blood group A and H-like antigens in germfree rats. J Exp Med 1965;122:1075–86.
897. Perlmann P, Hammarstrom S, Lagercrantz R, Gustafsson BE. Antigen from colon of germ-free rats and antibodies in human ulcerative colitis. Ann NY Acad Sci 1965;124:(Part I):377–94.
898. Lagercrantz R, Hammarstrom S, Perlmann P, Gustafsson BE. Immunological studies in ulcerative colitis. III. Incidence of antibodies to colon antigen in ulcerative colitis and other gastrointestinal disease. Clin Exp Immunol 1966;1: 263–76.
899. Cornelis W. Contribution a r'etude clinique et experimentale des da recto colite hemorragique. Paris Faculte Medecin, 1958. Cited by Kraft SC, Kirsner JB. The immunology of ulcerative colitis and Crohn's disease: Clinical and humoral aspects. In: Kirsner JB, Shorter RG, eds. Inflammatory bowel disease. Philadelphia: Lea and Febiger, 1975:60–80.
900. Bernier JJ, Lambling A, Cornelis W. Sur la presence d'anticorps anti-colon dans le serum de malades atteints de colite ulcereuse. Bull Mem Soc Hopitaux Paris 1960;28/29:1129–34.
901. Koffler D, Minkowitz S, Rothman W, Garlock J. Immunocytochemical studies in ulcerative colitis and regional ileitis. Am J Pathol 1962;41:733–46.
902. Polcak J, Vokurka V. Autoimmune reactions in the course of ulcerative colitis. Am J Dig Dis 1960;5:395–405.
903. Maratka Z, Wagner V. Recherche sur les auto-anticorps anticolon au cour: de la rectocolite hemorragique et de diverse affections digestives. Rev France Etudes Clin Biol 1961;6:182–5.
904. Nairn RC, Fothergill JE, McEntegart MG, Porteous IB. Gastrointestinal specific antigen – an immunohistological and serological study. Br Med J 1962;1:1788–90.
905. Nairn RC, Fothergill JE, McEntegart MG, Richmond HG. Loss of gastrointestinal specific antigen in neoplasia. Br Med J 1962;1:1791–3.
906. Klavins J. Cytoplasm of colonic mucosal cells as the site of antigen in ulcerative colitis. JAMA 1963;183:547–8.
907. McGiven AR, Datta SP, Nairn RC. Human serum antibodies against rat colon mucosa. Nature 1967;214:288–9.
908. Perlmann P, Hammarstrom S, Lagercrantz R, Campbell D. Autoantibodies to colon in rats and human ulcerative colitis: cross-reactivity with Escherichia Coli 0:14 antigen. Proc Soc Exp Biol Med 1967;125:975–80.
909. Lagercrantz R, Hammarstrom S, Perlmann P, Gustafsson BE. Immunological studies in ulcerative colitis. IV. Origin of autoantibodies. J Exp Med 1968;128: 1339–52.
910. Lagercrantz R, Perlmann P, Hammarstrom S. Immunological studies in ulcerative colitis. V. Family studies. Gastroenterology 1971;60:381–9.
911. Carlsson HE, Lagercrantz R, Perlmann P. Immunological studies in ulcerative colitis. viii. Antibodies to colon antigen in patients with ulcerative colitis, Crohn's disease and other diseases. Scand J Gastroenterol 1977;12:707–14.
912. Ford H, Kirsner JB. Iso antibodies to colon. Int Arch Allergy 1967;31:449–54.
913. Asherson GL, Holborow EJ. Autoantibody production in rabbits. VII. Autoantibodies to gut produced by the injection of bacteria. Immunology 1966;10: 161–7.

914. Cooke EM, Filipe MI, Dawson IM. The production of colonic auto-antibodies in rabbits by immunization with Escherichia Coli. J Pathol Bacteriol 1968;96:125–30.
915. Thayer, Jr. WR, Brown M, Sangree MH, Katz J, Hersh T. Escherichia Coli 014 and colon hemagglutinating antibodies in inflammatory bowel disease. Gastroenterology 1969;57:311–18.
916. Stefani S, Fink S. The ulcerative colitis-lymphocyte reaction to E. Coli 014 and colon antigens. Scand J Gastroenterol 1967;2:333–6.
917. Tabaqchali S, O'Donoghue DP, Bettelheim KA. Escherichia Coli antibodies in patients with inflammatory bowel disease. Gut 1978;19:108–13.
918. Marcussen H, Nerup J. Fluorescent anti-colon and organ-specific antibodies in ulcerative colitis. Scand J Gastroenterol 1973;8:9–15.
919. Heddle RJ, Shearman DJ. Serum antibodies to Escherichia Coli in subjects with ulcerative colitis. Clin Exp Immunol 1979;38:22–30.
920. Harrison WJ. Antibodies against intestinal and gastric mucous cells in ulcerative colitis. Lancet 1965;1:1346–50.
921. LeVeen HH, Falk G, Schatman B. Experimental colitis produced by anticolon sera. Ann Surg 1961;154:275–80.
922. Shean FC, Barker WF, Fonkalsrud EW. Studies in active and passive antibody induced colitis in the dog. Am J Surg 1964;107:337–9.
923. Bernier JJ, Lambling A, Terris G, Cornelis W. Autosensitization in hemorrhagic rectocolitis (ulcerative colitis) and experimental colitis induced by hetero- and auto-antibodies. Arch Mal App Dig 1962;51:1161–74.
924. Bernier JJ, Terris G, Lambling A. La reproduction experimentale des colites ulcereuses. Rev Fr d'Etudes Clin Biol 1963;8:598–613.
925. Nordstoga K. Fibrinous colitis in swine, a manifestation of Shwartzman reaction? Vet Rec 1973;92:698.
926. Sanarelli G. Le cholera experimentale. Ann Inst Pasteur 1924;38:11–72.
927. Chamovitz R, Valdes-Dapena A, Villardell F. Shwartzman-like phenomenon of the rabbit colon induced by a single injection of endotoxin. Proc Soc Exp Biol Med 1962;109:527–9.
928. Patterson M, Terrell II JC, O'Bryan BC. The Shwartzman reaction in the colon of rabbits. Texas Rep Biol Med 1962;20:658–64.
929. Richardson OS, Leskowitz S. An attempt at production of autoimmunity to tissue of the gastrointestinal tract. Proc Soc Exp Biol Med 1961;107:357–9.
930. McGiven AR, Ghose T, Nairn RC. Autoantibodies in ulcerative colitis. Br Med J 1967;2:19–23.
931. Rabin BS, Rogers SJ. Nonpathogenicity of anti-intestinal antibody in the rabbit. Am J Pathol 1976;83:269–78.
932. Rabin BS, Rogers SJ. A cell-mediated immune model of inflammatory bowel disease in the rabbit. Gastroenterology 1978;75:29–33.
933. Streilein JW. Inflammatory bowel disease: T lymphocytes may be the culprits (editorial). Gastroenterology 1978;75:150–2.
934. Shorter RG, Huizenga KA, Spencer RJ. A working hypothesis for the etiology and pathogenesis of nonspecific inflammatory bowel disease. Am J Dig Dis 1972;17:1024–32.
935. Whorwell PJ, Holdstock G, Whorwell GM, Wright R. Bottle feeding, early gastroenteritis and inflammatory bowel disease. Br Med J 1979;1:382.
936. Acheson ED, Truelove SC. Early weaning in the etiology of ulcerative colitis. A study of feeding in infants. Br Med J 1961;2:929–33.
937. Wright R, Truelove SC. A controlled therapeutic trial of various diets in ulcerative colitis. Br Med J 1965;2:138–41.

938. Wright R, Truelove SC. Auto-immune reactions in ulcerative colitis. Gut 1966; 7:32–40.
939. Thayer WR, Spiro HM. Persistence of serum complement in sera of patients with ulcerative colitis. J Lab Clin Med 1963;62:24–30.
940. Fletcher J. Serum complement in active ulcerative colitis. Gut 1965;8:172–6.
941. Ward M, Eastwood MA. Serum C_3 and C_4 complement components in ulcerative colitis and Crohn's disease. Digestion 1975;13:100–3.
942. Hodgson HJ, Potter BJ, Jewell DP. Complement in inflammatory bowel disease. Gut 1975;16:833–4.
943. Teisberg P, Gjone E. Humoral immune system activity in inflammatory bowel disease. Scand J Gastroenterol 1975;10:545–9.
944. Ross IN, Thompson RA, Montgomery RD, Asquith P. Significance of serum complement levels in patients with gastrointestinal disease. J Clin Pathol 1979; 32:798–801.
945. Kirsner JB. Observations on the etiology and pathogenesis of inflammatory bowel disease. In: Bockus HL, ed. Gastroenterology, 3rd edn, Vol. 2. Philadelphia: WB Saunders Co., 1976.
946. Fichtelius KE. The gut epithelium – a first level lymphoid organ? Exp Cell Res 1968;49:87–104.
947. Fichtelius KE, Sundstrom S, Kullgren B, Linna J. The lympho-epithelial organs of homo-sapiens revisited. Acta Pathol Microbiol Scand 1969;77:103–16.
948. Watson DW, Quigley A, Bolt RJ. Effect of lymphocytes from patients with ulcerative colitis on human adult colon epithelial cells. Gastroenterology 1966;51:985–93.
949. Shorter RG, Cardoza M, Spencer RJ, Huizenga KA. Further studies of in vitro cytotoxicity of lymphocytes from patients with ulcerative and granulomatous colitis for allogeneic colonic epithelial cells, including the effects of colectomy. Gastroenterology 1969;56:304–9.
950. Shorter RG, Cardoza M, Huizenga KA, ReMine SG, Spencer RJ. Further studies of in vitro cytotoxicity of lymphocytes for colonic epithelial cells. Gastroenterology 1969;57:305.
951. Shorter RG, Huizenga KA, Spencer RJ, Weedon D. Lymphotoxin in nonspecific inflammatory bowel disease lymphocytes. Am J Dig Dis 1973;18:79–83.
952. Shorter RG, McGill DB, Bahn RG. Cytotoxicity of mononuclear cells for autologous colonic epithelial cells in colonic diseases. Gastroenterology 1984; 86:13–22.
953. Kemler BJ, Alpert E. Inflammatory bowel disease study of cell mediated cytotoxicity for isolated human colon epithelial cells. Gut 1980;21:353–9.
954. James SP, Strober W. Cytotoxic lymphocytes and intestinal disease (editorial). Gastroenterology 1986;90:235–7.
955. Elson C. The immunology of inflammatory bowel disease. In: Kirsner JB, Shorter RG, eds. Inflammatory bowel disease. Boston: Williams and Wilkins, 1995:203–51.
956. Bicks RO, Kirsner JB, Palmer WL. Serum proteins in ulcerative colitis. I. Electrophoretic patterns in active disease. Gastroenterology 1959;37:256-262.
957. Soergel KH, Ingelfinger FJ. Proteins in serum and rectal mucus of patients with ulcerative colitis. Gastroenterology 1961;40:37–44.
958. Crabbe PA, Heremans JF. Presence of large numbers of plasma cells containing IgD in the rectal mucosa of a patient with ulcerative colitis. Acta Clin Belg 1966;21:73–83.
959. Gelzayd EA, Kraft SC, Fitch FW, Kirsner JB. Distribution of immunoglobulins in human rectal mucosa. II. Ulcerative colitis and abnormal mucosal control subjects. Gastroenterology 1968;54:341–7.

960. Brandtzaeg P, Baklien K, Fausa O, Hoel PS. Immunohistochemical characterization of local immunoglobulin formation in ulcerative colitis. Gastroenterology 1974;66:1123–36.
961. Brandtzaeg P, Baklien K. Immunopathology of the intestinal lesion in Crohn's disease. Zeitschr F Gastroenterologie 1979;17:(Suppl):77–82.
962. Rosenkrans PC, Meijer CJ, van der Wal AM, Cornelisse CJ, Lindeman J. Immunoglobulin-containing cells in inflammatory bowel disease of the colon: a morphometric and immunohistochemical study. Gut 1980;21:941–7.
963. Kett K, Rognum TO, Brandtzaeg P. Mucosal subclass distribution of immunoglobulin G-producing cells is different in ulcerative colitis and Crohn's disease of the colon. Gastroenterology 1987;93:919–24.
964. MacDermott RP, Stenson WF. Inflammatory bowel disease. In: Targan SR, Shanahan F. eds. Immunology and immunopathology of the liver and gastrointestinal tract. New York: Igaki-Shoin, 1990:459–86.
965. Brown WR, Lansford CL, Hornbrook M. Serum immunoglobulin E (IgE) concentrations in patients with gastrointestinal disorders. Am J Dig Dis 1973; 18:641–5.
966. Heatley RV, Calcraft BJ, Fifield R, Rhodes J, Whitehead RH, Newcombe RG. Immunoglobulin E in rectal mucosa of patients with proctitis. Lancet 1975;2: 1010–12.
967. Bendixen G. Specific inhibition of the in vitro migration of leukocytes in Ulcerative colitis and Crohn's disease. Scand J Gastroenterol 1967;2:214–21.
968. Sachar DB, Taub RN, Brown SM, Present DH, Korelitz BI, Janowitz HD. Impaired lymphocyte responsiveness in inflammatory bowel disease. Gastroenterology 1973;64:203–9.
969. Fixa B, Komarova O, Skaunic V, Nerad M, Kojecky Z, Benysek L. Inhibition of leucocyte migration by antigens from human colon and E. Coli 014 in patients with ulcerative colitis. Scand J Gastroenterol 1975;10:491–3.
970. Meuwissen SG, Schellekens PT, Huismans L, Tytgat GN. Impaired anamnestic cellular immune response in patients with Crohn's disease. Gut 1975;16:854–60.
971. Meuwissen SG. Impaired anamnestic cellular immune response in patients with Crohn's disease. In: Crohn's disease – clinical immunological and genetic aspects. Academic Thesis – University of Amsterdam, Drukkerij Daneele, Boerse, Belgium, 1977:37–47.
972. Asquith P, Kraft SC, Rothberg RM. Lymphocyte responses to nonspecific mitogens in inflammatory bowel disease. Gastroenterology 1973;65:1–7.
973. Bird AG, Britton S. No evidence for decreased lymphocyte reactivity in Crohn's disease. Gastroenterology 1974;67:926–32.
974. Kraft SC, Kirsner JB. Present status of immunological mechanisms in ulcerative colitis. Gastroenterology 1966;51:788–801.
975. Schwab JH. Suppression of the immune response by microorganisms. Bacteriological (Microbiological) Rev 1975;39:121–43.
976. Rhodes JM, Bartholomew TC, Jewell DP. Inhibition of leukocyte motility by drugs used in ulcerative colitis. Gut 1981;22:642–7.
977. Castro G. Immunological regulation of epithelial function. Am J Physiol 1981; 243:G321-9.
978. Kirsner JB. Inflammatory bowel disease – after 100 years – what next? Ital J Gastroenterol Hepatol 1999;31:651–8.
979. Kirsner JB. Inflammatory bowel disease: Overview of etiology and pathogenesis. In: Berk JE, Chief Editor. Bockus Gastroenterology. Philadelphia: WB Saunders Co., 1985:2093–126.

980. Elson CO. The immunology of inflammatory bowel disease. In: Kirsner JB, Shorter RG, eds. Inflammatory bowel disease. Philadelphia: Lea and Febiger, 1988:97–162.
981. Rogler G, Kullhann F, Rutgeerts P, Sartor RB, Scholmerick J, eds. IBD at the end of its first century (Falk Symposium 111). Dordrecht, Holland: Kluwer Academic Publishers, 2000.
982. Zinberg J, Vecchi M, Sakamaki S, Das KM. Intestinal tissue associated antigen in the pathogenesis of inflammatory bowel disease. In: Jarnerot G, ed. Inflammatory bowel disease. New York: Raven Press, 1987:67–76.
983. Das KM, Sakamaki S, Vecchi M. Ulcerative colitis: Specific antibodies against a colonic epithelial MR 40,000 protein. Immunol Invest 1989;18:459–72.
984. Das KM, Vecchi M, Squillante L, Dasgupta A, Henke M, Clapp N. MR 40,000 human colonic epithelial protein expression in colonic mucosa and presence of circulating anti-MR 40,000 antibodies in cottontop tamarins with spontaneous colitis. Gut 1992;33:48–54.
985. Sakamaki S, Takayanagi N, Yoshizaki N, Hayashi S, Takayama T, Kato J, et al. Autoantibodies against the specific epitope of human tropomyosin(s) detected by a peptide-based enzyme immunoassay in sera of patients with ulcerative colitis show antibody dependent cell mediated cytotoxicity against HLA-DPw9 transfected L cells. Gut 2000;47:236–41.
986. Kraft SC, Kirsner JB. The immunology of ulcerative colitis and Crohn's disease. Clinical and humoral aspects. In: Kirsner JB, Shorter RG, eds. Inflammatory bowel disease. Philadelphia: Lea and Febiger Co., 1975:60–80.
987. Kirsner JB. Inflammatory bowel disease. I. Nature and pathogenesis. Disease A Month, St. Louis: Mosby Yearbook, 1991.
988. Fiocchi C, Roche JK, Michener WM. High prevalence of antibodies to intestinal epithelial antigens in patients with inflammatory bowel disease and their relatives. Ann Int Med 1989;110:786–94.
989. Kraft SC, Kirsner JB. Ulcerative colitis. In: Samter M, ed. Immunological diseases, Vol. II. Boston: Little Brown and Company, 1971:1346–66.
990. Kraft SC. Inflammatory bowel disease (ulcerative colitis and Crohn's disease). In: Asquith P, ed. Immunology of the gastrointestinal tract. New York: Churchill Livingstone, 1979:95–128.
991. Matthews N, Mayberry JF, Rhodes J, Neale L, Munro J, Wensinck F, et al. Agglutinins to bacteria in Crohn's disease. Gut 1980;21:376–80.
992. Blaser MJ, Miller RA, Lacher J, Singleton JW. Patients with active Crohn's disease have elevated serum antibodies to antigens of seven enteric bacterial pathogens. Gastroenterology 1984;87:888–94.
993. Calabresi P, Thayer, Jr. WR, Spiro HM. Demonstration of circulating antinuclear globulins in ulcerative colitis. J Clin Invest 1961;40:2126–33.
994. Saxon A, Shanahan F, Landers C, Ganz T, Targan S. A distinct subset of antineutrophil cytoplasmic antibodies is associated with inflammatory bowel disease. J Allergy Clin Immunol 1990;86:202–10.
995. Targan SR, Landers CJ, King NW, Podolsky DJ, Shanahan F. Ulcerative colitis-linked antineutrophil cytoplasmic antibody in the cotton-top tamarin model of colitis. Gastroenterology 1992;102:1493–8.
996. Reumaux D, Colombel JF, Masy E, Duclos B, Heresbach D, Belaiche J, et al. Antineutrophil cytoplasmic auto-antibodies (ANCA) in ulcerative colitis: No relationship with disease activity. Inflamm Bowel Dis 2000;6:270–4.
997. Kraft SC. Approaches to the etiopathogenesis of inflammatory bowel disease: A University of Chicago perspective. In: Current Gastroenterology, Vol. 7. New York: Yearbook Medical Publishers, 1987:350–5.

998. Bienenstock J, McDermott M, Befus D, O'Neill M. A common mucosal immunologic system involving the bronchus, breast and bowel. Adv Exp Med Biol 1978;107:53–9.
999. Sachar D, Auslander MO, Walfish JS. Aetiological theories of inflammatory bowel disease. Clin Gastroenterol 1980;9:231–57.
1000. Targan SR, Karp LC, Shanahan F. Immunopathogenesis. In: Gitnick G, ed. Inflammatory bowel disease – diagnosis and treatment. New York: Igaku-Shoin, 1991:43–52.
1001. Mayer L, Eisenhardt D. Lack of induction of suppressor T cells by intestinal epithelial cells from patients with inflammatory bowel disease. J Clin Invest 1990;86:1255–60.
1002. McDermott RP, Elson CO. Mucosal immunology I. Basic principles. Gastroenterol Clin North Am 1991;20:3:Preface.
1003. Kagnoff MF. Immunology of the intestinal tract. Gastroenterology 1993;105: 1275–80.
1004. Elson CO. The immunology of inflammatory bowel disease. In: Kirsner JB, ed. Inflammatory bowel disease, 5th edn. Philadelphia: WB Saunders Co., 1999: 208–39.
1005. Tan EM. Interactions between autoimmunity and molecular and cell biology. Bridges between clinical and basic sciences. J Clin Invest 1989;84:1–6.
1006. Snook J. Are the inflammatory bowel diseases autoimmune disorders? Gut 1990;31:961–3.
1007. Kirsner JB, Shorter RG. Recent developments in "nonspecific" inflammatory bowel disease. N Engl J Med 1982;306:775–85, 837–48.
1008. Cantrell M, Prindiville T, Gershwin ME. Autoantibodies to colonic cells and subcellular fractions in inflammatory bowel disease: Do they exist? J Autoimmunity 1990;3(3):307–20.
1009. Seibold F, Scheurlen M. Autoantibodies in IBD. In: Emmeriel S, Liebe S, Stange EF, eds. Innovative concepts in inflammatory bowel disease. Falk Symposium 105. Dordrecht, Holland: Kluwer Academic Publishers, 1999:27–32.
1010. Rutgeerts P, Vermeire S. Serological diagnosis of inflammatory bowel disease (Letter to Editor). Lancet 2000;356:2117–18.
1011. Ducatelle R, Coussement W, Hoorens J. Sequential pathological study of experimental porcine adenovirus enteritis. Vet Pathol 1982;19:179–89.
1012. Shanahan F, Targan SR. Mechanisms of tissue injury in inflammatory bowel disease. In: MacDermott RP, Stenson WE, eds. Inflammatory bowel disease. New York: Elsevier, 1992:77–93.
1013. Schwartz M, Cohen IR. Autoimmunity can benefit self-maintenance. Immunol Today 2000;21:265–8.
1014. Weiner HL. Oral tolerance, an active immunologic process mediated by multiple mechanisms. J Clin Invest 2000;106:935–7.
1015. Posnett DN, Gottlieb A, Bussel JB, Friedman SM, Chiorazzi N, Li Y, et al. T Cell antigen receptors in autoimmunity. J Immunol 1988;141:1963–9.
1016. Hershberg RM, Mayer LF. Antigen processing and presentation by intestinal epithelial cells – polarity and complexity. Immunol Today 2000;21:123–8.
1017. Blumberg RS. Role of epithelial cells in IBD. In: Emmrich J, Liebe S, Stange EF, eds. Innovative concepts in inflammatory bowel disease. Dordrecht, Holland: Kluwer Academic Publishers, 1999:155–72.
1018. Blalock JE. A molecular basis for bidirectional communication between the immune and neuroendocrine systems. Physiological Rev 1989;69:1–32.
1019. Besedovsky HO, del Rey AE, Sorkin E. What do the immune system and the brain know about each other? Immunol Today 1983;4:342–6.

1020. James SP. The role of lymphokines and cytokines in mucosal immune function. Curr Opin Gastroenterol 1991;7:437–45.
1021. Atreya R, Mudter J, Finotto S, Mullberg J, Jostick T, Wirtz S, et al. Blockade of interleukin 6 trans signaling suppresses T-cell resistance against apoptosis in chronic intestinal inflammation: Evidence in Crohn's disease and experimental colitis in vivo. Nature Med 2000;6:583–8.
1022. Jafarian-Tehrani M, Sternberg EM. Animal models of neuroimmune interactions in inflammatory diseases. J Neuroimmunol 1999;100:13–20.
1023. Downing JE, Miyan JA. Neural immunoregulation: Emerging roles for nerves in immune homeostasis and disease. Immunol Today 2000;21:281–9.
1024. Klein J, Sato A. The HLA system. First of Two Parts N Engl J Med 2000;343:10:702–9, Second of Two Parts N Engl J Med 2000;343:11:782–6.
1025. Delves PJ, Roitt IM. The immune system. N Engl J Med 2000;343: Part I 37–49, Part II 108–17.
1026. Medzhitov R, Janeway, Jr. C. Innate immunity. N Engl J Med 2000;343:338–44.
1027. Papadakis KA, Targan SR. The role of chemokines and chemokine receptors in mucosal inflammation. Inflamm Bowel Dis 2000;6:303–13.
1028. Fujimura Y, Owen RL. The intestinal epithelial M cell – properties and functions. In: Kirsner JB, ed. Inflammatory bowel disease, 5th edn. Philadelphia: WB Saunders Co., 1999:33–54.
1029. Bye WA, Allan CH, Trier JS. Structure, distribution and origin of M cells in Peyer's patches of mouse ileum. Gastroenterology 1984;86:789–801.
1030. Wolf JL, Bye WA. The membranous epithelial (M) cell and the mucosal immune system. Ann Rev Med 1984;35:95–112.
1031. Kumagai K. Uber der resorptions vergang der corpuscularen bestaneteile in darm. Ber Gesamte Physiol Exp Pharmakologie 1923;17:414–15.
1032. Schmedtje JF. Some histochemical characteristics of lymphoepithelial cells of the rabbit appendix. Anat Record 1965;151:412–13.
1033. Owen RL, Jones AL. Epithelial cell specialization within human Peyer's patches. An ultrastructural study of intestinal lymphoid follicles. Gastroenterology 1974;66:189–203.
1034. Wolf JL, Rubin DH, Finberg R, Kauffman RS, Sharpe AH, Trier JS, et al. Intestinal M cells: a pathway for entry of reovirus into the host. Science 1981; 212:471–2.
1035. Nicoletti C. Unsolved mysteries of intestinal M cells (review). Gut 2000;47:735–9.
1036. Krachenbuhl JP, Neutra MR. Epithelial M cells. Differentiation and function. Ann Rev Cell Dev Biol 2000;16:301–32.
1037. Hartgers FC, Figdor CG, Adema GJ. Towards a molecular understanding of dendritic cell immunobiology. Immunol Today 2001;21:542–5.
1038. Ratner B, Gruehl HL. Passage of native proteins through the normal gastrointestinal wall. J Clin Invest 1934;13:517–32.
1039. Fordtran JS, Rector FC, Ewton MF, Soter N, Kinney J. Permeability characteristics of the human small intestine. J Clin Invest 1965;44:1935–44.
1040. Menzies IS. Absorption of intact oligosaccharide in health and disease. Biochem Soc Trans 1974;2:1042–7.
1041. Walker WA. Antigen absorption from the small intestine and gastrointestinal disease. Pediatr Clin North Am 1975;22:731–46.
1042. Pearson AD, Eastham EJ, Laker MF, Craft AW, Nelson R. Intestinal permeability in children with Crohn's disease and coeliac disease. Br Med J Clin Res Edn 1982;285:20–1.

1043. Madara JL, Sitaraman SV. Intestinal epithelial barrier function: Transepithelial migration. In: Kirsner JB, ed. Inflammatory bowel disease, 5th edn. Philadelphia: WB Saunders Co., 1999:20–32.
1044. Hollander D, Vadheim CM, Brettholz E, Peterson GM, Delahunty T, Rotter JI. Increased intestinal permeability in patients with Crohn's disease and their relatives. A possible etiologic factor. Ann Int Med 1986;105:883–5.
1045. Hollander D. The intestinal permeability barrier. Scand J Gastroenterol 1992; 27:721–6.
1046. Meddings JB, Swain MG. Environmental stress-induced gastrointestinal permeability is mediated by endogenous glucocorticoids in the rat. Gastroenterology 2000;119:1019–28.
1047. Soderholm JD, Perdue MH. Stress and the gastrointestinal tract. II. Stress and intestinal barrier function. Am J Physiol Gastrointest Liver Physiol 2001;280: G7–G13.
1048. Irvine EJ, Marshall JK. Increased intestinal permeability precedes the onset of Crohn's disease in a subject with familial risk. Gastroenterology 2000;119: 1740–4.
1049. Bjarnason I, MacPherson A, Hollander D. Intestinal permeability – an overview. Gastroenterology 1995;108:1566–81.
1050. Cereijido M, Shoshani L, Contreras RG. Molecular physiology and pathophysiology of tight junctions. I. Biogenesis of tight junctions and epithelial polarity. Am J Physiol Gastrointest Liver Physiol 2000;279:G473–82.
1051. Burns JL, Griffith A, Barry JJ, Jons M, Chi EY. Transcytosis of gastrointestinal epithelial cells by Escherichia Coli K1. Pediatr Res 2001;49:30–7.
1052. Garcia-Lafuente A, Antolin M, Guarner F, Crespo E, Salas A, Forcoda P, et al. Derangement of mucosal barrier function by bacteria colonizing the rat colonic mucosa. Eur J Clin Invest 1998;28:1019–26.
1053. Metchnikoff E. Untersuchungen uber die intracellularle verdauung bei wirbellosen thieren. Arbeit Zool Inst Univ Wien 1883;5:141–68. (See also Metchnikoff O. Life of Elie Metchnikoff. New York: Houghton Mifflin Co., 1921)
1054. Stenson WF. The tissue reaction in inflammatory bowel disease. In Kirsner JB, ed. Inflammatory Bowel Disease, 5th edn. Philadelphia: WB Saunders Co., 1999:179–90.
1055. Menkin V. Studies on inflammation: Mechanisms of fixation by inflammatory reaction. J Exp Med 1931;53:171–7.
1056. Menkin V. Further studies on the leukocytosis-promoting factor and on necrosin in inflammatory exudates. Am J Med Sci 1944;208:290–7.
1057. Menkin V. Modern views on inflammation. Int Arch Allergy 1953;4:131–68.
1058. McCord JM, Fridovich I. Superoxide dismutase. An enzymatic function for erythrocuprein (hemocuprein). J Biol Chem 1969;244:6049–55.
1059. Babior BM, Kipnes RS, Curnutte JT. Biological defense mechanisms. The production by leukocytes of superoxide, a potential bactericidal agent. J Clin Invest 1973;52:741–4.
1060. Henson PM, Johnston Jr. RB. Tissue injury in inflammation. J Clin Invest 1987; 79:669–74.
1061. Southorn PA, Powis G. Free radicals in medicine. I. Chemical nature and biologic reactions. Mayo Clin Proc 1988;63:381–9. II. Involvement in human disease. Mayo Clin Proc 1988;63:390–408.
1062. Granger DN, Rutili G, McCord JM. Superoxide radicals in feline intestinal ischemia. Gastroenterology 1981;81:22–9.
1063. McCafferty DM. Peroxynitrite and inflammatory bowel disease (review). Gut 2000;46:436–9.

1064. Grisham MB, Granger DN. Neutrophil-mediated mucosal injury. Role of reactive oxygen metabolites. Dig Dis Sci 1988;33:(Suppl 3):6S–15S.
1065. Gould SR. Prostaglandins, ulcerative colitis, and sulphasalazine. Lancet 1975;2: 988.
1066. Sharon P, Ligumsky M, Rachmilewitz D, Zor U. Role of prostaglandins in ulcerative colitis. Enhanced production during active disease and inhibition by sulfasalazine. Gastroenterology 1978;75:638–40.
1067. Sharon P, Stenson WF. Enhanced synthesis of leukotriene B4 by colonic mucosa in inflammatory bowel disease. Gastroenterology 1984;86:453–60.
1068. Cominelli F, Nast CC, Llerena R, Dinarello CA, Zipser RD. Interleukin-1 suppresses inflammation in rabbit colitis. Mediation by endogenous prostaglandins. J Clin Invest 1990;85:582–6.
1069. Slifka ML, Whitton JL. Clinical implications of dysregulated cytokine production. J Mol Med 2000;78:74–80.
1070. Gery I, Gershon RK, Waksman BH. Potentiation of the T-lymphocyte response to mitogens. I. The responding cell. J Exp Med 1972;136:128–42.
1071. Atkins E. Pathogenesis of fever. Physiol Rev 1960;40:580-646.
1072. Paetkau V, Mills G, Gerhart S, Monticone V. Proliferation of murine thymic lymphocytes in vitro is mediated by the concanavalin-A-induced release of a lymphokine (co-stimulator). J Immunol 1976;117:1320–4.
1073. Chen DM, di Sabato G. Further studies on the thymocyte stimulating factor. Cell Immunol 1976;22:211–24.
1074. Majno G. Inflammatory mediators – where are they going? In: Higgs GA, Williams TJ, eds. Inflammatory mediators. Federal Republic of Germany: Weinheim, 1985:1–6.
1075. Barbara G, Xing Z, Hogaboam CM, Gauldie J, Collins SM. Interleukin-10 gene transfer prevents experimental colitis in rats. Gut 2000;46:344–9.
1076. Ouellette AJ, Selsted ME. Paneth cell defensins: Endogenous peptide components of intestinal host defense. FASEB J 1996;10:1280–9.
1077. Bevins CL, Martin-Porter E, Ganz T. Defensins and innate host defence of the gastrointestinal tract. Gut 1999;45:911–15.
1078. Dinarello CA. Interleukin-1 and Interleukin-1 antagonism. Blood 1991;77: 1627–52.
1079. Lilja I, Gustafson-Svard C, Franzen L, Sjodahl R. Tumor necrosis factor – alpha in ileal mast cells in patients with Crohn's disease. Digestion 2000;6:1:68–76.
1080. Jobin C, Sartor RB. The IκB/NFκB system: A key determinant of mucosal inflammation and protection. Am J Physiol 2000;278:C451–62.
1081. Romagnani S. Th1/Th2 cells. Inflamm Bowel Dis 1999;5:285–94.
1082. Chen Q, Ghilardi N, Wang H, Baker T, Xie MH, Gurney A, et al. Development of Th1-type immune responses requires the Type I Cytokine Receptor TCCR. Nature 2000;407:916–20.
1083. Mossman TR, Coffman RI. Heterogeneity of cytokine secretion patterns and functions of helper T cells. Adv Immunol 1989;46:111–46.
1084. Strober W, Ludviksson BR, Fuss IJ. The pathogenesis of mucosal inflammation in murine models of inflammatory bowel disease. Ann Int Med 1998;128:848–56.
1085. Doe W. Workshop I – New developments in inflammation – summary. In: Tytgat GNJ, Bartelsman JFM, Van Deventer SJH, eds. Inflammatory bowel disease. Dordrecht, Holland: Kluwer Academic Publishers, 1995:49–51.
1086. Sen R, Baltimore D. Inducibility of K immunoglobulin enhancer-binding protein NFκB by a posttranslational mechanism. Cell 1986;47:921–8.
1087. Baldwin Jr. AS. The transcription factor NFκB and human disease. J Clin Invest 2001;107:3–6.

1088. Fiocchi C. Autoantibodies and cytokines in IBD: First mediators or secondary markers? In: Rachmilewitz D, ed. V. International symposium on inflammatory bowel isease. Part I: IBD: What was achieved by the last 50 years? Dordrecht, Holland: Kluwer Academic Publishers, 1998:46–56.
1089. Reinshagen M, Rohn H, Lakshmanan J, Eyssgleim VE. Neuroimmune interactions in the gut. In: Emmrich J, Lieb S, Stange EF, eds. Innovative concepts in inflammatory bowel disease. Dordrecht, Holland: Kluwer Academic Publishers, 1999:43–6.
1090. Standiford TJ. Anti-inflammatory cytokines and cytokine antagonists. Curr Pharm Design 2000;6:633–49.
1091. Bregenholt S. Cells and cytokines in the pathogenesis of inflammatory bowel disease: New insights from mouse T cell transfer models. Exp Clin Immunogenetics 2000;17:115–29.
1092. Papadakis KA, Targan SR. Tumor necrosis factor: Biology and therapeutic inhibitors. Gastroenterology 2000;119:1148–57.
1093. Kubes P, McCafferty DM. Nitric oxide and intestinal inflammation. Am J Med 2000;109:150–8.
1094. Podolsky DK, Fiocchi C. Cytokines, chemokines, growth factors, eicosanoids and other bioactive molecules. In: Kirsner JB, ed. Inflammatory bowel disease – 5th edn. Philadelphia: WB Saunders Co., 1999:191–207.
1095. Hodgson HJF. What has science provided over the last 50 years? In: International symposium on inflammatory bowel disease. Dordrecht, Holland: Kluwer Academic Publishers 1998:25–32.

Genetic Aspects

1096. Sherlock P, Bell BM, Steinberg H, Almy TP. Familial occurrence of regional enteritis and ulcerative colitis. Gastroenterology 1963;45:413–20.
1097. Barker WF. Familial history of patients with ulcerative colitis. Am J Surg 1962; 103:25–6.
1098. Singer HC, Anderson JG, Frischer H, Kirsner JB. Familial aspects of inflammatory bowel disease. Gastroenterology 1971;61:423–30.
1099. Kirsner JB. Genetic aspects of inflammatory bowel disease. Clin Gastroenterol 1973;2:557–76.
1100. McConnell RB. Crohn's disease and ulcerative colitis. In: McConnell RB. The genetics of gastrointestinal disorders. London: Oxford University Press, 1966:128–42. Cited by McConnell RB. Genetics of gastrointestinal disorders. Clin Gastroenterol 1973;2:487–724.
1101. Morl M, Koch H, Rosch W, Fruhmorgen P, Zeus J. Familiare enterocolitis regionalis Crohn. Dtsch Med Wochschr 1976;101:493–6.
1102. Morichau-Beauchant M, Matuchansky C, Dofing JL, Yver L, Morichau-Beauchant J. Enterite regionale chez des jumeaux homozygotes. Revue de la litterature a propos de lle cs rapporte. Gastroenterol Clin Biol 1977;1:783–8.
1103. Lewkonia RM, McConnell RB. Familial inflammatory bowel disease – heredity or environment? Gut 1976;17:235–41.
1104. Freysz H, Haemmerli A, Kartagener M. Ileitis regionalis bei einem weibichen zqillingspaar. Gastroenterologia 1958;89:75–82.
1105. Crismer R, Dreze C, Dodinval P. Maladie de Crohn a localisation ileo-cecale chez des jumeaux univitellins. Arch Mal d-APP Dig Mal Nutr 1963;52:957–69.
1106. Bisordi W, Lightdale CJ. Identical twins discordant with ulcerative colitis with colon cancer. Am J Dig Dis 1976;21:71–3.

1107. Moltke O. Familial occurrence of non-specific ulcerative colitis. Acta Med Scand 1936;78:Supplement 72:426–32.
1108. Feder IA. Chronic ulcerative colitis – an analysis of 86 cases. Am J Dig Dis Nutr 1938;5:239–45.
1109. Hommes M, Lemmans AM. Engeval van familiaire colitis gravis. Ned Tijdschr Geneesk 1936;80:5131–4.
1110. Jackman RJ, Bargen JA. Familial occurrence of chronic ulcerative colitis (thrombo ulcerative colitis). Am J Dig Dis Nutr 1942;9:147–9.
1111. Paulson ME. Nonspecific or indeterminate colitis. In: Portis SA, ed. Diseases of the digestive system, 3rd edn. Philadelphia: Lea and Febiger, 1953:783.
1112. Banks BB, Korelitz BI, Zetzel L. The course of nonspecific ulcerative colitis: Review of twenty years experience and late results. Gastroenterology 1957;32:983–1012.
1113. Bacon H. Ulcerative colitis. Philadelphia: JB Lippincott Co., 1958.
1114. Schlesinger B, Platt J. Ulcerative colitis in childhood and a follow-up study. Proc Royal Soc Med 1958;51:733–5.
1115. Gassaniga AB, Gassaniga DA. Carcinoma of the colon following chronic ulcerative colitis. Report of two unusual cases in brothers. Dis Colon Rectum 1962;5:437–43.
1116. Aronson AR, Ruoff M. Regional enteritis – occurrence in a father and both siblings. JAMA 1969;201:267–9.
1117. Kuspira J, Bhambhani R, Singh SM, Links H. Familial occurrence of Crohn's disease. Hum Heredity 1972;22:239–42.
1118. de Matteis V. L'aspetto familiare della malattia di Crohn. Ann Ital Chir 1963;39:936–1006.
1119. Rosenberg JL, Kraft SC, Kirsner JB. Inflammatory bowel disease in all three members of one family. Gastroenterology 1976;70:759–60.
1120. Zetzel L. Crohn's disease in a husband and wife. Lancet 1978;2:583.
1121. Morris PJ. Familial ulcerative colitis. Gut 1965;6:176–8.
1122. Niederle B. Ileite regionale chez des jumelles univitellines. Arch Mal Appar Dig 1961;50:1245–6.
1123. Purrmann J, Bertrams J, Borchard F, Miller B, Cleveland S, Stolze T, et al. Monozygotic triplets with Crohn's disease of the colon. Gastroenterology 1986;91:1553–9.
1124. Acheson ED. An association between ulcerative colitis, regional enteritis and ankylosing spondylitis. Q J Med 1960;29:489–99.
1125. Macrae I, Wright V. A family study of ulcerative colitis. Ann Rheum Dis 1973;32:16–20.
1126. Price WH. A high incidence of chronic inflammatory bowel disease in patients with Turner's syndrome. J Med Genet 1979;16:263–6.
1127. Knudtzon J, Svane S. Turner's syndrome associated with chronic inflammatory bowel disease – a case report and review of the literature. Acta Med Scand 1988;223:375–8.
1128. Ishii E, Matui T, Iida M, Inamitu T, Ueda K. Chediak-Higashi syndrome with intestinal complication – report of a case. J Clin Gastroenterol 1987;9:556–8.
1129. Lee FI, Bellary SV, Francis C. Increased occurrence of psoriasis in patients with Crohn's disease and their relatives. Am J Gastroenterol 1990;85:8:962–3.
1130. Sheehan RG, Necheles TF, Lindeman RJ, Meyer HJ, Patterson JF. Regional enteritis and granulomatous colitis associated with erythrocyte glucose-6-phosphate dehydrogenase deficiency. N Engl J Med 1967;277:1124–7.
1131. Katsaros D, Truelove SC. Regional enteritis and glucose-6-phosphate dehydrogenase deficiency. N Engl J Med 1969;281:295–6.

1132. Schinella RA, Greco MA, Cobert BL, Denmark LW, Cox RP. Hermansky-Pudlak syndrome with granulomatous colitis. Ann Int Med 1980;92:20–3.
1133. Binder V, Weeke E, Olson JH, Anthonisen P, Riis P. A genetic study of ulcerative colitis. Scand J Gastroenterol 1966;1:49-56.
1134. Burch PR, deDombal FT, Watkinson G. Ulcerative colitis. II. A new hypothesis. Gut 1969;10:277–84.
1135. Cho JH, Nicolae DL, Gold LH, Fields CT, LaBuda MC, Rohal PM, et al. Identification of novel susceptibility loci for inflammatory bowel disease on chromosomes 1p, 3q, and 4q: Evidence for epistasis between 1p and IBD1. Proc Natl Acad Sci USA 1998;95:7502–7.
1136. deDombal FT, Burch PR, Watkinson G. Aetiology of ulcerative colitis. I. A review of past and present hypotheses. Gut 1969;10:270–7. II. A new hypothesis. Gut 1969;10:277–84.
1137. Kuster W, Pascoe L, Purrmann J, Funk S, Majewski F. The genetics of Crohn's disease – complex segregation analysis of a family study with 265 patients with Crohn's disease and 5387 relatives. Am J Med Genet 1989;32:105–8.
1138. Monsen U, Iselius L, Johansson C, Hellers G. Evidence for a major additive gene in ulcerative colitis. Clin Genet 1989;36:411–14.
1139. Posnett DN, Schmelkin I, Burton DA, August A, McGrath H, Mayer LF. T cell antigen receptor V gene usage. J Clin Invest 1990;85:1770–6.
1140. Hammer RE, Maika SD, Richardson JA, Tang JP, Taurog JD. Spontaneous inflammatory disease in transgenic rats expressing HLA-B27 and human B_2m: An animal model of HLA-B27-associated human disorders. Cell 1990; 63:1099–112.
1141. Farmer RG, Michener WM, Mortimer EA. Studies of family history among patients with inflammatory bowel disease. Clin Gastroenterol 1980;9:271–7.
1142. Kirsner JB. Inflammatory bowel disease – clinical, etiological and genetic aspects. In: Rotter JI, Samloff IM, Rimoin DL, eds. Genetics and heterogeneity of common gastrointestinal disorders. New York: Academic Press, 1980:261–80.
1143. Rotter JI, Yang H. Resolving the genetics of IBD – the challenge for the 90s. Prog Inflamm Bowel Dis 1993;14:1–7.
1144. Satsangi J, Parkes M, Jewell DP, Bell JI. Genetics of inflammatory bowel disease. Clin Sci 1998;94:473–6.
1145. Cho JH, Nicolae DL, Ramos R, Fields CT, Rabenau K, Corradino S, et al. Linkage and linkage disequilibrium in chromosome band 1p36 in American Chaldeans with inflammatory bowel disease. Hum Mol Genet 2000;9:1425–32.
1146. Brant ST. Evaluation of IBD candidate genes and the case of NRAMP2 (Editorial). Inflamm Bowel Dis 2000;6:99-102.
1147. Vermeire S, Peeters M, Vlietinck R, Parkes M, Satsangi J, Jewell D, et al. Exclusion of linkage of Crohn's disease to previously reported regions on chromosomes 12, 7 and 3 in the Belgian population indicates genetic heterogeneity. Inflamm Bowel Dis 2000;6:165–70.
1148. Brant SR, Panhuysen CIM, Bailey-Wilson JE, Rohal PM, Lee S, Mann J, et al. Linkage heterogeneity for the IBD1 locus in Crohn's disease pedigrees by disease onset and severity. Gastroenterology 2000;119:1483–90.
1149. Forabosco P, Collins A, Latiano A, Annese V, Clementi M, Andriulli A, et al. Combined segregation and linkage analysis of inflammatory bowel disease in the IBD1 region using severity to characterize Crohn's disease and ulcerative colitis. Eur J Hum Genet 2000;8:846–52.
1150. de la Concha EG, Fernandez-Arquero M, Lopez-Nava G, Martin E, Allcock RJ, Conejero L, et al. Susceptibility to severe ulcerative colitis is associated with

polymorphism in the central MHC gene IKBL. Gastroenterology 2000;119: 1491–5.
1151. Weiss A. Structure and function of the T cell antigen receptor. J Clin Invest 1990;86:1015–22.
1152. Persing DH. Polymerase chain reaction: Trenches to benches. J Clin Microbiol 1991;29:1281–5.
1153. Randall T. Mitochondrial DNA: A new frontier in acquired and inborn gene defects. JAMA 1991;266:1739–40.
1154. Guo SW. Familial aggregation of environmental risk factors and familial aggregation of disease. Am J Epidemiol 2000;151:1121–31.
1155. Sartor RB. Microbial stimuli in IBD; specific agent or host response. In: Rachmilewitz D, ed. V. International symposium on inflammatory bowel disease. Dordrecht, Holland: Kluwer Academic Publishers, 1998:35–45.
1156. Motulsky AG. Some future directions in medical genetics. Am J Hum Genet 2000;66:1190–1.
1157. Schreiber S, Hampe J, Eickhoff H, Lehrach H. Functional genomics in gastroenterology. Gut 2000;47:601–7.

Concluding Commentary

1158. Demling L. Is Crohn's disease caused by antibiotics? Hepato-Gastroenterology 1994;41:549–51.
1159. Wurzelmann JI, Lyles CM, Sandler RS. Childhood infections and the risk of inflammatory bowel disease. Dig Dis Sci 1994;39:555–60.
1160. Persson PG, Ahlbom A, Heller G. Diet and inflammatory bowel disease. Epidemiology 1992;3:47–52.
1161. Greenstein AJ, Janowitz HD, Sachar DB. The extraintestinal manifestations of ulcerative colitis and Crohn's disease – a study of 700 patients. Medicine 1976; 55:401–12.
1162. Rosenberg IH, Bengoa JM, Sitrin MD. Nutritional aspects of inflammatory bowel disease. Ann Rev Nutr 1985;5:463–84.
1163. James AH. Breakfast and Crohn's disease. Br Med J 1977;1:943–5.
1164. Martini GA, Brandes JW. Increased consumption of refined carbohydrates in patients with Crohn's disease. Klin Wochschr 1976;54:367–71.
1165. Heaton KW, Thornton JR, Emmett PM. Treatment of Crohn's disease with an unrefined carbohydrate fibre-rich diet. Br Med J 1979;2:764–6.
1166. Jewett DL, Fein G, Greenberg MH. A double blind study of symptom provocation to determine food sensitivity. N Engl J Med 1990;323:429–33.
1167. Hanasu K, Masuda K, Shimada S, et al. Regional enteritis in Japanese. A review of 548 cases. Int J Surg 1967;47:497–502.
1168. Shiratori T, Nakano H. Inflammatory bowel disease. Tokyo, Japan: University of Tokyo Press, 1984.
1169. Bernstein CN, Blanchard JF, Rawsthorne P, Wajda A. Epidemiology of Crohn's disease and ulcerative colitis in a central Canadian province: A population-based study. Am J Epidemiol 1999;149:916–24.
1170. Gent AE, Hellier MD, Grace RH, Swarbrick ET, Coggon D. Inflammatory bowel disease and domestic hygiene in infancy. Lancet 1994;343:766–7.
1171. Fox JG, Beck P, Dangler CA, Whary MT, Wang TC, Shi HN, et al. Concurrent enteric helminth infection modulates inflammation and gastric immune responses and reduces Helicobacter-induced gastric atrophy. Nature Med 2000;6:536–42.

1172. Elliott DE, Li J, Crawford C, Blum A, Metwali A, Qader K, and Others, incl. J.V Weinstock. Exposure to helminthia parasites protects mice from intestinal inflammation (Abstract). Gastroenterology 1999;116:Part 2:A706.
1173. van den Biggelaar AHJ, van Ree R, Rodrigues LC, Lell B, Deelder AM, Krimsner PG, et al. Decreased atopy in children infected with Schistosoma Haematobium: A Role for parasite-induced Interluekin 10. Lancet 2000;356:1723–7.
1174. Shi HN, Ingui CJ, Dodge I, Nagler-Anderson C. A Helminth-induced mucosal Th2 response alters nonresponsiveness to oral administration of a soluble antigen. J Immunol 1998;160:2449–55.
1175. Gutensohn N, Cole P. Childhood social environment and Hodgkin's disease. N Engl J Med 1981;304:135–40.
1176. Gilat T, Hacohen D, Lilos P, Langman MJ. Childhood factors in ulcerative colitis and Crohn's disease. An international cooperative study. Scand J Gastroenterol 1987;22:1009–24.
1177. Duggan AE, Usmani I, Neal KR, Logan RFA. Appendicectomy, childhood hygiene, helicobacter pylori status and risk of inflammatory bowel disease: Case control study. Gut 1998;43:494–8.
1178. Ekbom A. Appendicectomy and childhood hygiene: different sides of the same coin? (Editorial Comment) Gut 1998;43:451.
1179. Rutgeerts P, D'Haens G, Hiele M, Geboes K, Vantrappen G. Appendectomy protects against ulcerative colitis. Gastroenterology 1994;106:1251–3.
1180. Russel MG, Dorant E, Brummer RJ, van de Kruijs MA, Muris JW, Bergers JM, et al. Appendectomy and the risk of developing ulcerative colitis or Crohn's disease: Results of a large case-control study. Gastroenterology 1997;113:377–82.
1181. Andersson RE, Olaison G, Tysk C, Ekbom A. Appendectomy and protection against ulcerative colitis. N Engl J Med 2001;344:808–14.
1182. Mizoguchi BA, Mizoguchi E, Chiba C, Bhan AK. Role of appendix in the development of inflammatory bowel disease in TCR-a mutant mice. J Exp Med 1996;184:707–15.
1183. DiSebastiano P, Fink T, di Mola FF, Weihe E, Innocenti P, Friess H, et al. Neuroimmune appendicitis. Lancet 1999;354:461–6.
1184. Greenstein AJ, Sachar DB, Pasternack BS, Janowitz JD. Reoperation and recurrence in Crohn's colitis and ileocolitis – crude and cumulative rates. N Engl J Med 1975;293:685–90.
1185. Rutgeerts P, Geboes K, Vantrappen G, Kerremans R, Coenegrachts JL, Coremans G. Natural history of recurrent Crohn's disease at the ileocolonic anastomosis after curative surgery. Gut 1984;25:665–72.
1186. Olaison G, Smedh K, Sjodahl R. Natural course of Crohn's disease after ileocolonic resection: Endoscopically visualized ileal ulcers preceding symptoms. Gut 1992;33:331–5.
1187. Shivananda S, Hordijk ML, Pena AS, Mayberry JF. Inflammatory bowel disease. One condition or two? Digestion 1987;38:187–92.
1188. Jenkins D, Goodall A, Scott B. Ulcerative colitis: One disease or two (quantitative histological differences between distal and extensive disease). Gut 1990;31:426–30.
1189. Ward M. The pathogenesis of Crohn's disease. Lancet 1977;2:903–5.
1190. Fessel WJ. The nature of illness and diagnosis. Am J Med 1983;75:555–60.
1191. Spiegel D. Healing words: Emotional expression and disease outcome (Editorial). JAMA 1999;281:1328–9.
1192. Carpenter HA, Talley NJ. The importance of clinicopathological correlation in the diagnosis of inflammatory conditions of the colon. Histological patterns with clinical implications. Am J Gastroenterol 2000;95:878–96.

1193. Targan S, Saxon A, Landa SC. Serum antineutrophil cytoplasmic autoantibodies to distinguish ulcerative colitis from Crohn's disease patients. Gastroenterology 1989;96(Suppl):A505.
1194. Duerr RH, Targan SR, Landers CJ, Sutherland LR, Shanahan F. Perinuclear antineutrophil cytoplasmic antibodies in ulcerative colitis, comparison with other colitides/diarrheal illnesses. Gastroenterology 1991;100:1590–6.
1195. Seibold F, Brandwein S, Simpson S, Terhorst C, including C. O. Elson. pAnca represents a cross-reactivity to enteric bacterial antigens. J Clin Immunol 1998; 18:153-92.
1196. Jaszewski R, Tolia V, Ehrinpreis MN, Bodzin JH, Peleman RR, Korlipara R, et al. Increased colonic mucosal angiotensin I and II concentrations in Crohn's colitis. Gastroenterology 1990;98:1543-8.
1197. Sawyer AM, Pottinger BE, Wakefield AJ. Serum anti-endothelial cell antibodies are present in Crohn's disease but not ulcerative colitis. Gut 1990;31:A1169.
1198. Seibold F, Weber P, Jenss H, Wiedmann KH. Antibodies to a trypsin sensitive pancreatic antigen in chronic inflammatory bowel disease: Specific markers for a subgroup of patients with Crohn's disease. Gut 1991;32:1192–7.
1199. Lindberg E, Magnusson KE, Tysk C, Jarnerot G. Antibody (IgG, IgA and IgM) to baker's yeast (saccharomyces cerevisiae), yeast mannan, gliadin, ovalbumin and betalactoglobulin in monozygotic twins with inflammatory bowel disease. Gut 1992;33:909–13.
1200. Sendid B, Quinton JF, Charrier G, Goulet O, Cortot A, Grandbastien B, et al. Anti-saccharomyces cerevisiae mannan antibodies in familial Crohn's disease. Am J Gastroenterol 1998;93:1306–10.
1201. Reddy KR, Colombel JF, Poulain D, Krawitt EL. Anti-saccharomyces antibodies in autoimmune liver disease (Letter to Editor). Am J Gastroenterol 2001;96: 252–3.
1202. Machella TE. Problems in ulcerative colitis. Am J Med 1952;13:760–76.
1203. Dignass AU. Mechanisms and modulation of intestinal epithelial repair. Inflamm Bowel Dis 2001;7:68–77.
1204. Hooper LV, Wong MH, Thelin A, Hansson L, Falk PJ, incl. JI Gordon. Molecular analysis of commensal host – microbial relationships in the intestine. Science 2001;291:881–4.
1205. Ouellette AJ, Bevins CL. Paneth cell defensins and innate immunity of the small bowel. Inflamm Bowel Dis 2001;7:43–50.
1206. Relman DA. The search for unrecognized pathogens. Science 1999;284:1308–10.
1207. Hecht G, Savkovic SD. Review article: Effector role of epithelia in inflammation – interaction with bacteria. Aliment Pharmacol Ther 1997;11:(Suppl 3):64–9.
1208. Mayer L. Current concepts of inflammatory bowel disease: Etiology and pathogenesis. In Kirsner JB, ed. Inflammatory bowel disease, 5th edn. Philadelphia: WB Saunders and Co., 1999:280–96.
1209. Beck PL, Podolsky DK. Growth factors in inflammatory bowel disease. Inflamm Bowel Dis 1999;5:44–60.
1210. Maratka Z. Pathogenesis and aetiology of inflammatory bowel disease. In: deDombal FT, Myren J, Bouchier IAD, eds. Inflammatory bowel disease, 2nd edn. London: Oxford University Press, 1986:42–95.
1211. Gorbach SL. Summary – interactions of intestinal microflora luminal content and the host in IBD. In: Tytgat GNJ, Bartelsman JFM, van Deveter IJH, eds. Inflammatory bowel disease (Falk Symposium 85). Dordrecht, Holland: Kluwer Academic Publishers, 1995:517.

1212. Duchmann R, Neurath MF, zum Buschenfelde KHM. Responses to self and nonself intestinal microflora in health and inflammatory bowel disease. Res Immunol 1997;148:589–94.
1213. Cong Y, Brandwein SL, McCabe RP, Lazenby A, Birkenmeier EH, Sundberg JP, et al. CD^{4+} T cells reactive to enteric bacterial antigens in spontaneously colitic C3H/HejBir mice: Increased T helper cell Type 1 response and ability to transfer disease. J Exp Med 1998;187:855–64.
1214. Ringel Y, Drossman DA. Psychosocial aspects of Crohn's disease. Surg Clin North Am 2001;81:231–52.
1215. Elson CO, Cong Y, Brandwein S. What can be learned from animal models? In Rachmilewitz D, ed. Falk symposium – International symposium on inflammatory bowel disease. Dordrecht, Holland: Kluwer Academic Publishers, 1995:65-72.

Appendix

*The Early Treatment of Inflammatory Bowel Disease –
Joseph Kirsner*

*Pharmacologic Development of Aminosalicylates –
Ulrich Klotz*

Additional Early IBD Publications

The Early Treatment of Inflammatory Bowel Disease

Joseph B. Kirsner
M.D., Ph.D., D.Sci. (hon.)
The Louis Block Distinguished Service Professor of Medicine,
Department of Medicine, University of Chicago, Chicago, IL, USA

Past therapeutic approaches to ulcerative colitis and Crohn's disease reflected prevailing limitations in the understanding of human illness and scarce therapeutic resources. Early in the 1900s the treatment of IBD included "slop diets," three pints daily of milk soured by lactic acid (Sydenham's treatment), "bacterial vaccines," astringents, antiseptics, calomel, starch and opium, tincture of hamamelis, tincture of iodine, and rectal instillations of boracic acid, silver nitrate, creolin, iron pernitrate, or kerosene.[1] Strange therapy to physicians in the year 2002, but hardly as bizarre as the approach of earlier times to diarrhea and the associated problems as described in the following:[2]

> Once upon a time, a King, following a large repast, experienced a sudden abdominal cramping pain followed by severe watery diarrhea and then lapsed into a coma. The following treatment was employed by the royal physicians: A pint of blood was extracted from his right arm; then eight ounces from the left shoulder; next an emetic, two physics, and an enema consisting of 15 substances were administered. Then his head was shaved and a blister raised on the scalp. To purge the brain, a sneezing powder was given; then cowslip powder to strengthen it. Meanwhile more emetics, "soothing" drinks, and more bleeding; also a plaster of pitch and pigeon dung applied to the royal feet. Not to leave anything undone, the following substances were taken orally: melon seeds, manna, slippery elm, black cherry water, extract of lily of the valley, peony, lavender, pearls dissolved in vinegar, gentian root, nutmeg and finally 40 drops of an extract of human skull. As a last resort, a bezoar stone was applied. But the royal patient died. The unfortunate patient was Charles II, King of England.

UNUSUAL DISCARDED TREATMENTS

The intense search for effective therapeutic agents for IBD also is represented in such earlier, now discarded, treatments as the intracolonic insufflation of oxygen,[3] zinc peroxide rectally,[4] hypnosis,[5] narco-analysis,[6] roentgen (600 rads) irradiation of the right lower quadrant of the abdomen (Crohn's disease),[7] gentian violet, tincture of iodine,[8] thiouracil drugs,[9] copper sulfate ("ionization"),[10] liver extracts,[11] artificial fever therapy[12] (Kettering hypertherm), hot (120°F) water enemas, azochloramid as an "antibacterial" agent,[13] Bacille Calmette-Guerin vaccine orally[14,15] (Crohn's disease), the detergent sodium lauryl sulfate[16] to "destroy" trypsin or lysozyme, "vaccines,"[17-19] horse serum,[20] "extracts" of hog intestine, stomach, and colon[21-24] to "restore" an "intestinal protective agent," and injections of a "posterior pituitary peptide"[25] ("Coherin") to "adjust" an intestinal motor dysfunction in Crohn's disease.

"Pelvic autonomic neurectomy"[26] in 1951 and distal vagotomy[27] were futile surgical efforts to correct an alleged "parasympathetic overactivity." Thymectomy[28] was utilized for ulcerative colitis in the 1960s, presumably to adjust an "immune abnormality." Nobel prize-winning selective electro-coagulation of the "prefrontal lobes"[29] in the 1950s, disrupting connections between the cortex of the frontal lobe and the thalamo-hypothalamic region to remove a "harmful neurogenic factor" in the prefrontal area of the brain, allegedly causing serious emotional disorders, reflected unusual, unconvincing and fortunately short-lived support for psychogenically-related ulcerative colitis in France and elsewhere.

Diet

Foods always have been implicated in human illness, and IBD was no exception.[30-33] The reasons varied: "allergy" (milk, eggs, wheat), "cytotoxicity" of chemically processed fats (margarine), and increases in the gut microflora (refined sugar[34]). Dietary programs included bland, high-fiber,[35] low-fiber, gluten-free, low-fat,[36] low-carbohydrate, "purified" (crystalline amino acids), "allergy-free diets" and food allergy elimination diets.[37] The symptomatic benefit experienced by some patients in eliminating milk probably represented instances of lactose or casein intolerance. The temporary elimination of raw fruits and vegetables nonspecifically decreased the number of bowel movements because of the decreased intake of "rough fiber"; and the avoidance of fruit juices diminished the intake of potentially irritating sorbitol, fructose, and sucrose. The etiologic implications of an increased intake of processed foods rich in food additives, preservatives, and coloring and hydrogenated fats (margarine) used in the production of shortenings, candies, cookies, corn flakes, and bran were highly speculative. Granting individual variations in the response to foods and the symptomatic benefit in their removal, dietary beliefs as etiologic hypotheses have been unconvincing in their subjectivity, lack of controls, and the inadequacy of recollected information on past eating habits. The many chemical additives[38] utilized today in the processing of foods preclude a realistically valid assessment of "food intolerance."

Nutritional deficiencies were suggested as possible causes of IBD 50 years ago, partly because of the clinically evident undernutrition among patients and partly because of the colonic ulcerations observed in animals made deficient in such nutritional elements as pantothenic acid, pyridoxine, folic acid, and vitamin A.[39] Vitamin deficiencies occur in patients with ulcerative colitis or Crohn's disease who are severely malnourished, but not in most patients with IBD. Knowledge of nutrition and its role in health and disease during the 1920s to 1940s was limited. Adequate food supplements were not available, and the early preparations were not well tolerated. Kirsner et al.[40,41] in 1953 found that, despite fecal loss of proteins, protein metabolism was essentially normal in uncomplicated ulcerative colitis and Crohn's disease and demonstrated that high-quality protein foods were utilized more efficiently than the hydrolyzed protein preparations of the time. Early attempts at intravenous hyperalimentation were limited by the methodology and the crude preparations.[42,43] Hyperalimentation with protein hydrolysates administered orally via a Miller-Abbott tube into the distal small bowel was utilized by Machella and Miller[44] in 1948 in the treatment of ulcerative colitis, based upon the concept of providing nutrition but not burdening the diseased colon. The alimentation consisted of a solution of equal parts of an enzymatic casein digest and of dextrimaltose containing 225–450 g of the protein digest and an equivalent amount of carbohydrates given daily for varying periods of time. A remission was induced in 11 of the 12 patients treated and was prolonged in 9. Today, oral and parenteral hyperalimentation therapy[45–47] with improved nutritional preparations is a valuable therapeutic adjunct, especially in Crohn's disease, with beneficial effects attributed in part to "bowel rest," decreased intestinal secretion, local restorative effects on the intestinal mucosa (as in the supply of nutrients such as glutamine), and diminished antigenic stimulation of the gut-associated immune system. The use of fish oil rich in omega-3 fatty acids to produce leukotriene LTB_5,[48] less chemotactic and less inflammatory than the LTB_4, demonstrated in the IBD tissue reaction, while helpful experimentally, was not useful clinically. The concept of a deficit in a tissue protective factor continues in the possible role of glutathione depletion.[49]

Psychotherapy

Psychotherapy and occasionally psychoanalysis were major approaches to patients with ulcerative colitis and less so in Crohn's disease during the 1930–50s,[50–54] based largely upon the prevailing psychiatric thought and uncontrolled clinical observations. Therapeutic evaluations ranged widely from dramatically successful to ineffective and even harmful. In retrospect, the supportive psychotherapy of the 1930–60s, a time when little was known of ulcerative colitis, medical therapy was limited, and surgical intervention was hazardous, seemed reasonable then and, in my experience, helped patients to cope with illness, though the long-term course usually was unchanged. On the other hand, irrespective of the role of psychogenic disturbances and their contribution to the severity of IBD, the use of psychoanalysis in patients seriously ill with ulcerative colitis was unwise practically. Subsequent controlled studies[55–58] indicated that the psychogenic disturbances were responses to chronic recurrent illness and the psychological problems eased when the IBD was treated successfully, medically or surgically.

Sulfonamides

IBD therapy always included some form of "antibacterial" treatment even though microbiological concepts and antimicrobial resources were limited. In the 1900s, "antiseptics," "astringents," and rectal instillation of silver nitrate were followed in the 1920s and 1930s by injections of polyvalent antidysentery serum, autologous vaccines of fecal diplostreptococci, and typhoid vaccine. After World War I, antibacterial treatment included the rectal instillation of Dakin's solution, 1:10,000 solution of potassium permanganate, cod liver oil and nisulfazole enemas, and the rectal insufflation of oxygen to "decrease or eliminate anaerobic organisms," without significant benefit.

The discovery of Prontosil rubrum (the source of sulfanilamide) by Domagk et al.[59] in Germany in 1935 initiated the modern antibacterial era, beginning in 1938 with sulfanilamide and followed by neoprontosil, sulfapyridine, sulfadiazine, sulfaguanidine, nisulfazole, gantrisin, sulfathalidine, and sulfasuxidine. Each of these compounds was tested in patients with ulcerative colitis and to a lesser extent with Crohn's disease in open uncontrolled therapeutic trials, and included the measurement of the aerobic flora in the feces, with the usual initial enthusiasm and subsequent disappointment. Although the sulfonamides were perceived and prescribed in the 1940s and 1950s as antibacterial compounds,[60–62] little was known of the microflora of the gut, and the few studies of the antibacterial effects of the sulfonamides on the fecal flora in patients with ulcerative colitis were unimpressive.

Sulfasalazine, the most important of the sulfonamide preparations in the 1940s, was created by Karolinska biochemists (E. Askelof and P.H. Willstaedt) in cooperation with N. Svartz of Stockholm in 1940, uniting the prevailing sulfonamide sulfapyridine and 5-aminosalicylic acid (5-ASA) by a chemical azo bond.[63–66] The preparation was named salicylazosulfapyridine or salazopyrine. Svartz, for four years, had been involved in experiments on the treatment of rheumatic polyarthritis with combinations of sulfanilamide and salicylate preparations. Svartz, in studies with Lindberg in the Institute of Pathology (Karolinska Institute), had been impressed with the changes "in the connective tissue below the muscularis mucosae" in ulcerative colitis and their resemblance to the histological changes in the joints of patients with rheumatoid arthritis; and "a pronounced affinity for connective tissue everywhere in the body." A salicylate was selected because of its beneficial effect on the joints and surrounding tissues. The choice of a sulfonamide was influenced by Svartz's acceptance of the concept attributing rheumatoid arthritis to a streptococcal infection, the continuing emphasis upon the possible role of the Bargen diplostreptococcus in ulcerative colitis, and the assumption of an anti-streptococcal effect of the sulfonamide sulfapyridine. Discussions in 1938 with Domagk had focused upon the stimulation of phagocytosis by sulfa drugs and the demonstration by L. Whitby (1938) of the effectiveness of sulfapyridine against various types of cocci. Initial use of the combination in animals (rabbits, rats, mice) indicated no toxicity. In cooperation with Helander, studies indicated "a definite affinity for connective tissue." Autoradiography by S. Ullberg of the Veterinary School of Stockholm confirmed the concentration of sulfasalazine in the connective tissue of the intestine, joint capsule, skin, blood vessels, and liver. The original purpose of this combination, therefore, was to deliver 5-ASA to the synovial tissues surrounding joints in the expectation that the local concentration of salicylate would relieve joint pain. When this compound proved helpful in patients with arthritis and ulcerative colitis, as reported in 1941 and 1942, its use was extended to ulcerative colitis alone, with initially favorable results (75–80% of patients). The recommended dose was two 500-mg tablets four to six times daily. Side effects included nausea, vomiting, fever, "cyanosis" (methemoglobin), liver injury, hematologic changes and skin rash. Bargen,[67] supporting the use of salazopyrine in the treatment of ulcerative colitis, in 1949 noted the similarity between rheumatic fever (caused by streptococci) and "chronic ulcerative colitis of the streptococcic type" and encouraged the use of sulfasalazine.

Kirsner et al.[60,68,69] studied the antibacterial effects of these sulfonamides on the aerobic flora of the feces in patients with ulcerative colitis during the 1940s and demonstrated decreases in total bacterial counts, including hemolytic coliforms. However, the antimicrobial effects were temporary, disappearing after several months despite continued sulfonamide administration. Furthermore, the decreases in fecal bacteria did not correlate with the clinical course. In one patient, sulfaguanidine, on repeated intermittent administration, became a "growth factor" for enteric bacteria. While helpful in the control of associated infections, antibacterial agents did not have the curative effects in IBD as anticipated initially. Complete eradication of the bacterial flora of the gut proved impossible (and probably would have been unwise), and initial antibacterial effects diminished after several months, as the flora was replaced by "new" bacteria and fungi. The subsequent 50-year worldwide experience with sulfasalazine confirmed its benefit in many patients with ulcerative colitis and in some with Crohn's colitis. Extensive studies of sulfasalazine's efficacy, safety, pharmacokinetics, and toxicity were made during the last half-century.[70,71] Clinical trials at the University of Chicago in the 1940s (not known to Svartz) had shown the ineffectiveness of sulfapyridine as treatment of ulcerative colitis and also had documented the weak antibacterial capacity of sulfasalazine. The 1977 studies of Azad-Khan et al.[72] demonstrated the efficacy of the 5-ASA component alone and its safety in patients intolerant of sulfasalazine. The details of this important pharmacotherapeutic development are described in the accompanying supplement by Professor U. Klotz. Preparations of 5-ASA (mesalamine, mesalazine) today are prescribed for ulcerative proctitis, ulcerative colitis, and also Crohn's colitis, not as antibacterial agents as in the 1950s though decreasing colonic bacterial sulfide production, but rather for their capacity to disrupt the superoxide anion radical, prevent hydroxyl radical formation, inhibit proinflammatory molecules of the lipoxygenase pathways, and for their ability to lower neutrophil chemotaxis, natural killer cell cytotoxicity, and activated lamina propria lymphocytes.[73] Favoring the continued use of sulfasalazine is its capacity to suppress NFκB activity, a very potent proinflammatory mediator, by directly inhibiting IκB kinases A and B. 5-aminosalicylic acid apparently lacks this capacity.

Antibiotics

The re-discovery of penicillin by Fleming[74,75] in 1928 (not available for medical use until 1940) inaugurated the antibiotic era after World War II. Earlier, Burdon-Sanderson (1871) and Lister (1892) apparently had noted the potentially beneficial antibacterial effects of penicillium mold but were in no position to capitalize on the observation. Subsequent antibiotics, in addition to penicillin, included streptomycin, neomycin, aureomycin, chloramphenicol, and tetracycline. The not infrequent relapses or intensifications of ulcerative colitis or Crohn's disease after the oral administration of penicillin and other antibiotics (e.g. aureomycin), often prescribed for respiratory illness. presented another problem. Handicapped by insufficient knowledge of the vast anaerobic flora of the gut and the commensal microbial flora associated with the intestinal epithelium, the use of antibiotics in the management of IBD and their capacity to consistently modify the enteric flora remains controversial.

Adrenocorticotropic Hormone, Steroids

The discovery of adrenocorticotropic hormone (ACTH) by Hench et al.[76] of the Mayo Clinic and the subsequent development of the glucocorticoids, cortisone, hydrocortisone, prednisone, prednisolone, and methylprednisolone, ushered in the steroid IBD therapy era late in 1950. The striking, at times dramatic, effects of ACTH in ulcerative colitis and Crohn's disease in the 1950s for a brief period suggested an adrenocortical deficiency as a possible etiology, a hypothesis soon discarded. The open observations of Kirsner and Palmer[77] in 1951 and the later controlled studies of Truelove and Witts[78] rapidly documented the immediate, often dramatically beneficial, effects of ACTH and later hydrocortisone. Many studies were made of virtually all aspects of these compounds, and the results subsequently were reported at the 1952 and 1953 National Conferences on ACTH and Adrenal Steroids organized by Mote of Chicago and the Wilson Company. The initial experience with cortisone was not encouraging, but hydrocortisone proved effective. Subsequent early studies included prednisone, prednisolone, and methylprednisolone. With more experience, the early dosage problems and the complications of steroid therapy[79] diminished, and their use in IBD, together with sulfasalazine, became virtually routine. Additional observations soon related the beneficial effects of the corticosteroid compounds to reductions in inflammatory cells (lymphocytes, plasma cells), decreased capillary permeability, and neutralization of the biochemical expressions of inflammation. Recent studies indicate that steroids (glucocorticoids) inhibit synthesis of most cytokines and of several cell surface molecules required for immune function. Glucocorticoids also are potent inhibitors of nuclear factor kappa B (NF-κK), a major component of their anti-inflammatory activity.[80] (However, continued experience with steroids in IBD demonstrated that the benefits of steroids often were temporary, and their intermittent use occasionally induced an unexplained "tolerance," with diminishing clinical efficacy and increasing side effects,[80] including harmful effects on bones.

Immunosuppressant Medication

As related by Schwartz,[81] "Within a few years of its discovery the immune response was tested for its susceptibility to chemical agents," beginning in 1898 with Salmonsen and Madsen.[82] Up to 1965, more than 100 different chemical agents had been utilized in attempts to suppress the immune response, dating back to Hektoen[83,84] in 1911. Studies of 6-mercaptopurine were initiated in 1950 by Hitchings and Elion[85,86] of Burroughs-Wellcome and continued in 1954 with papers on the fate of 6-mercaptopurine (6-MP) in mice and in humans.[87,88] In 1958 Schwartz et al.[89] demonstrated that 6-MP, a purine analogue, administered to rabbits in a dosage of 6 mg/kg body wt/day, completely blocked the primary immune response to a soluble protein antigen. 6-MP and its analogues presumably acted by blocking the conversion of inosinic acid to adenylic acid, a central biochemical process whose disruption led to wide-spread intracellular effects, especially the synthesis of nucleic acids. In 1962 Page et al.[90] found that 6-MP "markedly altered the inflammatory cycle in rabbits, virtually eliminating the participation of hematogenous mononuclear cells in the process." In 1962 and 1966 Bean[91,92] of Australia utilized 6-MP in the treatment of IBD. In 1966 Bowen, Kirsner et al.[93] administered azathioprine, an analogue of 6-MP, to 10 patients with severe IBD (9 ulcerative colitis, 1 Crohn's disease of the colon) in a dosage of 6 mg/kg body wt/day. The toxic effects of this dosage (including bone marrow toxicity) were too severe to evaluate therapeutic benefits. Subsequent dosage schedules of 2–3 mg/kg body wt/day virtually eliminated the acute side effects. Extensive open clinical therapeutic trials with 6-MP and azathioprine were undertaken subsequently, especially in Crohn's disease. Controlled trials with azathioprine in Crohn's disease and in ulcerative colitis by Rosenberg, Kirsner et al.[94,95] demonstrated its efficacy in facilitating reductions or complete elimination of steroids. Present, Korelitz et al.,[96] in particular, have demonstrated the usefulness of 6-MP in the management of Crohn's disease. A brief trial of nitrogen mustard in IBD[97] was limited by the drug's toxicity.

Cyclosporine (cyclosporin A) is a cyclosporin immunosuppressive agent produced by Tolypocladium inflatum genus (formerly Trichoderma polysporum) or Clindrocarpin lucidum, Booth. The drug is a nonpolar, cyclic polypeptide antibiotic consisting of 11 amino acids. Cyclosporine is one of several biologically active antibiotics (cyclosporins) produced by these fungi; cyclosporin A and C are the major metabolites. Petcher et al.[98] and Ruegger et al.[99] in 1976 first described the potent immunosuppressive activity of cyclosporine A involving T-lymphocytes, including inhibiting helper T-cells and decreasing the production of interleukin 2 and other lymphokines. Exactly what is being suppressed in IBD, the degree of immunosuppression and the duration of immunosuppressive therapy are not known. The proinflammatory molecules now being discovered (e.g. TNF-α) are important recent developments.

SURGICAL TREATMENT OF IBD

Ulcerative Colitis

The surgical approach to ulcerative colitis throughout the years reflected the insufficient knowledge of the disease and the limitations of abdominal surgery. The operative procedures of the early 1900s, appendicostomy,[100] cecostomy,[101] and colostomy, with and without "colonic irrigations," represented attempts to eliminate a "noxious substance" and perhaps to "rest" the diseased bowel. Brown[102] of the United States, based upon an experience with one ulcerative colitis patient, proposed the ileostomy as early as 1913 for such a purpose. Actually, these procedures had been performed earlier under varying circumstances. In 1850 Pennell[103] created a surgical opening in the sigmoid colon for a rectovesical fistula presumed to be related to an IBD. Franke[104] (cited by Bacon[105]) in 1889 performed an ileostomy before resecting part of the ascending colon. According to Strombeck[106] of Sweden, Follet of France and Novaro of Italy had first performed a cecostomy. Strauss et al.[107,108] of Chicago also as early as 1917 had advocated ileostomy and since 1923 had recommended this procedure "as soon as the diagnosis of ulcerative colitis is made." A.A. Strauss performed an ileostomy in a patient with severe ulcerative colitis named Koenig, an artist, chemist and adept mechanically. Koenig, under the guidance of Strauss, developed an adherent appliance to contain the ileal content and in partnership with A.M.P.

Rutzen produced the Strauss–Koenig–Rutzen bag, commonly used during the 1930s, 40s and 50s.[109] During the period 1930–50, construction of the ileostomy was associated with many technical problems and complications including ulcerative enteritis, peristomal ulceration, and intestinal obstruction.[110] In addition, the diseased bowel did not rest as had been assumed; the inflammation persisted and remained a threat to the patient. The mucosal modification of the ileostomy procedure (maturation of the ileostomy stoma at the time of surgery), independently by B.N. Brooke[111,112] of London and R. Turnbull[113] of Cleveland in the 1950s, improved the operation dramatically. According to Bacon,[105] the procedure (of simple eversion of the exposed ileum on itself and suturing the mucosal edge to the skin) had been suggested by Campbell in 1950. In 1951 Patey[114] of England had sutured the mucosa of a colostomy to the skin. Other significant early contributions to the surgery of ulcerative colitis as noted by Bacon include those of Coffey.[115] In 1943 Devine of Melbourne, Australia, described a multiple-stage procedure of partial colectomy for seriously ill patients with ulcerative colitis. In 1944 Strauss of Chicago introduced an improved ileostomy appliance, consisting of a short circular metal disk covered with rubber with a central hole for the ileostomy. A flat rubber pouch with an outlet at the bottom was attached to the disk for the collection and the elimination of the intestinal content. As related by Bacon,[105] this was the first of numerous modifications of ileostomy appliances and came to be known as the Koenig–Rutzen or the Strauss–Koenig–Rutzen bag. In 1948 Cattell of the Lahey Clinic in Boston described a three-stage surgical approach: ileostomy, subtotal colectomy, and finally an abdominoperineal resection of the rectum. In 1949 Miller of Montreal recommended a two-stage ileostomy and proctocolectomy, and in 1951 Ravitch and Handelman accomplished the procedure in one stage.

The reluctance during these early years (1930–60) to promptly resect the diseased bowel of severe ulcerative colitis complicated by toxic megacolon and the issue of "intractability" was a matter of vigorous debate between surgeons and gastroenterologists, reflecting concerns with the hazards of bowel surgery, early unfamiliarity with the long-term consequences of the ileostomy, patient reluctance to wear an ill-fitting, malodorous, and uncomfortable bag, and the lingering hope of reversibility of the disease. As a consequence, some patients ultimately were referred for surgery in a seriously debilitated state with a severely diseased bowel, depleted of blood, protein, and electrolytes. The high mortality in this group of patients subsequently encouraged earlier referrals to surgery for poorly responding patients, and the indications for operative intervention are much clearer today. Partial colon resection (Devine operation) was discontinued in the United States because of recurrent colonic disease. Subtotal colectomy with ileorectal anastomosis, despite favorable reports by Aylett[116] of London, was discarded during the 1960s and 1970s because of continuing disease but has regained some popularity. The procedure of procto-colectomy and ileal (Kock) pouch for ulcerative colitis, popular in the 1970s,[117] has been replaced by the ileoanal operation, with and without J pouch.[118,119]

Today, ileostomy and total proctocolectomy, proctocolectomy with ileo-pouch-anal anastomosis, and ileorectostomy and ileal pouch distal rectal anastomosis are successful operations for ulcerative colitis, especially among young women.[120,121] However, the development of pouchitis in 30% or more of patients is a major problem. The "diversion colitis"[122,123] after colostomy presumably resulting from defective oxidation of short-chain fatty acids (butyric acid) in the colon and its response to short-chain fatty acids[124] has directed attention to the insufficiently studied metabolic activities[125] of the colon.

Crohn's Disease

The earliest (infrequent) operations for regional enteritis (1890–1930) were abdominal explorations for preoperative diagnoses of "malignant tumor" and more often in the 1920s and 1930s for "acute appendicitis." Crohn wrote on the treatment of regional ileitis in 1941: "A specific conservative or medical approach does not exist; the long, slowly downward course cannot be interfered with or changed by any method now known. Vaccines and specific and nonspecific protein therapy have not been of any avail."[30] He strongly recommended surgical resection of diseased bowel, but already was aware of the recurrences. As reported by Leonardo[126] in 1937, a simple ileostomy proved highly effective in the resolution of an extensive ileocecal Crohn's disease. The surgical treatment of regional enteritis (Crohn's disease) during the 1940–60 period consisted of extensive resection of diseased intestine and re-anastomosis, attempting to remove all histologically detectable disease. Recurrences were common and the radical operations resulted in the short-bowel syndrome with significant physiologic consequences. The intestinal bypass operation, performed at New York Mt. Sinai Hospital in the 1950s and 1960s, though associated with healing of the bypassed loop, was discarded because of the bacterial overgrowth and the increased potential for later development of cancer. The absence of recurrence of Crohn's disease after intestinal resection and re-anastomosis when accompanied by a diverting ileostomy in contrast to the frequent recurrences when bowel continuity was restored is of particular interest. Surgeons and gastroenterologists, increasingly aware of the futility of extensive bowel resection for Crohn's disease, have recognized the physiologic and nutritional importance of preserving as much small bowel as possible by more limited bowel resections.

Operations for Crohn's colitis now include total proctocolectomy and ileostomy and subtotal colectomy and ileorectal anastomosis. Other procedures are strictureplasty in selected instances of small bowel narrowing and gastroenterostomy and vagotomy for Crohn's disease of the gastric antrum and proximal duodenum.[127] Significant scientific progress has been made toward the goal of transplantation of small intestine despite the formidable immunologic problems.

CONCLUDING COMMENTS

The current treatment of IBD, though much improved over earlier programs, remains variable rather than uniform and supportive rather than curative. The differing therapeutic practices result from the fact that the etiologies of the IBD are obscure, from limited knowledge of the biological and pharmacological actions of drugs commonly prescribed (sulfasalazine, 5-ASA compounds, steroids, 6-MP, and azathioprine), from an inadequate understanding of genetic factors influencing drug metabolism, from insufficient awareness of the factors involved in drug availability (concurrent use of antimotility drugs, cigarette smoking, food combinations), from variability of the patient groups studied (extent and severity of disease), and from incomplete documentation of the clinical status of patients at the time of therapeutic trial.[128]

From the standpoint of pathogenesis, the various therapeutic modalities and clinical responses have not provided significant etiologic clues to IBD. Nutritional support improves body defenses, enhances healing of the inflamed bowel, and facilitates the clinical response to medication, nonspecifically. The emotional support of the patient with IBD decreases the "burden of disability" but is not exclusive to IBD. No single drug is curative. The anti-inflammatory capacities of sulfasalazine and the 5-ASA preparations are not specific to IBD. Antibiotics decrease the enteric microflora temporarily, but whether or not this effect is beneficial is unknown. Furthermore, none of the antibiotics permanently heals IBD. The temporary favorable responses to ACTH and the adrenal corticosteroids are observed in other diseases. The "immunosuppressive" compounds 6-MP, azathioprine and cyclosporine, helpful especially in patients with Crohn's disease, require continued administration for effect. Total proctocolectomy and ileostomy and colectomy with ileoanal anastomosis for ulcerative colitis are ablative procedures. The operations for Crohn's disease of the small intestine and colon, though helpful, are not necessarily curative.

Future advances in treatment, including anti-inflammatory and immunotherapy and multiple drug programs, will depend on new information about the nature of IBD and of drug pharmacology and bioavailability, derived from collaborative studies by clinicians, clinical investigators, and basic scientists. Decisive multicenter therapeutic studies require agreement on definitions of ulcerative colitis and Crohn's disease, recognition of clinically variable subtypes, accurate characterization and stratification of patient groups, acceptable objective criteria of IBD severity and activity, and reliable indicators of therapeutic response. Since evaluations based on trials of 4–6 weeks reflect early, often transient effects, trials should continue for at least 1 year. These approaches, facilitating the acquisition of comparable data and more definitive therapeutic evaluations, will accelerate our understanding of the IBDs. Investigation of the molecular mechanisms of intestinal inflammation have identified pro- and anti-inflammatory molecules and has made possible the concept of targeted biological therapy of the inflammatory bowel diseases typified by the recent success with anti-tumor necrosis alpha in Crohn's disease,[129] and the potential of NFκB signalling proteins[130] and stem cell transplantation.[131]

REFERENCES

1. Allchin WH. Ulcerative colitis. An address introductory to the subject. Proc Roy Soc Med 1909;2:59–75.
2. Haggard H. The doctors in history – New Haven 1934. In: MacKinney LC, ed. Baltimore: Johns Hopkins Press, 1937:33–4.
3. Dack GM, Dragstedt LR. Effect of introducing oxygen into isolated colon of patient with chronic ulcerative colitis. Am J Dig Dis 1938;5:84–6.
4. Meleney FL. In discussion of L. R. Dragstedt, G. M. Dack, J. B. Kirsner. Chronic ulcerative colitis. Ann Surg 1941;114:653–62.
5. Curtius F. Hypnotische behandlung schwerer colitiden. Dtsch Arch Klin Med 1943;190:444–56.
6. Dorfman W. Narco analysis in ulcerative colitis. NY State J Med 1952;52:2019–21.
7. Popp WC, Bargen JA, Dixon CF. Regional enteritis – roentgen therapy. Proc Mayo Clin 1950;25:1–5.

8. Logan AH. Three cases of chronic ulcerative colitis cured by iodine. Med Clin North Am 1923;7:105–12.
9. Herfort RA, Livingston H. Thiouracil drugs in treatment of chronic ulcerative colitis. NY State J Med 1952;52:431–6.
10. Burnford J. Ulcerative colitis – its treatment by ionization – summary of twenty eight cases. Br Med J 1930;2:640–1.
11. Cheney G. Injection of highly concentrated liver extract in treatment of idiopathic ulcerative colitis. Arch Intern Med 1939;63:813–29.
12. Ferguson LK, Fetter K, Schnabel TG. Artificial fever in the treatment of ulcerative colitis: A preliminary report. Am J Dig Dis 1937;4:487–8.
13. Schmelkes FD, Marks HC. N,N-Dichloro-azao-dicarbomidine (azochloramid), an n-chloro deriviatve of oxidant in an oxidation-reduction system. J Am Chem Soc 1934;56:1610–13.
14. Goffrey Y, Colin R, Hacketsweiler PH, Segrestin M. Traitement de la maladie de Crohn per le BCG. Arch Mal l'Appareil Dig 1971;64:299–308.
15. Burnham WR, Lennard-Jones JE, Hecketsweiler P, Colin R, Geffroy Y. Oral BCG vaccine in Crohn's disease. Gut 1979;20:229–33.
16. Portis S, Block L, Necheles H. Studies on chronic ulcerative colitis and some biological effects of detergents. Gastroenterology 1944;3:106–13.
17. Horgan E, Horgan J. Chronic ulcerative colitis – results of treatment with vaccine in 5 cases. JAMA 1929;93:263–6.
18. Lups S. Vaccine therapy in ulcerative colitis. Am J Dig Dis Nutr 1935;2:65–90.
19. Maratka Z, Wagner F. The treatment of nonspecific ulcerative colitis by autogenous vaccine: correlated bacteriological and immunological studies. Gastroenterology 1948;113:34–49.
20. Kalk H. Therapie der colitis gravis durch erzeugung von anaphylaxis und mit bluttransfusionen. Ztsch f Klin Med 1931;118:560–83.
21. Gill AM. Chronic ulcerative colitis clinical experiments with pig's intestine. Lancet 1944;246:536–7.
22. Ehrlich R. Treatment of chronic ulcerative colitis with fractional component of hog's stomach. Am J Dig Dis Nutr 1950;17:1–4.
23. Streicher MH, Grossman MI, Ivy AC. Preliminary report of a clinical trial of orally administered hog duodenum powder in the treatment of chronic ulcerative colitis. Gastroenterology 1949;12:371–4.
24. Friedman MHF, Haskell BF. Treatment of nonspecific ulcerative colitis for one year with extracts of intestinal mucosa. Gastroenterology 1946;11:833–41.
25. Hiatt B. Abnormal intestinal motility as an etiological factor in inflammatory bowel disease. J Clin Gastroenterol 1984;6:201–3.
26. Schlitt RJ, McNally JJ, Shafiroff BGP, Hinton JW. Pelvic autonomic neurectomy for ulcerative colitis. Gastroenterology 1951;19:812–16.
27. Dennis C, Eddy FD. Response to vagotomy in idiopathic ulcerative colitis. Ann Surg 1948;128:479–86.
28. Cesnick H. Thymectomy in ulcerative colitis: Promising results in seven patients. Langenbecks Arch Klin Chir 1968;321:86–98.
29. Sanpanet R, Bucaille M. Procaine injection of the prefrontal lobe of the brain – technic and present indications. Ann Surg 1955;141:388–97.
30. Crohn BB. Regional ileitis. In: Portis SA, ed. Diseases of the digestive system. Philadelphia: Lea and Febiger, 1941:722–9.
31. Paulson M. Nonspecific or indeterminate ulcerative colitis. In: Portis SA, ed. Diseases of the digestive system. Philadelphia: Lea and Febiger, 1941:844–71.
32. Casten D. Nutritional disturbances in regional enteritis. Surgery 1939;6:708–16.
33. James AH. Breakfast and Crohn's disease. Br Med J 1977;1:943–5.

34. Martini GA, Brandes JW. Increased consumption of refined carbohydrates in patients with Crohn's disease. Klin Wochenschr 1976;54:367–71.
35. Heaton KW, Thornton JR, Emmett PM. Treatment of Crohn's disease with an unrefined carbohydrate, fibre rich diet. Br Med J 1979;2:764–6.
36. Guthy E. Aetiologie der morbus Crohn. Deutsch Med Wochenschr 1983;45:1729–33.
37. Andresen AFR. Ulcerative colitis – an allergic phenomenon. Am J Dig Dis 1942;9:91–8.
38. Carstensen J. Food additives and their possible role in Crohn's disease. Z Gastroenterol 1979;(Suppl)17:145–53.
39. Tilden E, Miller E. The response of the monkey to the withdrawal of vitamin A from the diet. J Nutr 1930;3:121–40.
40. Kirsner JB, Sheffner AL, Palmer WL. Studies on amino acid excretion in man. V. Chronic ulcerative colitis and regional enteritis. J Clin Invest 1950;29:874–80.
41. Kirsner JB, Brandt MB, Sheffner AL. Diet and amino acid utilization in gastrointestinal disorders. J Am Diet Assoc 1953;29:1103–8.
42. Elman R, Weiner DO. Intravenous alimentation – with special reference to protein (amino acid) metabolism. JAMA 1939;112:796–802.
43. Remington JH, Bargen JA, Lundy JS. Amino acid alimentation in gastrointestinal diseases. Gastroenterology 1946;7:442–9.
44. Machella TE, Miller TG. Treatment of idiopathic ulcerative colitis by means of a "medical ileostomy" and an orally-administered protein hydrolysate-dextrimaltose mixture. Gastroenterology 1948;10:28–45.
45. Dudrick SJ, Wilmore DW, Vars HM, Rhoads JE. Longterm total parenteral nutrition with growth, development and positive nitrogen balance. Surgery 1968;64:134–42.
46. Dudrick SJ, Wilmore DW, Vars HM, Rhoads JE. Can intravenous feeding as the sole means of nutrition support growth in the child and restore weight loss in an adult? An affirmative answer. Ann Surg 1969;169:974–84.
47. Fisher JE, Foster GS, Abel RM, Abbott WM, Ryan JA. Hyperalimentation as primary therapy for inflammatory bowel disease. Am J Surg 1973;125:165–75.
48. Vilaseca J, Salas A, Guarner F, Rodriquez R, Martinez M, Malagelada JR. Dietary fish oil reduces progression of chronic inflammatory lesions in rat model of granulomatous colitis. Gut 1990;31:539–44.
49. Koch TR, Yuan LX, Fink JG, Petro A, Opara EC. Induction of enlarged intestinal lymphoid aggregates during acute glutathione depletion in a murine model. Dig Dis Sci 2000;45:11:2115–21.
50. Alexander F. The influence of psychologic factors upon gastrointestinal disturbances. A symposium. Psychoanal Q 1934;3:501–39.
51. Grace WJ, Pinsky RH, Wolff H. Treatment of ulcerative colitis. Gastroenterology 1954;26:462–8.
52. Karush A, Daniels GE, Flood CF, O'Connor JF, with the assistance of Druss R, Sweeting J. Psychotherapy in chronic ulcerative colitis. Philadelphia: W.B. Saunders, 1977.
53. Almy TP. Psychosocial aspects of chronic ulcerative colitis and Crohn's disease. In: Kirsner JB, Shorter RG, eds. Inflammatory bowel disease. Philadelphia: Lea and Febiger, 1980:44–54.
54. von Curtius F, Ruhrmoser HG. Zur pscyhotherapie der colitis ulcerosa. Deutsche Med Wochschr 1955;8033:105–8.
55. Feldman F, Cantor D, Soll S, Bachrach W. Psychiatric study of a consecutive series of 34 patients with ulcerative colitis. Br Med J 1967;3:14–17.

56. Helzer JE, Stillings WA, Chammas S, Norland CC, Alpers DH. A controlled study of the association between ulcerative colitis and psychiatric diagnoses. Dig Dis Sci 1982;27:513–18.
57. North CS, Clouse RE, Spitznagel EL, Alpers DH. The relation of ulcerative colitis to psychiatric factors: A review of findings and methods. Am J Psychiatry 1990; 147:974–81.
58. Helzer JE, Chammas S, Norland CC, Stillings WA, Alpers DH. A study of the association between Crohn's disease and psychiatric illness. Gastroenterology 1984;86:324–30.
59. Domagk G. Ein beitrag zur chemotherapie der bakteriellen infektionen. Dtsch Med Wochenschr 1935;61:250–3.
60. Rodaniche EC, Kirsner JB, Palmer WL. Effect of oral administration of sulfonamide compounds in the fecal flora of patients with nonspecific ulcerative colitis. Gastroenterology 1943;1:133–9.
61. Marshall HC, Palmer WL, Kirsner JB. Effects of chemotherapeutic agents on fecal bacteria in patients with chronic ulcerative colitis. JAMA 1950;144:900–3.
62. Cooke EM. Fecal flora of patients with ulcerative colitis during treatment with salicylazosulphapyridine. Gut 1967;10:565–8.
63. Svartz N, Kallner S. Sulfonamide preparations and continued investigations on complications after treatment with brief report on new therapeutic experiments. Forsatta undersokningar over biverkningar vid behandling med sulfonamidpreparat samt en kort redogorelse fur nya terapeutiska forsok. Nord Med 1940; 8:1935–40.
64. Svartz N. Salazopyrin – a new sulfanilamide preparation. A. Therapeutic result in rheumatoid arthritis. B. Therapeutic results in ulcerative colitis. C. Toxic manifestations on treatment with sulfanilamide preparations. Acta Med Scand 1942;110:577–90. (also Nord Med 1941;11:2261–2.)
65. Bachrach WH. Sulfasalalzine. I. An historical perspective. Am J Gastroenterol 1988;83:487–96.
66. Svartz N. Sulfasalazine: II. Some notes on the discovery and development of salazopyrin. Am J Gastroenterol 1988;83:497–503.
67. Bargen JA. Treatment of ulcerative colitis with salicylazosulfapyridine (salazopyrin). Med Clin North Am 1949;33:935–42.
68. Kirsner JB, Rodaniche EC, Palmer WL. The use of sulfaguanidine in non-specific ulcerative colitis and other infections of the bowel. Am J Dig Dis 1942;9:229–33.
69. Rodaniche EC, Palmer WL, Kirsner JB. The streptococci present in the feces of patients with nonspecific ulcerative colitis and the effect of oral administration of sulfonamide compounds upon them. J Infect Dis 1943;72:222–7.
70. Klotz U, Maier K, Fischer C, Heinkel K. Therapeutic efficacy of sulphasalazine and its metabolites in patients with ulcerative colitis and Crohn's disease. N Engl J Med 1980;303:1499–502.
71. Peppercorn MA. Distribution studies of salicylazosulfapyridine and its metabolites. Gastroenterology 1973;64;240–5.
72. Azad-Khan AK, Piris J, Truelove SC. An experiment to determine the active therapeutic moiety of sulphasalazine. Lancet 1977;2:892–5.
73. Gaginella TS, Walsh RE. Sulfasalazine – multiplicity of action. Dig Dis Sci 1992; 37:801–12.
74. Fleming A. The 1928 discovery of penicillin. Br Med Bull 1944;2:4–5.
75. Fleming A. On the antibacterial action of a penicillium with special reference to their use in the isolation of B. Influenzae. Br J Exp Pathol 1929;10:226–38.
76. Hench PS, Kendall EC, Slocumb CH, Polley HF. The effect of a hormone of the adrenal cortex (17-hydroxy-11 Dehydrocorticosterone) (compound E) and of

pituitary adrenocorticotropic hormone on rheumatoid arthritis – preliminary report. Proc Staff Meet Mayo Clin 1949;24:181–97.
77. Kirsner JB, Palmer WL. Effect of corticotropin (ACTH) in chronic ulcerative colitis. JAMA 1951;147:541–9.
78. Truelove SC, Witts IJ. Cortisone in ulcerative colitis. Report on therapeutic trial. Br Med J 1955;2:1041–8.
79. Goldstein MJ, Gelzayd EA, Kirsner JB. Some observations on the hazards of corticosteroid therapy in patients with inflammatory bowel disease. Trans Am Acad Ophthal Otolaryngol 1967;71:254–61.
80. Auphan N, DiDonato JA, Rosette C, Helmberg A, including Karin M. Immunosuppression by glucocorticoids: inhibition of NF-kappa B activity through induction of IκB synthesis. Science 1995;270:286–90.
81. Schwartz RS. Immunosuppressive drugs. Prog Allergy 1965;9:246–303.
82. Salmonsen CJ, Madsen T. Sur la reproduction de la substance antitoxique apres de fortes saignees. Ann Inst Pasteur 1898;12:763–73.
83. Hektoen L. Effect of toluene on production of antibodies. J Infect Dis 1911;19:737–45.
84. Hektoen L, Corper HJ. Effect of mustard gas on antibody formation. J Infect Dis 1921;28:279–85.
85. Hitchings GH, Elion GB, Falco EA, Russell PB, VanderWerff H. Studies on analogs of purines and pyrimidines. Ann NY Acad Sci 1950;52:1318–35.
86. Hitchings GH, Elion GB, Falco EA, Russell PB, Sherwood MB, VanderWerff H. Antagonists of nucleic acid derivatives: lactobacillus casei model. J Biol Chem 1950;183:1–9.
87. Elion GB, Bieber S, Hitchings GH. The fate of 6 Mercaptopurine in mice. Ann NY Acad Sci 1954;60:297–302.
88. Hamilton L, Elion GB. The rate of 6 Mercaptopurine in man. Ann NY Acad Sci 1954;60:304–14.
89. Schwartz RS, Stack J, Dameshek W. Effect of 6 Mercaptopurine on antibody production. Proc Soc Exp Biol Med 1958;99:164–7.
90. Page AH, Condie RM, Good RA. Effect of 6 Mercaptopurine on inflammation. Am J Pathol 1962;40:519–30.
91. Bean RHD. The treatment of chronic ulcerative colitis with 6 Mercaptopurine. Med J Aust 1962;1:592–3.
92. Bean RHD. Treatment of ulcerative colitis with anti-metabolites. Br Med J 1966;1:1081–4.
93. Bowen GE, Irons Jr. GV, Rhodes JB, Kirsner JB. Early experiences with Azathioprine in ulcerative colitis – a note of caution. JAMA 1966;195:460–4.
94. Rosenberg JL, Levin B, Wall AJ, Kirsner JB. A controlled trial of Azathioprine in Crohn's disease. Dig Dis 1975;20:721–6.
95. Rosenberg JL, Wall AJ, Levin B, Binder HJ, Kirsner JB. A controlled trial of Azathioprine in the management of chronic ulcerative colitis. Gastroenterology 1975;69:96–9.
96. Present DH, Korelitz BI, Wisch N, Glass JL, Sachar DB, Pasternack BS. Treatment of Crohn's disease with 6 Mercaptopurine – a long term randomized double blind study. N Engl J Med 1980;302:981–7.
97. Winkelman EI, Brown CH. Nitrogen mustard in the treatment of chronic ulcerative colitis and regional enteritis. Cleveland Clinic Q 1965;32:165–74.
98. Petcher TJ, Weber HP, Ruegger A. Crystal and molecular structure of an iodo-derivative of the cyclic undecapeptide Cyclosporin A. Helv Chim Acta 1976;59:1480–9.

99. Ruegger A, Kuhn M, Lichti H, Loosli HR, Huguenin R, Quiquerez C, et al. Cyclosporin A ein immunosuppressio wirksauer peptimetabolit aus trichoderma polysporium (Link ex Pers.) rifai. Helv Chim Acta 1976;59:1075–92.
100. Weir RF. A new use for the useless appendix in surgical treatment of obstinate colitis. Med Rec 1902;62:201–2.
101. Allison CC. Cecostomy: the operation of choice for temporary drainage of the colon. JAMA 1909;53:1562.
102. Brown JY. The value of complete physiological rest of large bowel in treatment of certain ulcerative and obstructive lesions of this organ. Surg Gynecol Obstet 1913;16:610–13.
103. Pennel JWC. Stricture of rectum – artificial anus established in left lumbar region. Med Chir Trans 1850;33:255–60.
104. Franke K. Colectomy or resection of the large intestine for malignant disease. Med Chir 1889;72:211–32. In: Bacon HE. Ulcerative colitis. Philadelphia: Lippincott, 1958.
105. Bacon HE. Ulcerative colitis. Philadelphia: Lippincott, 1958.
106. Strombeck JF. Surgical treatment of ulcerative colitis. Acta Chir Scand 1949;98:414–27.
107. Strauss AA. Ulcerative colitis. Surg Clin North Am 1923;3:1033–42.
108. Strauss AA, Friedman J, Block L. Colectomy for ulcerative colitis. Surg Clin North Am 1924;4:667–86.
109. Hill JL. Ileostomy: surgery, physiology and management. New York: Grune and Stratton, 1976:1–11.
110. Whittaker LD. Observation on the human being following colectomy or colonic exclusion with ileostomy. Proc Staff Meet Mayo Clin 1937;12:183–7.
111. Brooke BN, Cooke WT. Ulcerative colitis: diagnostic problems and therapeutic warning. Lancet 1951;2:462–4.
112. Brooke BN. The management of an ileostomy including its complications. Lancet 1952;2:102–4.
113. Turnbull RB. Management of an ileostomy. Am J Surg 1953;86:617–24.
114. Patey DH. Primary epithelial apposition in colostomy. Proc Roy Soc Med 1951;44:423–4.
115. Coffey RC. Two stage operation in abdominal surgery – making and closing an ileostomy opening. Trans West Surg Assoc 1916;26:159–72.
116. Aylett S. Diffuse ulcerative colitis and its treatment by ileorectal anastomosis. Ann Roy Coll Surg Engl 1960;27:260–5.
117. Kock NG. Continent ileostomy. Progress Surg 1973;12:180–201.
118. Ravitch MM, Sabiston DC. Anal ileostomy with preservation of the sphincter. A proposed operation on patients requiring total colectomy for benign lesions. Surg Gynecol Obstet 1947;84:1095–9.
119. Parks AG, Nicholls RJ, Belliveau P. Proctocolectomy with ileal reservoir and anal anastomosis. Br J Surg 1980;67:533–8.
120. Dozois RR, Kelly K. Newer operations for ulcerative colitis and Crohn's disease. In: Kirsner JB, Shorter RG, eds. Inflammatory bowel disease. Philadelphia: Lea and Febiger, 1988:655–83.
121. Kelly KA. Anal sphincter-saving operations for chronic ulcerative colitis. Am J Surg 1992;163:5–11.
122. Glotzer DJ, Glock ME, Goldman H. Proctitis and colitis following diversion of the fecal stream. Gastroenterology 1981;80:438–41.
123. Korelitz BI, Cheskin LJ, Sohn N, Sommers SC. Proctitis after fecal diversion in Crohn's disease and its elimination with re-anastomosis – implications for surgical management. Gastroenterology 1984;87:710–13.

124. Harig JM, Soergel KH, Komorowski RA, Wood CM. Treatment of diversion colitis with short chain fatty acid irrigation. N Engl J Med 1989;320:23–8.
125. Roediger WE. Role of anaerobic bacteria in the metabolic welfare of the colonic mucosa in man. Gut 1989;21:793–8.
126. Leonardo RA. Intestinal obstruction due to non-specific ileocecal granulomas (combined "regional ileitis" and colitis). Am J Surg 1937;35:607–8.
127. Block GE. Surgical management of Crohn's colitis. N Engl J Med 1980;302:1068–70.
128. Kirsner JB. Limitations in the evaluation of therapy for inflammatory bowel disease – suggestions for future research. J Clin Gastroenterol 1990;12:516–24.
129. Sandborn WJ, Hanauer SB. Antitumor necrosis factor therapy for inflammatory bowel disease: a review of agents, pharmacology, clinical results and safety. Inflamm Bowel Dis 1990;5:119–33.
130. Jobin C, Sartor RB. NFκB signalling proteins as therapeutic targets for inflammatory bowel disease. Inflamm Bowel Dis 2000;6:206–13.
131. Hawkey CJ, Snowden JA, Lobo A, Beglinger C, Tyndall A. Stem cell transplantation for inflammatory bowel disease. Practical and ethical issues. Gut 2000;46:869–72.

Pharmacological Development of Aminosalicylates for the Treatment of Inflammatory Bowel Disease

Ulrich Klotz, Ph.D.
Professor of Pharmacology, Dr Margarete Fischer-Bosch-Institut für Klinische Pharmakologie, Stuttgart, Germany

Metabolic experiments with labelled SASP, 5-ASA and SP in mice demonstrated that the azo-link was split by bacterial reduction and unchanged SASP was excreted in minor amounts. 5-ASA and acetyl-5-ASA (Ac-5-ASA) as well as SP and acetylated SP could be identified in urine. Besides the two major acetylated metabolites, other unidentified products appeared in negligible quantities.[1,2] This metabolic pattern also was found in man. The major pathways of all three compounds are summarized in Figure 1.[3,4]

Clinical studies subsequently were performed to determine whether the therapeutic properties of SASP resided in the parent molecule or in the primary metabolites SP and/or 5-ASA. Since orally administered SP and 5-ASA are absorbed almost totally from the small intestine,[3] the agents were first used in the form of retention enemas in patients with mild or moderately active UC to determine topically effective drug levels. In random order, three groups of patients received nightly for two weeks enemas with SASP (2 g), 5-ASA (0.7 g) or SP (1.3 g). Most of the tested patients (87%) already were on oral maintenance treatment with 2 g SASP, which was continued during the trial. Pronounced histological improvement was observed in approximately 30% of patients receiving SASP or 5-ASA and only in 5% of those receiving SP, indicating that the active therapeutic moiety of SASP is 5-ASA, with SP functioning as a carrier, facilitating the release of 5-ASA within the colon.[5]

The second trial was performed in 45 patients with active idiopathic proctitis who were randomly assigned to three groups treated double-blindly for four weeks with suppositories twice daily containing either 200 mg 5-ASA, 300 mg SP or placebo. Complete clinical remission with healing of the rectal mucosa as noted sigmoidoscopically occurred in 60% of patients given 5-ASA but in only 13% and 27% of those receiving SP or placebo, respectively. Again, this study identified 5-ASA as the active therapeutic moiety of SASP.[6]

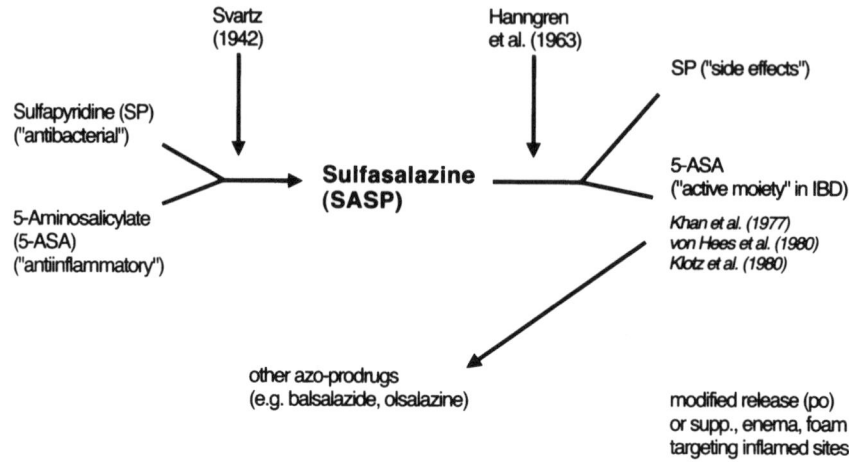

Figure 1. The development of sulfasalazine (SASP) and aminosalicylates (5-ASA).

At the same time, 23 patients with active UC and 9 patients with active CD were treated (tid) in a randomized, controlled trial with 1 g SASP (po), 0.5 g SP orally or with 0.5 g 5-ASA suppositories for six weeks. A significant ($p < 0.001$) decrease in an activity index and improvement in stool quality was achieved with only SASP and 5-ASA. Significantly higher remission rates were observed with 5-ASA (86%) and SASP (64%), compared with SP (14%). As 5-ASA was at least as effective as SASP, this metabolite was regarded as a therapeutic alternative to the parent drug.[7]

These favorable clinical results initiated numerous comparative studies with 5-ASA (now known as mesalazine or mesalamine) in different dosages and formulations either for inducing or maintaining remission in patients with IBD, especially UC. In addition, most of the observed side effects of SASP could be attributed to SP and an association was found with the plasma concentrations of SP, which were especially high in genetically determined slow acetylators of SP.[8,9] In contrast, 5-ASA was well tolerated, allowing even higher dosage than initially selected (1.5 g/day).

Since 5-ASA acts from the luminal site of the intestine, it appeared rational to develop delivery systems which would favor a topical action in the small and/or large bowel. Consequently, for UC different rectal forms (e.g. suppositories, enemas, foam) were utilized, whereas for CD special slow release preparations were developed. Moreover, other azo-prodrugs of 5-ASA were synthesized (Figure 2), which, like SASP, depend upon an effective reductive cleavage of the azo-bond by colonic bacteria. In the prodrug ipsalazide, the carrier SP was replaced by p-aminohippurate (4-aminobenzoylglycine), in balsalazide by 4-aminobenzoyl-β-alanine,[10] in HB-313 by p-aminobenzoate[11] or by a non-absorbable sulphanilamido-ethylene polymer in poly-ASA.[12] In azodisalicylate (olsalazine) two molecules of 5-ASA were connected.[13]

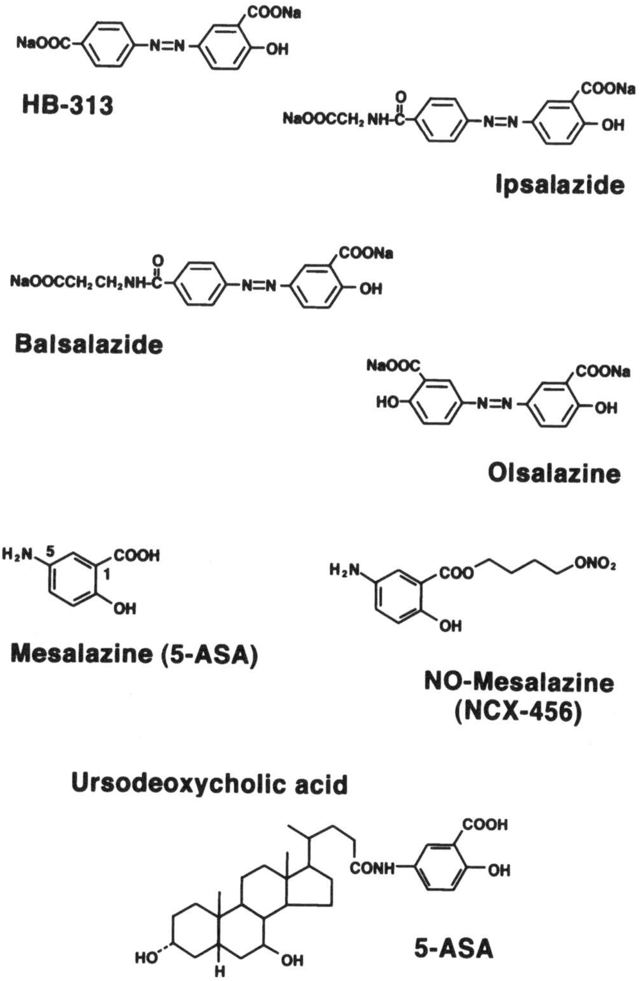

Figure 2. Structure and metabolic pathways of sulfasalazine (SASP).

Early in the 1980s, three different slow-release preparations of 5-ASA were developed,[14–16] which were prescribed orally for the treatment of UC and CD.[17–19] The first marketed 5-ASA preparations were Salofalk® suppositories (March 1984 in Germany), Asacol® tablets (November 1984 in Switzerland) and Salofalk® tablets (January 1985 in Germany).[20] The administration of 5-ASA itself seemed to be simpler, less toxic (no carrier or azo-bond mediated side effects) and less vulnerable to interference by drug interactions and/or pathophysiological conditions.[4] 5-ASA gained wide clinical acceptance. In contrast, 4-ASA or PAS (p-aminosalicylate), also with clinical efficacy in IBD, received less attention.[21]

Numerous studies and meta-analyses established the clinical value of 5-ASA in IBD.[22–26] In active UC, 5-ASA was clearly superior to placebo and slightly better than corticosteroids in inducing remission. In general, remission rates for 5-ASA ranged between 40 and 75% and today rectal administration of 5-ASA can be regarded as first choice for the treatment of active UC and for maintenance of remission. In several controlled studies of active Crohn's disease, results were variable and somewhat conflicting. Consequently, the benefit of 5-ASA in CD is only modest (probably doses of ≥3 g/day are desirable) and further clinical studies are needed to determine whether subgroups of patients will show a better response.[22,23,27,28] Similarly, maintenance of remission by oral 5-ASA appeared equivocal and benefit apparently was achieved mainly after surgery in patients with ileitis and in patients with prolonged disease.[22–24,28,29]

Different preparations (with various time or pH-dependent release patterns) and varying dosages will influence the concentrations of active 5-ASA at target sites in the inflamed mucosa. Following oral or rectal administration, the released 5-ASA is taken up by the epithelial cells in the small and large bowel. During the absorption processes, presystemic acetylation to the inactive Ac-5-ASA occurs (see Figure 3). Both 5-ASA and Ac-5-ASA are actively secreted into the lumen by membrane-bound drug efflux pumps. Thus, intra- and inter-individual variability in the expression and activity of both N-acetyltransferase and the drug transporting proteins will affect topical concentrations of 5-ASA in the mucosa.[30] Recent studies indicate that sufficiently high mucosal 5-ASA levels are needed for a positive response. Apparently, a relationship exists between tissue concentrations of 5-ASA and inflammatory manifestations.[31,32]

The exact mode of action of 5-ASA remains obscure. Aminosalicylates exert several biochemical actions *in vitro* and *in vivo*. The inhibitory effect of 5-ASA on cyclooxygenase and 5-lipoxygenase initially favored blocking

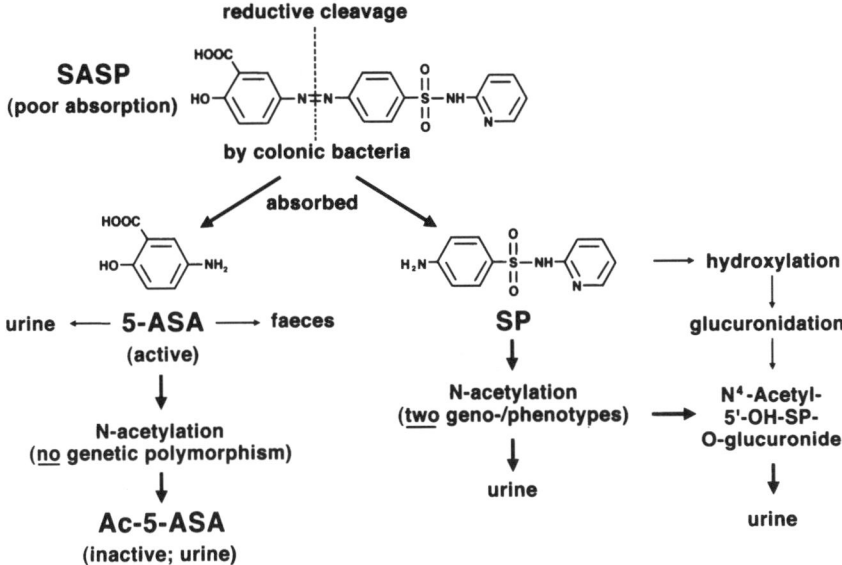

Figure 3. Structures of various old prodrugs which were developed to deliver the active 5-ASA into the large bowel and two novel conjuates of 5-ASA with therapeutic potential.

the synthesis of prostaglandins and leukotrienes as the key factor.[33] Subsequently, it was learned that 5-ASA is one of the most potent free radical scavengers and antioxidants.[34,35] More recently, the inhibitory effect of 5-ASA on various immunological processes has attracted attention, including inhibition of T cell proliferation, antibody production, IgG_1-induced phagocytosis and cytotoxicity, chemotaxis and adhesion, production of interleukin (IL)1 and IL8 or tumor necrosis factor α (TNF-α). It now appears that many of the actions of 5-ASA can be related to the inhibition of nuclear factor-κB (NFκB), a central regulator of immunological and inflammatory processes.[36,37]

With increasing knowledge of the mode of action of 5-ASA, its therapeutic indications might be extended. Mesalazine can induce apoptosis and decrease proliferation in colorectal mucosa in patients with sporadic polyps of the large bowel.[38] Moreover, it selectively induces apoptosis of tumor cells in patients with colorectal cancer,[39] observations suggesting that 5-ASA may be useful in the chemoprevention of colorectal cancer.[40]

CONCLUSIONS AND FUTURE PERSPECTIVES

Multiple therapeutic options for IBD now have become available but the "poly-potent" aminosalicylates remain among the first line drugs.[41,42] More knowledge in this area, as well as in the etiopathogenesis of IBD, will contribute to identifying the "best" 5-ASA preparation. Perhaps NO releasing derivatives of mesalazine[43] or new conjugates (see Figure 2) of 5-ASA with ursodeoxycholic acid[44] might contribute to further therapeutic efficacy. Such novel conjugates with dual action could represent a renewal of the aminosalicylate story which began in 1942 with SASP.

Acknowledgement

This work was supported by the Robert Bosch Foundation, Stuttgart, Germany.

REFERENCES

1. Hanngren A, Hansson E, Svartz N, Ullberg S. Distribution and metabolism of salicyl-azo-sulfapyridine. I. A Study of C^{14}-salicyl-azo-sulfapyridine and C^{14}-5-amino-salicylic acid. Acta Med Scand 1963;173:61–72.
2. Hanngren A, Hansson E, Svartz N, Ullberg S. Distribution and metabolism of salicyl-azo-sulfapyridine. II. A study with S^{35}-salicyl-azo-sulfapyridine and S^{35}-sulfapyridine. Acta Med Scand 1963;173:391–9.
3. Schröder H, Campbell DES. Absorption, metabolism and excretion of salicylazosulfapyridin in man. Clin Pharmacol Ther 1972;13:539–51.
4. Klotz U. Clinical pharmacokinetics of sulphasalazine, its metabolites and other prodrugs of 5-aminosalicylic acid. Clin Pharmacokinet 1985;10:285–302.
5. Azad Khan AK, Piris J, Truelove SC. An experiment to determine the active therapeutic moiety of sulphasalazine. Lancet 1977;II:892–5.
6. Van Hees PAM, Bakker JH, Van Tongeren JHM. Effect of sulphapyridine, 5-aminosalicylic acid, and placebo in patients with idiopathic proctitis: a study to determine the active therapeutic moiety of sulphasalazine. Gut 1980;21:632–5.
7. Klotz U, Maier K, Fischer C, Heinkel K. Therapeutic efficacy of sulfasalazine and its metabolites in patients with ulcerative colitis and Crohn's disease. N Engl J Med 1980;303:1499–502.
8. Das KM, Eastwood MA, McManus JPA, Sircus W. Adverse reactions during salicylazosulfapyridine therapy and the relation with drug metabolism and acetylator phenotype. N Engl J Med 1973;289:491–5.
9. Fischer C, Klotz U. Is plasma level monitoring of sulfasalazine indicated in the treatment of Crohn's disease or ulcerative colitis? Ther Drug Monit 1980;2:153–8.
10. Chan RP, Pope DJ, Gilbert AP, Sacra PJ, Baron JH, Lennard-Jones JE. Studies of two novel sulfasalazine analogs, ipsalazide and balsalazide. Dig Dis Sci 1983;28:609–15.
11. Bartalsky A. Salicylazobenzoic acid in ulcerative colitis. Lancet 1982;I:960.
12. Garretto M, Riddell RH, Winans CS. Treatment of chronic ulcerative colitis with poly-ASA: A new nonabsorbable carrier for release of 5-aminosalicylate in the colon. Gastroenterology 1983;84:1162.

13. Willoughby CP, Aronson JK, Agback H, Bodin NO, Truelove SC. Distribution and metabolism in healthy volunteers of disodium azodisalicylate, a potential therapeutic agent for ulcerative colitis. Gut 1982;23:1081–7.
14. Dew MJ, Hughes P, Harries AD, Williams G, Evans BK, Rhodes J. Maintenance of remission in ulcerative colitis with oral preparations of 5-amino salicylic acid. Br Med J 1982;285:1012.
15. Rasmussen SN, Bondesen S, Hvidberg EF, Hansen SH, Binder V, Halskov S, et al. 5-Aminosalicylic acid in a slow-release preparation: bioavailability, plasma levels and excretion in humans. Gastroenterology 1982;83:1062–70.
16. Klotz U, Maier KE, Fischer C, Bauer KH. A new slow-release form of 5-aminosalicylic acid for the oral treatment of inflammatory bowel disease. Arzneimittelforschung 1985;35:636–9.
17. Dew MJ, Harries AD, Evans N, Evans BK, Rhodes J. Maintenance remission in ulcerative colitis with 5-aminosalicylic acid in high doses by mouth. Br Med J 1983;287:23–4.
18. Rasmussen SN, Binder V, Maier K, Bondesen S, Fischer C, Klotz U, et al. Treatment of Crohn's disease with peroral 5-aminosalicylic acid. Gastroenterology 1983;85:1350–3.
19. Maier K, Frühmorgen P, Bode JC, Heller T, von Gaisberg U, Klotz U. Successful acute management of chronic inflammatory intestinal diseases with oral 5-aminosalicylic acid. Dtsch Med Wochenschr 1985;110:363–8.
20. Kirsner JB. The influence of 20th century biomedical thought on the origins of inflammatory bowel disease therapy. In: Rogler G, Kullmann F, Rutgeerts P, Sartor RB, Schölmerich J, eds. IBD at the end of its first century. Dordrecht/Boston, London: Kluwer Academic Publishers, 2000:145–59.
21. Allgayer H, Klotz U, Böhne P, Schmidt M, Kruis W. Recent therapeutic modalities in chronic inflammatory bowel diseases: 4- or 5-aminosalicylic acid. Z Gastroenterol 1994;32:647–50.
22. Klotz U. The role of aminosalicylates at the beginning of the new millennium in the treatment of chronic inflammatory bowel disease. Eur J Clin Pharmacol 2000;56:353–62.
23. Sutherland LR. Aminosalicylates in the treatment of ulcerative colitis and Crohn's disease. In: Rutgeerts P, Colombel J-F, Hanauer SB, Schölmerich J, Tytgat GMH, van Gossum A, eds. Advances in inflammatory Bowel Diseases. Dordrecht: Kluwer Academic Press, 1999:201–9.
24. Solomon P, Kornbluth A, Aisenberg J, Janowitz HD. How effective are current drugs for Crohn's disease? A meta-analysis. J Clin Gastroenterol 1992;14:211–15.
25. Camma C, Giunta M, Rosselli M, Cottone M. Mesalamine in the maintenance treatment of Crohn's disease: a meta-analysis adjusted for confounding variables. Gastroenterology 1997;113:1465–73.
26. Cohen RD, Woseth DM, Thisted RA, Hanauer SB. A meta-analysis and overview of the literature on treatment options for left-sided ulcerative colitis and ulcerative proctitis. Am J Gastroenterol 2000;95:1263–76.
27. Colombel JF, Lemann M, Cassagnou M, Bouhnik Y, Duclos B, Dupas JL. A controlled trial comparing ciprofloxacin with mesalazine for the treatment of active Crohn's disease. Am J Gastroenterol 1999;94:674–8.
28. Sutherland LR. Maintenance of remission in ulcerative colitis and Crohn's disease. In: Rogler G, Kullmann F, Rutgeerts P, Sartor RB, Schölmerich J, eds. IBD at the end of its first century. Dordrecht: Kluwer Academic Publishers, 2000: 258–64.
29. Sutherland LR. Mesalamine for the prevention of post-operative recurrence: Is nearly there the same as being there? Gastroenterology 2000;118:436–8.

30. Schwab M, Klotz U. Pharmacokinetic considerations in the treatment of inflammatory bowel disease (IBD). Clin Pharmacokinet 2001;40(9).
31. Frieri G, Pimpo MT, Palumbo G, Tonelli F, Annese V, Sturniolo GC, et al. Anastomotic configuration and mucosal 5-aminosalicylic acid (5-ASA) concentrations in patients with Crohn's disease: A GISC study. Am J Gastroenterol 2000; 95:1486–90.
32. Frieri G, Giacomelli R, Pimpo M, Palumbo G, Passacantando A, Pantaleoni G. Mucosal 5-aminosalicylic acid concentration inversely correlates with severity of colonic inflammation in patients with ulcerative colitis. Gut 2000;47:410–14.
33. Stenson WF. Role of eicosanoids as mediators of inflammation in inflammatory bowel disease. Scand J Gastroenterol 1990;172(suppl):13–18.
34. Ahnfelt-Ronne I, Nielsen OH, Christensen A, Langholz E, Binder V, Riis P. Clinical evidence supporting the radical scavenger mechanism of 5-aminosalicylic acid. Gastroenterology 1990;98:1162–9.
35. Fischer C, Klotz U. Radical-derived oxidation products of 5-aminosalicylic acid and N-acetyl-5-aminosalicylic acid. J Chromatogr B 1994;661:57–68.
36. Bantel H, Berg C, Vieth M, Stolte M, Kruis W, Schulze-Osthoff K. Mesalazine inhibits activation of transcription factor NK-κB in inflamed mucosa of patients with ulcerative colitis. Am J Gastroenterol 2000;95:3452–7.
37. McDermott RP. Progress in understanding the mechanisms of action of 5-aminosalicylic acid. Am J Gastroenterol 2000;95:3343–5.
38. Reinacher-Schick A, Seidensticker F, Petrasch S, Reiser M, Philippou S, Theegarten D, et al. Mesalazine changes apoptosis and proliferation in normal mucosa of patients with sporadic polyps of the large bowel. Endoscopy 2000;32:245–54.
39. Bus PJ, Nagtegaal ID, Verspaget HW, Lamers CB, Geldof H, Van Krieken JH, et al. Mesalazine-induced apoptosis of colorectal cancer: on the verge of a new chemopreventive era? Aliment Pharmacol Ther 1999;13:1397–402.
40. Eaden J, Abrams K, Ekbom A, Jackson E, Mayberry J. Colorectal cancer prevention in ulcerative colitis - a case-control study. Aliment Pharmacol Ther 2000;14:145–53.
41. Sands BE. Therapy of inflammatory bowel disease. Gastroenterology 2000;118: S68–82.
42. Kho YH, Pool MO, Jansman FGA, Harting JW. Pharmacotherapeutic options in inflammatory bowel disease: An update. Pharm World Sci 2001;23:17–21.
43. Wallace JL, Vergnolle N, Muscara MN, Asfaha S, Chapman K, McKnight W. Enhanced anti-inflammatory effects of a nitric oxide-releasing derivative of mesalamine in rats. Gastroenterology 1999;117:557–66.
44. Batta AK, Tint GS, Xu G, Shefer S, Salen G. Synthesis and intestinal metabolism of ursodeoxycholic acid conjugate with an anti-inflammatory agent, 5-aminosalicylic acid. J Lipid Res 1998;39:1641–6.

Additional Early Publications on Inflammatory Bowel Disease

Wilks S, Moxon W. Lectures on pathologic anatomy. London: Churchill, 1875.

Bonorino UC. Les colites ulceroses chroniques. Paris: G Doin, 1929.

Rankin FW, Bargen JA, Buie LA. Chronic ulcerative colitis. In: Rankin FW, Bargen JA, Buie LA. The colon, rectum and anus. Philadelphia: WB Saunders Co., 1932: 217–86.

Coste J. Les rectocolitis ulcéreuses de cause inconnue. Paris: G. Doin, 1937.

Bensaude R, Rachet J. Recto-colite hemorragico purulente. In: Bensaude R, ed. Maladies de l'intestin. Paris: Masson et cie. 1939

DaMura P. La rettocolite ulcerosa criptogenetica. Bologna: Capelli, 1942.

Paulson M. Non-specific or indeterminate ulcerative colitis. In: Portis SA, ed. Disorders of the digestive system. Philadelphia: Lea and Febiger, 1944.

Brooke BN. Ulcerative colitis and its surgical treatment. London: Livingstone, 1954.

Rachet J, Busson A. Maladies de l'intestin. Paris: Flammarion Ed., 1955.

Placitelli G, Franchini A, Mini M et al. La colite ulcerosa. Rome: EMES (Edizioni Mediche E. Scientifiche), 1958.

Lindenberg J (Denmark). Ulcerative colitis. Acta Chir Scand Suppl. 1958;236: 1–106.

Bacon HE. Ulcerative colitis. Philadelphia: JB Lippincott Co., 1958.

Curtius F. Die colitis ulcerosa and its conservative treatment. Berlin: Springer-Verlag, 1962.

Lippi M, Corso P. La rectocoliti cryptogenica. Rome: Leonardo Edizioni Scientifiche, 1963.

Goligher JC, de Dombal FT, Watts JMcK, Watkinson G, Morson BC. Ulcerative colitis. Baltimore: Williams and Wilkins Co., 1968.

Feiereis H. Klinik und therapia der colitis ulcerosa. Munchau: Hans Marseille Verlag (an extensive bibliography mostly published between 1930 and 1974), 1970.

Kirsner JB. Ulcerative colitis 1970 – recent developments. Scand J Gastro-enterol Suppl. 1970;6:63–91.

Thayer WR. Crohn's disease (regional enteritis) – a look at the last few years. Scand J Gastroenterol Suppl. 1970;6:165–85.

Mottet NK. Histopathologic spectrum of regional enteritis and ulcerative colitis. Philadelphia: WB Saunders Co., 1971.

Engel A, Larsson T. Regional enteritis (Crohn's disease). Stockholm: Nordiska Uokhandelns Forlag, 1971.

Bercowitz ZT, Kirsner JB, Lindner AE, Marshak RH, Menguy RB, Sommers SC. Ulcerative and granulomatous colitis. Springfield: IL: CC Thomas, 1973.

Brooke BN, Cave DR, Gurry JF, King DW. Crohn's disease. New York: Oxford University Press, 1977.

Goodman MJ, Sparberg M. Ulcerative colitis. New York: J Wiley and Sons, 1978.

Julien M, Vignal J. La maladie de Crohn recto-colique. Paris: Masson, 1979.

Langman MJS. The epidemiology of chronic intestinal disease. Bath, UK: Edward Arnold, 1979.

Brooke BN, Wilkinson AW. Inflammatory disease of the bowel. Bath, UK: Pitman Medical, 1980.

Gebbers JO. Colites ulcerosa: Immun- und ultrastrukturpathologie. Stuttgart: G Thieme Verlag, 1981.

Ottenjann R, Fahrländer H. Entzundliche erkrankungen der dick darms. Berlin, Germany: Springer-Verlag, 1983.

Shiratori T, Nakano H, eds. Inflammatory bowel disease. Tokyo, Japan: University of Tokyo Press, 1984.

Janowitz HD. Inflammatory bowel disease – a personal view. New York: Field, Rich and Associates Inc., 1985.

McConnell R, Rozen P, Langman M, Gilat T. The genetics and epidemiology of inflammatory bowel disease. Frontiers of gastrointestinal research, Vol. 11. Basel, Switzerland: Karger, 1986.

Goebell H, Peskar BM, Malchow H, eds. Inflammatory bowel disease. Lancaster, UK: MTP Press, 1988.

deDombal FT, Myren J, Bouchier IAD, Watkinson G, Softley A, eds. Inflammatory bowel disease, 2nd edn. Oxford: Oxford University Press, 1993.

Lindenberg J. Ulcerative colitis. Acta Chir Scand Suppl 236, 1958.

Gebbers JO. Ulcerative colitis. Boca Raton, Florida: CRC Press, 1991.

O'Morain C. Crohn's disease-treatment and pathogenesis. Boca Raton, Florida: CRC Press, 1987.

Weterman IT, Pena AS, Booth CC. The management of Crohn's disease. Amsterdam: Excerpta Medica, 1976.

Index

Aaronson, RM 82
abdominal trauma 66–7
abdominoperineal resection 216
Abercrombie, J 55
acantholysis 32
acetyl-5-ASA (Ac-5-ASA) 227
Acheson, ED 146
achylia gastrica 67
Activated Eosinophils in IBD: Do They Matter? 38
acute toxic arthritis 28
additives 208
Adenovirus 126
adrenocortical deficiency 213
adrenocorticotrophic hormone (ACTH) 4, 25, 213–14
Advisory Council of the National Institute for Arthritis, Metabolic and Digestive Diseases of the NIH 6
Aerobacter aerogenes 122, 127
Aeromonas hydrophila 128
Aerosol OT 121
Ahlberg, J 130
Airs, Waters and Places (Hippocrates) 103
Alcaligenes fecalis 122
Alexander, F 114
Allchin, WH 17, 19
allergy-free diets 208
Almy, TP 9, 115, 161
Alpert, E 147
American College of Gastroenterology 10
American Gastroenterological Association 9–10
aminosalicylates 227–31
5-aminosalicylic acid (5-ASA) 3, 157, 218, 227, 228 (fig.)
  administration 230–1
  azo-prodrugs 229 (fig.)
Ammann, RW 83
Andersen, AFR 134–5
angioneurotic edema, pylorus 134
angiotensin I/II, colon tissue levels 170
ankylosing spondylitis 112, 164, 168
annexins 158

anthropometric measurements 109
anti-endothelial cell antibodies 170
anti-erythrocyte antibodies 136
anti-neutrophil cytoplasmic antibodies 170
anti-tumor necrosis α 219
antibiotics 131, 167
antibodies against goblet cells 170
antibodies to a trypsin-sensitive antigen 170
anticolon autoantibodies 140
anticolon serum 144
antimicrobial therapy 3
antimotility drugs 218
antineutrophil cytoplasmic IgG antibodies 150–1
antinuclear cytoplasmic antibodies 152
antinuclear globulins 150
antioxidants 231
antiseptics 207, 210
Antopol, W 69
appendicectomy 169, 215
appendicitis fibroplastica 60
aquaporins 158
arachidonic acid, cascade 157
Aranson, AR 162
Archer, GT 33
Aretaeus 14
arthritis
  treatment 3
  ulcerative colitis, associated with 28
4-ASA 230
asacol 212, 230
Asquith, P 149
astringents 19, 207, 210
atopic adult individuals 135
atopic diseases 133
Auer, J 137
Auer–Kirsner "immune complex colitis" 5
Auer–Kirsner reaction 137
aureomycin 213
Auslander, MO 151
autoallergic disease 138
autoimmune hemolytic anemia 112, 168
autoimmune liver disease 171
azathioprine 218

237

azochloramid 208
azotemic colitis 23

Babior, B 157
Bacille Calmette-Guerin vaccine 208
Bacillus acidophilus 132
Bacillus coli 122
Bacillus lactis aerogenes 122
Bacillus morgagni 124
Bacillus proteus 122
Bacillus pyocyaneus 122
Bacillus vulgatus 127
backwash ileitis 77–8
"bacterial vaccines" 207
Baird, A 110
balsalazide 228–9 (figs)
Bargen diplostreptococcus 21, 122, 124, 211
Bargen, JA 2, 9, 22, 122–3
Barker, WF 161
Baron, JH 55
Bartholomew, TC 149
Bass, C 120
Bassler, A 20
von Behring, E 133
Bendixen, G 148–9
Bensaude, A 23
Berg, AA 69–70, 72
Bernier, JJ 55, 144
Bienenstock, J 120, 134
Bifidobacteria 127, 132
Binder, V 164
biogenic amines 39
Bisell, AD 62
bismuth 18, 22
Blastocystis hominis 128
blood transfusions 2
bloody flux 14
Boas, I 18, 19
Bockus, HL 70, 83
Boeck's sarcoidosis 81, 127
Boller, R 109
Bolton, PM 129
boracic acid 18, 19
  rectal instillation 207
Boston Collaboration Drug Surveillance
  program 110–11
Bourne, G 21
bowel rest 209
bradykinin 156
Brandtzaeg, P 148
Bregenholt, S 161
Bregman, E 138
Bright, R 18–19
Bright's disease 23
Bristowe, JS 57
Broberger, O 138–9
Brooke, BN 5, 26–7, 33, 77–8, 84
Brown, JY 20
Brunner's glands 83

Budd, W 103
Buie, L 21
Bulmer, E 22
Burch, PR 164
Burnett, FM 136
Burns, JL 156
Busson, A 124
Buttiaux, R 123
butyric acid 42, 217

C3H/HEj Bir mice 42
Cabanis, PJG 112–13
Calabresi, P 150
Calcraft, BJ 148
Calkins, BM 107, 112
calomel 207
Campbell, D 141–2
Campylobacter fetus ssp. jejuni 127
Cannon, WB 113
Carlsson, HE 142
Carpenter, HA 170
carrageenans 41
casein, intolerance 208
catarrhal intestinal ulcus 15
catarrhal ulcerative colitis 17
Cave, DR 129
cecostomy 215
celiac disease 111
cellular hyporesponsiveness 170
CGO disease 88
CGO paper 67, 71
Chandler, CA 113
Chediak–Higashi syndrome 112, 164
Chen, Q 159
Chiba, M 132
Chlamydia trachomatis 126
chloramphenicol 213
*Chronic Cicatrizing Enteritis of the Ileum
  Regional Enteritis (Crohn's)* 87
chronic infectious granuloma 67
chronic phlegmonous ileitis 67
chronic stenosing terminal ileitis 60–1
cicatrizing enteritis 61, 88
claudins 158
Clindrocarpin lucidum 215
Clostridium difficile 124, 141
Cobb, S 113
Cocksackie A and B 126
cod liver oil 210
Coffen, TH 61
Coffman, RI 159
Coggeshal, LT 8
coherin 208
Cohn, V 9
Cohnheim, J 113
Cole, P 169
colectomy, subtotal 217–18
coli vaccine 19
coliforms 122, 128

colitic arthritis 28
colitis gravis 25
colon
    catarrhal inflammation 15
    partial resection 217
colon tissue-bound disease specific IgG 180
colonic autoimmunity 170, 171
colonic irrigation 215
colonic rest 20
colonoscope, fiberoptic 84
colony stimulating factor 158
colostomy 215
Combe, C 55
Cominelli, F 42
Cooke, EM 125
Cooke, WT 77
copper sulphate 208
coproantibodies 133, 135
Coprococcus 127
Corbett, RS 20, 37
Cornelis, W 144
cortisone 213
Counsell, PB 37
Crabbe, PA 147
creolin 19, 207
Crispinn, EL 134
Crohn, B 61–2, 70–1
Crohn–Dalziel disease 88
Crohn's and Colitis Foundation of America 10
Crohn's disease 1–5, 55–89
    20th century reports 71–7
    abdominal trauma 66–7
    animal 63–6
    clinical recognition, early 58–63
    colon-delayed recognition 77–81
    electron microscopy 84–7
    eponym, origin of 87–9
    etiopathogenesis, stages 171–2
    experimental 63–6
    experimental models 4
    familial patterns 162–3
    genetic aspects 162
    IgA, salivary 76
    microbial aspects 126–33
    microscopic description, first 56
    Mt. Sinai (NY) experience 67–71
    origins 55–8
    pathology, early 81–4
    psychogenic aspects 119–20
    psychotherapy 210
    recognition pattern 13
    surgical treatment 5, 217–18
    "transmissible agents" 129–30
    twins 163–4
Crohn's disease activity index 77
cyclosporine 215
cytokines 156–61
cytomegalovirus 126

Daft, FS 8
Dakin's solution 2, 210
Dalziel, TK 59–60, 77
Daniels, GE 115
Darfeuille-Michaud, A 155–6
Darwin, C 113
Das antigen 150
Datta, SP 141
deDombal, FT 164
defensins 158
Devine operation 217
dextran sodium sulphate 42
diarrhoea
    forms 14
    nervous system, connection between 113
    summer 122
    traveller's 131
    yin-yang balance 14
diets 208–10
    allergy-free 208
    elimination 25, 135
    food allergy elimination 208
    milk-free 15
    slop 19
Digestive Disease Foundation 9
Diggle, R 110–11
dipentum 212
diplostreptococcus 122
diplostreptococcus vaccine 2
disease, deviation from normal 13
disodium chromoglycate 35
diversion colitis 217
DNA hybridization 132
Dobbins, WO 85
Doe, W 159
Donnellan, WL 39
Dourmashkin, RR 85
Duchmann, R 172
Dukes, CE 37
Dvorak, A 39–40
dysbiosis 125
dysentery
    amebic 1
    bacillary 14–15, 19, 102
    epidemics, colonial America 14
    Flexner 122

Eastwood, MA 147
Epstein–Barr virus 126
Echo virus 126
Ehrlich, P 133, 156
eicosanoids 161
Eighth International Congress of
    Gastroenterology (Prague, 1968) 88–9
Eisenhardt, D 151
Eisenhower, D 9
electrocoagulation, selective 208
Elson, CO 152, 153–4, 172–3
endo-anal anastomosis, J pouch with 5

endotoxins 128
enemas 228
Entameba histolytica 1, 19, 124
enteric nervous system 154
Enzer, N 21
eosinophils 38
epithelial permeability 155–6
erythrocyte glucose-6-phosphate
    dehydrogenase deficiency 164
Escherichia coli 124
Escherichia coli (Nissle strain) 132
Escherichia coli 0157.H7 128
Eubacteria strains (Me46, Me47) 127

F-met-leu-phc (FMLP) 172
Fabry, Wilhelm (Guilhelmus Fabricius
    Hildanus 55–6
Falk, H 1
familial inflammatory bowel disease in twins
    161
fast foods 167
fat(s)
    hydrogenated 209
    processed 168, 208
febrile epidemic dysentery 17
Fenwick, S 57
Fernandez-Herlihy study 28
fever therapy 208
fiber
    dietary 168
    rough 208
fibrinolytic agents 156
fibroblasts 154
Fichtelius, KE 146–7
Fielding, J 55–6
Fifield, R 148
Fink, S 143
Fiocchi, C 160–1
fish oil 209
Fiterman, M 6–7, 9
Fixa, B 149
Fleck, L 121
Fleming, AB 120, 213
Fletcher, J 146
Flexner, S 122
fluorescent antiglobulin technique 150
foam 228
folic acid 168, 209
food intolerance 209
food protein-induced enterocolitis 135
food sensitivity 134
food supplements 209
Fordtran, J 155
Forsman antigen 141
frei skin tests 126
Freud, S 114
Freund's adjuvant 42
Fridovich, I 157
fructose 208

Gallart-Mones, F 33
gamma globulins 147
gantricin 210
Garcia-Lafuente, A 156
Gassaniga, AB 162
Gassaniga, DA 162
Gastro-Intestinal Research Foundation 6–7
gastroenterostomy 218
gastrointestinal endoscopy 84
Gear, J 138
Gebbers, JO 137–8
Gelzayd, EA 134, 147–8
gene clusters 165–6
General Medicine Study Section of the NIH 8
genomic finger printing 132
gential violet 208
Ghose, T 144
giant cell systems 82
Ginsberg, RS 40
Ginzburg, L 61–2, 67, 69–70, 80
Gjone, E 146
glucocorticoids 214
glutamine 209
Goldstein, HI 58
Goodman, MJ 87
Gorbach, SL 172
Gould, SR 157
Graber, P 133
Granger, DN 157
granular proctitis 25
Granulomatous Disease of the Intestinal Tract
    (Crohn's Disease) 79
Gray, BK 62
Gray–Walzer experiment 136
Grisham, MB 157
Guilhelmus Fabricius Hildanus (Wilhelm
    Fabry) 55–6
Gutensohn, N 169

Hale-White, W 17–18, 19
hamamelis, tincture 18, 19, 207
Hamburger, M 23
Hammarstrom, S 141–2
Hardy, TL 22
Harries, AD 110
Harris, FI 62, 87
Harvey Lecture on Hypersensitivity in Disease
    133
Hashimoto's thyroiditis 112, 136
Hass, GM 62
Hawkins, HP 20
HB-313 229 (fig.)
heat 208
Heatley, RV 148
Hellers, G 58
Helmholz, HZ 21
helminthic infestation 169
Helzer, JE 118
hemagglutination inhibition 141

Henderson, E 125
heparin 34
Heremanns, JF 134, 147
Hermansky–Pudlak syndrome 112, 164
Hern, JRB 22
herpes 126
Hidden Flame – Ulcerative Colitis, The 9
Hijmans, J 21
Hippocrates 14
histamine 33–4, 156
Historical Background of Immunology in Basic and Clinical Immunology 133
History of Immunology in Fundamental Immunology 133
History of Regional Enteritis 58
HLA (human leukocyte Ceptum A) gene complex 165
Hodgson, HJF 146, 161
hog intestine, "extracts" 208
Hollander, D 155
Homans, J 62
horse serum 208
Houghton-Naish families 162
Hurley Type I suspension 129
Hurst, A 20
hydrocortisone 213
5-hydroxytryptamine 156
hyperalimentation therapy 209
hypnosis 208

IBD: T Lymphocytes may be the Culprits 145
idiopathic proctocolitis 25
IκB 159
ileal pouch 217
ileorectal anastomosis 5, 217–18
ileorectostomy 217
ileostomy 215–17
  clubs 7
  continent 5
"iliac passion" 55
immune mechanisms 133–54
immunoglobulin A, secretory 134
immunosuppressant medication 214
indeterminate ulcerative colitis 25
inflammation 156–61
Inflammatory Abdominal Masses Stimulating Malignant Growths 59
inflammatory bowel disease
  adrenocorticotrophic hormone 3
  aminosalicylates 227–31
  catabolic effects 4
  colonic injury 4–5
  epidemiology 103–9
    Ashkenazi Jews 104
    ethnic groups, worldwide 105
    United Kingdom 108
    USA 107–8
  genetic aspects 161–7
  genetic factors, role of 167

immune-mediated inflammatory response 154–5
incidence 168
protein metabolism 3–4
rarity, third world countries 168
smoking 109–12
treatment 207–19
influenza virus 126
Ingelfinger, FJ 147
inguinal colostomy 18
integrins 158
interferon-γ 42, 158
interleukin(s) 35
interleukin-1β 158
interleukin-2 154, 158
interleukin-4 154, 158
interleukin-6 154, 158
interleukin-6R 154
interleukin-6S 154
interleukin-7 159
interleukin-8 158
interleukin-10 158, 159
interleukin-11 158
interleukin-12 159
interleukin-15 159
interleukin-16 159
interleukin-18 159
interleukin-19 159
International Congress of Gastroenterology (Brussels, 1935) 23
intestinal bacteria 168
intestinal bypass 9
intestinal permeability 155
"intestinal toxin" 31
intestinal tuberculosis 61
intestine, barrier function 155
intimins 158
iodine, tincture 207
ipsalazide 229 (fig.)
iritis 168
iron deficiency anemia 25
iron pernitrate 207
Irvine, EJ 156
Ivy, AC 40

J pouch 217
Jackman, RJ 62
Jankelson, I 124–5
Janowitz, HD 10, 69, 80
Jenner, E 133
Jewell, DP 149
Johne's disease 60, 127
Jones, AL 155

Kagnoff, MF 128
Kantor, JL 20, 103
Karp, LC 151
Karush, A 118
Kemler, BJ 147

kerosene 207
Kett, K 148
Kettering hypertherm 208
Kienbock, R 20
Kirsner, JB 1–11, 126, 134, 138, 161–2, 207–19
Klebsiella pneumoniae 124
Klemperer, P 70
Klotz, U 227–31
Knutti, R 8
Koch, R 121, 133
Kock pouch 217
Koenig–Rutzen bag 216
Kraft, SC 134, 149
Krawitt, EL 14–15
van Kruiningen, HJ 109
Kumagai, K 154–5
Kveim test 81, 129

lactic acid 207
Lactobacillus 132
lactose, intolerance 208
Lagercrantz, R 21, 140–2
Lambling, A 144
laminins 158
Lartigan, AJ 58–9
Läwen, A 60
Lawrence, J 9
Leskowitz, S 144
Lesniowski, A 87–8
Lesniowski–Crohn's disease 87–8
leukopexin 156
leukotoxin 156
leukotriene B$_4$ 111, 157
leukotriene B$_5$ 209
Lewis, HW 9
lidocaine 39
Lilja, I 159
Lindemann, E 115
lipo-oxygenase pathway 171
lipopolysaccharides 128, 172
Lister, TD 18
Lium, R 115
liver extracts 208
Lloyd, G 35
Lockhart-Mummery, JP 18–19, 62, 78
Logan, AH 20
Logan, RF 128
London Symposium on "sporadic" ulcerative colitis (1909) 19
lymphocyte cytotoxicity 170
lymphokines 156–61
lymphopathia venereum 124, 126
lysozyme 120–1

MacDermott, RP 148, 152
McKeown, T 109
McConnell, R 161
McCord, JM 157
McEwen–Kirsner study 28

McGiven, AR 141, 144
McGovern, VJ 33–4
Machella, T 3
Mackie, TT 24
Madara, J 155
Majno, G 158
malnutrition 168
Manson Bahr, PH 30–1
Mantoux reaction 127
Maratka, Z 140
Marcussen, H 143
margarine 208–9
Marin, ML 86–7
Marshak, R 62–3, 78–9
Marshall, JK 156
mast cells 33, 38, 154–5, 169
  hypersensitivity reaction 34–5
Mathieu, A 20
Mayer, EA 118–19
Mayer, L 151
Medawer, P 133
Medical History of the War of the Rebellion 17
Medical and Surgical History of the Rebellion USA 15
Meijer, CJ 148
Melrose, AG 104
Mendeloff, AI 9, 106–7, 112
Menzies, IS 155
6-mercaptopurine (6-MP) 214–15, 218
mercury 82
mesalamine 228
mesalazine 212, 228–30
Metchnikoff, E 133, 156
methemoglobin 212
methylene blue (5% solution) 18
methylprednisolone 213
Meukin, V 156
Meuwissen, SG 149
Meyer, A 113
microcins 158
microsatellite mapping technology 166–7
mid-arm circumference 109
milk, allergy 168, 208
Miller, N 120
Miller–Abbot tube 209
Mirvish, L 34
Mitchell, DN 129–30
Mizoguchi, BA 169
Modell, W 10
Modern Immunology in Perspective 133
Moeller, HC 135
"Mohawk Baron" 14
Moltke, O 161
monoclonal antibody methodology 166
Morbid Anatomy of Some of the Most Important Parts of the Human Body 15
Moreau, A 113
Morgagni, GB 55, 57
Morson, BC 36–7, 62, 84

Moschowitz, E 67–8, 77, 80
Mossman, TR 159
Moxon, G 16–17
Mr-40,000 protein 150
Mt. Sinai (NY) experience 67–71
Mt. Sinai (NY) study (1962) 24
mucosal colitis 25
mumps 126
Murray, C 113–14
Mycobacterium avium paratuberculosis 127
Mycobacterium linda 128

Nagel, E 87
Nagler-Anderson, C 124
Nairn, RC 141, 144
narco-analysis 208
National Foundation for Ileitis and Colitis 10
National Foundation for Research in Ulcerative Colitis 9
National Institute of Arthritis and Metabolic Diseases 8
natural resistance associated macrophage protein 2 166
neomycin 213
neoprontosil 210
Nerup, J 143
nerve growth factor 120
neuroimmune appendicitis 169
neuropeptides 120
Nickerson–Kveim skin test 127
nicotine, actions 110–11
Nielsen, MH 85, 137–8
nisulfazole 210
   enemas 210
nitric oxide 35, 111, 154, 159
nitrogen, urinary 4
NK cells 147
NO-mesalazine 229 (fig.)
NOD/it mouse model 42
non-immunologically-related food sensitivity 135
non-specific colitis 25
non-steroidal anti-inflammatory drugs 155–6, 167
Nonspecific Granulomata of the Intestines (Inflammatory Tumors and Strictures of the Bowel) 69
Nordstroga, K 144
nuclear factor kappa B (NF-κB) 159–60, 214, 231
nutritional deficiencies 171, 209

oligopeptides 128
olsalazine 228–9 (figs)
omega-3 fatty acids 209
One Hundred Cases with Albuminous Urine 19
opium 19, 207
Oppenheimer, G 61–2, 69–70, 80
oral contraceptive pill 167

Osler, WM 18
Otto, HF 137–8
Owen, RL 155
oxygen
   intracolonic insufflation 208
   rectal insufflation 210
   transanally 2

Paetkau, V 158
Palmer, WL 9, 126
pancreatic dystrophy 31
Paneth cell biology 171
pantothenic acid 168, 209
Papadakis, KA 161
Paris Congress of Medicine (1913) 20
Parkinson's disease 111
PAS (p-aminosalicylate) 230
Pasteur, L 121, 133
Paulley, JW 115
Paulson, M 126
Pavlov, IP 113
Pearson, AD 155
pelvic autonomic neurectomy 208
penicillin 25, 120, 213
peptidoglycan polysaccharide (PG-PS) complex 42, 172
peptidoglycans 128
Peptostreptococcus 127
Perlmann, P 138–9, 141–2
phagocytosis 156
phospholipase A 156–7
von Pirquet, CE 133
platelet activating factor 158
Plato 112
Platt, J 162
Plesiomonas shigelloides 128
Podolsky, DK 161
Podolsky–Isselbacher (Boston) Study 33
polymerase chain reaction 132, 166
polyvalent antidysenteric serum 20, 122
potassium permanganate 2, 210
pouchitis 217
prednisolone 213
prednisone 213
preservatives 208
probiotics 132–3
procto-colectomy 217–19
proctosigmoidoscope, electrically illuminated 18–19
prontosil rubrum 210
prostaglandin E2 158
prostigmine 28
"proteolytic substance" 32
Proteus vulgaris 124
pseudoallergy 135
Pseudomonas aeruginosa 124
Pseudomonas maltophlia 124
psoriasis 164
psychosomatic illness 171

psychotherapy 2, 210
Purrmann, J 16
pyoderma gangrenosum 25, 168
pyostomatitis vegetans 28–9
pyrexin 156
pyridoxine 168, 209

Rabin, BC 145
Rachet, J 124
radical scavenger 231
Ranlov, P 85
rectocolite haemorrhagique 25
rectocolitis ulcerosa cryptogenetica 25
Rees, RJ 129–30
regional enteritis 3–4, 9, 58, 61–2, 71
   surgical treatment 217
regional migrating colitis 77
Reinshagen, M 160
restriction fragment length polymorphism
   analysis 166
Rhodes, JM 33, 109–10, 149, 168
Rich, AR 133
Richardson, OS 144
Richet, C 113
Rider, JA 135
right-sided ulcerative ileocolitis 72
Roberts, CJ 110–11
Robertson, DJ 128
Robson, M 18
Rodaniche, E 126
Roediger, WE 41
roentgen, irradiation 208
Rogers, SJ 145
Rognum, TO 148
Rokitansky, K 15
Rosenkrans, PC 148
Rosenow, EC 123
Rosenthal, I 10
Rothberg, RM 149
Rotter, JI 166
Roux, JC 20
Rowe, AH 134–5
Rowe's elimination diet 135
Ruffine, JM 9
Ruoff, M 162
Rutgeerts, P 152–3

Sachar, D 151
salazopyrine 211–12, 212
salicylazosulfapyridine 211
Salmonella typhi 19
Salofalk 230
Sammons, HG 32, 120–1
Samuelsson, SM 109
Sanarelli–Shwartzman reaction 144
Sandler, M 7
Sandler, RS 112, 128
Sartor, RB 167
Saunders, W 55

Saunders–Abercrombie–Crohn's ileitis 88
Scheffner, L 3
Schesinger, B 162
Scheurlen, M 152
Schmedtje, JF 155
Schmidt, A 20–1
Schwab, J 149
SCID mice 42
sclerosing cholangitis 27
segmental enteritis 71
Seibold, F 152
selectins 158
Selye, H 113
Seneca, H 125
Sevin, A 123
Shanahan, F 151, 153
Shannon, J 8
Shapiro, R 59
Sharon, P 157
Sherlock, P 161
Shiga bacillus infection 133
Shiga toxin 122
Shigella dysenteriae 19
short-bowel syndrome 215
Shorter, R 145–6
Siemers, PT 85
Siltzbach, LE 129
silver nitrate 18, 19, 20, 22, 207
   rectal installation 210
Silverstein, AM 133
Skinner, JM 87
sleep therapy 2
small intestine, transplantation 218
smoking 167, 218
   association with
      Crohn's disease 111
      inflammatory bowel disease 109–11
      ulcerative colitis 111
   body weight, changes 109
Snow, J 103
sodium lauryl sulfate detergent 208
Soergel, KH 147
Solomon, GF 113, 120
Soltis, RD 138
somatic illness, neuro-psychogenic
   disturbances, association with 113
somatostatin 120
Soranus of Ephesus 14
sorbitol 208
sour milk 132
SP 227, 228 (fig.)
spherophorus necrophorus 124
Spiro, HM 82, 146
Sprints, H 113
Standiford, TJ 161
Stanisz, AM 120
Staphylococci 122
Staphylococcus aureus S209 141
starch 207

statins 158
Stead, RH 120
Stefani, S 143
stem cell transplantation 219
Stenson, WF 156, 157
Sternberg, E 118–19
steroids 213–14
Stierlin, E 20
Stone, CT 9
Stoughton, RB 31–2
Strauss, H 20, 22
Strauss–Koenig–Rutzen bag 216
streptococcal colitis 25
streptococci 122
Streptococcus aureus 63
Streptococcus hemoliticus 29, 63
Streptococcus viridans 29, 63
streptomycin 120, 213
stress 119–20, 170
  human illness, relationship to 120
  intestinal permeability, effect on 156
strictureplasty 218
Strober, W 42, 159–60
substance P 120
sucrose 208
sugar
  overuse 168
  refined 208
sulfadiazine 210
sulfaguanidine 210, 212
sulfanilamide 3, 25, 210
sulfapyridine 3, 210, 228 (fig.)
sulfasalazine 3, 211, 213, 218, 228 (fig.)
sulfasuxidine 210
sulfathalidine 210
sulfonamides 3, 210–12
Sullivan, AJ 113–14
superoxide dismutase 157
suppositories 228–30
Swartz, JH 124–5
Sweet, JE 122
Sydenham, T 14
Sydenham's remedy 19
Sydenham's treatment 207
systemic lupus erythematosus 112, 136
Syverton, JT 126

T cell antigen receptors 154
Talley, NJ 170
tannic acid solution 20
tannin 22
Targan, Sr 151, 153, 161
Taub, RN 129
Taylor, KB 135
Teisberg, P 146
Terris, G 144
tetanus antitoxin 133
tetracycline 213
Th1/2 cells 159–60

Thayer, WR 146
Thaysen, TEH 22
thiouracil drugs 208
Thomas, CH 17
thrombo-ulcerative colitis 25
thrombocytosis 168
thymectomy 208
Tolypocladium inflatum genus 215
Tomasi, TB 134
total colectomy 5
transforming growth factor β 154, 158
transforming growth factors 158
Trichoderma polysporum 215
Truelove, SC 29, 87, 135, 146
trypsin 156
Tulin, M 115
tumor necrosis factor α 35, 42, 158, 231
tumor necrosis factor β 158
tumor necrosis factors 158–9
tunnelling electron microscopy 166
Turnbull, PR 5, 9
Turner's syndrome 164
twins 163–4
typhoid vaccine 2, 122, 210
typical ulcerative colitis 124

ulcerative colitis 1–4, 13–43
  anemia, microangiopathic hemolytic 28
  antimicrobial therapy 3
  appendicectomy, protective effect 169
  beginnings 14–23
  children, retarded growth and development 24
  clinical recognition 24–30
  colonic motility 27–8
  colorectal cancer, risk of 30
  complications 30
    colonic cancer 21
    hepatic insufficiency, associated with 24
    nephrolithiasis 24
    ocular 21
    thrombosis, arterial and venous 24
  early IBD-related events 13–14
  electron microscopy 39–40
  epithelial hypersensitivity 25
  etiopathogenesis, stages 171–2
  experimental 40–3
  experimental models 4
  familial 23
  familial patterns 162–3
  genetic aspects 161–2
  geographic distribution 25–6
  impact description 16
  microbial aspects 121–6
  "natural" 40–3
  origins 14
  oxygen, transanally 2
  pathology and pathogenetic implications 30–9

personality 114
pregnancy, impact on and vice versa 22–3
protein balance 4
psychoanalysis 115–18
psychogenic aspects 112–19
psychogenic hypothesis 27–8
psychogenic illness 2
psychosomatic hypothesis 33
psychotherapy 2, 210
radiologic appearance 20
recognition pattern 13
 simple 15, 17
sleep therapy 2
smoking 109
surgical treatment 5, 215–17
twins 163–4
Yellow Emperor's canon 14
ulcerative colo-ileitis 72
United States Co-operative Crohn's Disease Study 77
University of Chicago Study 1
ursodeoxycholic acid 229 (fig.)

vagotomy 218
 distal 208
Valenti, J 7
valvular cecostomy 20
Varro, MT 121
vascular endothelial cells 154
vasoactive intestinal peptide 120
Vermeire, S 152–3
Virchow, R 15
vitamin A 168, 209
vitamin deficiencies 209

Wagner, V 140
Wakefield, AJ 128
van der Wal, AM 148
Walfish, JS 151
Walker, WA 155
Wallach, L 6
Wangensteen, OH 9
Wanstrup, J 85
Ward, M 146, 169
Warren, S 31–2
water enemas 208
Watkinson, G 164
Weil, RF 18
Weinstein, L 122
Weinstock, HI 115
Weinstock, JV 82
Wells, C 77, 114
Wensinck, F 127
Whalen, G 108–9
wheat, allergy 168
Whitehead, R 82
Whorwell, PJ 146
Wilbur, DL 9
Wilensky, AO 67–8, 77, 80
Wilks, S 16, 57
Wilson, AG 18
Wiskott–Aldrich syndrome 112
Wittkower, E 115
Wolf, SG 112–13
Wolf, SG Jr 9
World Congress of Gastroenterology (1958) 26

Yang, H 166
yatren 22
Yeomans, FC 20
Yersinia enterocolitica 127
yin-yang balance 14

zinc peroxide, rectally 208